Germaine Riccardo
Rm 217 McHale Hall

Printed in the United States of America

Library of Congress Catalog Card No. 81-86210

ISBN: 0-913590-80-0

Published by:

SLACK Incorporated
6900 Grove Road
Thorofare, NJ 08086

Last digit is print number 8 7 6 5 4 3 2

Barbara J. Hemphill
M.S., O.T.R., Editor

The Evaluative Process
In Psychiatric
Occupational Therapy

*Dedicated
to my
Parents
and to
Betty, and Mary,
who influenced my career*

For the ease of those who read
The Evaluative Process, male gender pronouns
have been used throughout the book,
unless female gender is specified.
We regret there are no concise or appropriate
unisex terms that could have been used instead;
the invention of these are awaited with impatience.

Foreword

It has been said that the future gives meaning to the present and the past. In the design and development of this book, Barbara Jo Hemphill has paid tribute to the past, provided resources and a stimulus to the present, and recognized possibilities for the future.

For occupational therapy students, this book provides a resource for developing knowledge and skills in the evaluation process, and an appreciation of the importance of a theoretical base and systematized methods for establishing the reliability and validity of evaluation instruments. For the practicing clinician, it provides a clear set of alternative possibilities to explore and to use. For the learner who exists in all of us, it is a stimulus to further develop and refine our bases of knowledge and skills.

It has long been a major concern to occupational therapists to develop the means to do accurate assessments of the strengths and needs of their clients, so that clearly relevant goals and plans for treatment can be developed. Early in the history of psychiatric occupational therapy, goals and treatment plans were based on the physician's assessment of the client as translated into a "prescription." At that time, the occupational therapist's own approaches to therapeutic intervention, beyond the often-limited physician's prescription, were largely intuitive. During the past three decades, therapists have become increasingly aware of the need to assume a greater measure of professional responsibility themselves, and have worked to develop assessment tools and systematized ways of organizing information about their clients. Many of these tools and systems have been kept local, serving the needs of the therapists who developed them. Some have been published or presented to the profession through workshops or papers, but heretofore there have been minimal efforts to compile them into a single, manageable publication.

Concepts of evaluation in psychiatric occupational therapy finally seem to have come of age. The purpose and value of methods of research into the bases of our practice have now been recognized. The impetus which Barbara Hemphill must have felt when she began to survey the field three years ago, attests to this fact.

The authors of the chapters have provided an important service to the profession by delineating the processes and theoretical frameworks through which they developed their evaluation methods. By sharing, in detail, the protocols for the administration of their tools, the current status of research with regard to their reliability, validity, and standardization, they have raised questions which have heuristic value for the profession.

For the profession as a whole, and especially for the therapists of the future whose ability to apply their knowledge and skills will have been enhanced by and built upon the bases provided here, we are grateful to Barbara Hemphill and the 20 contributing authors.

December, 1980   *Elizabeth G. Tiffany*
Philadelphia, Pa.

Preface

The purpose of this textbook is to provide the occupational therapy student with information relevant to understanding the evaluation process in psychiatric occupational therapy, to provide the clinician with current and accurate information about assessment tools developed for evaluating the psychiatric client, and to generate research for the further development of evaluations produced by occupational therapists.

By using the techniques of therapeutic interviewing and applying appropriate assessments, the student can learn to engage in the activities of the professional occupational therapist. This material is intended to assist the student in identifying pertinent data from interviewing and testing procedures that are relevant to occupational therapy. The mark of a professional evaluator is one who uses learned techniques to evaluate specialized patterns of behaviors for a specific purpose that focuses on a specific content area. Thus, the major theme of this textbook is to provide a framework for proceeding from the interview, to the application of appropriate instruments in evaluating the functioning of psychiatric clients.

Therefore, this textbook is organized into four major sections: 1) the interviewing process; 2) the projective instruments used in occupational therapy; 3) the observation scales, questionnaires, and performance evaluations developed by occupational therapists; and 4) the research methodology used in developing assessment tools. Each author will discuss the following information about his or her instrument.

A. The theoretical base will include the:
   1. historical development
   2. reason for its development
   3. behaviors being assessed
   4. types of clients appropriate for its use
   5. review of the literature

B. The administration of the evaluation will include the:
   1. procedure
   2. problems with administering
   3. materials used

C. The utilization of the evaluation will include the:
   1. presentation
   2. interpretation of results

3. statistical analysis and recent studies
4. case presentation if studies have not been completed

D. Suggestions for further research

The material is not intended to present a particular theoretical frame of reference, but a compilation of psychiatric assessment tools that have been developed and reported on in journals, workshops, conferences, and unpublished manuscripts. This textbook brings together updated information about assessment tools that were developed by occupational therapists for clinical therapists. Thus, it was written through a collaborative effort by originators of appropriate occupational therapy assessments.

Many of the assessments are in the beginning stages of research development. As the need for research is recognized for continued growth of the occupational therapy profession, I hope to provide the reader with the impetus to further develop the assessment tools in psychiatric occupational therapy. Thus, each author critiques his or her own instrument and discusses implications for further research. The last chapter is designed to provide the clinician and student with the research methodology employed when developing or improving assessment tools in psychiatric occupational therapy.

I would like to acknowledge JoAnne H. Wallis, M.A., instructor of English, Cuyahoga Community College West, Cleveland, Ohio, for her editorial expertise during the writing of this textbook. And thanks are due to Anne Bailey-Spruance, my editor at Charles B. Slack, who patiently guided this book through the publishing process. Also, I wish to extend my gratitude to uncounted occupational therapists for their support and encouragement; without their help this textbook could not have become a reality. Finally, I would like to extend my appreciation to Caroline Brayley, F.A.O.T.A. for her support and encouragement.

Barbara J. Hemphill

Table of Contents

Preface
Foreword
Table of Contents
List of Contributors

List of Contributors

Azima, Fern, J. Cramer, Ph.D.
  Associate Professor
  Department of Psychiatry
  McGill University
  Montreal, Canada

Black, Maureen, Ph.D., O.T.R.
  Psychologist
  University of Maryland Medical Center
  Department of Pediatrics
  Baltimore, Maryland

Block, Marjorie Papke, O.T.R.
  Staff Therapist
  Mesa Vista Hospital
  San Diego, California
  Masters Degree Student

Bloomer, Judith, M.S.W., O.T.R.
  Former staff therapist at Langley Porter
    Psychiatric Institute
  University of California
  San Francisco, California
  Currently in private practice
  Doctoral Student
    Department of Psychology
  Florida State University
  Tallahassee, Florida

Brayman, Sara J., M.S., O.T.R.
  Director of Occupational Therapy
  Greenville Hospital Center
  Greenville, South Carolina

Clark, Nelson E., O.T.R., Lt. U.S. Navy
  Head
  Occupational Therapy Branch
  Naval Regional Medical Center
  Clinical Faculty of Occupational Therapy
  Medical University of South Carolina
  Charleston, South Carolina

Cross, Michael S., Ph.D., Lt. U.S. Navy
   Clinical Psychologist
   National Naval Medical Center
   Bethesda, Maryland

Ehrenberg, Frances, O.T.R.
   Assistant Director of Occupational Therapy
   Psychiatric Occupational Therapy Program
   Hanna Pavilion
   University Hospitals of Cleveland
   Cleveland, Ohio

Evaskus, Marsha Goodman, O.T.R.
   Clinical Instructor
   Department of Occupational Therapy
   College of Associated Health Professions
   University of Illinois at the Medical Center
   Chicago, Illinois

Fidler, Gail, F.A.O.T.A.
   Assistant Hospital Administrator Programming
   Greystone Park Psychiatric Hospital
   Morris Plains, New Jersey
   Curriculum Development Consultant
   Department of Occupational Therapy
   School of Education, Health, Nursing, and Art Professions
   New York University
   New York, New York

Garfield, Mary, Ph.D., O.T.R.
   Army Specialist Corps, U.S. Army
   Chief, Occupational Therapy Department
   Landstuhl Army Regional Medical Center
   Landstuhl, Germany

Hemphill, Barbara J., M.S., O.T.R.
   Assistant Professor
   Department of Occupational Therapy
   Western Michigan University
   Kalamazoo, Michigan

King, Lorna Jean, F.A.O.T.A.
   President
   Center for Neurodevelopmental Studies
   Phoenix, Arizona

Kirby, Thomas, F., Ph.D.
   Psychologist
   Director of Licensing and Certification
   Piedmont Region/Whitten Center
   Clinton, South Carolina

Lerner, Carole, O.T.R.
   Charge Occupational Therapist
   Department of Psychiatry
   Mt. Sinai Hospital
   Toronto, Ontario, Canada

Schroeder, Carolyn Van, O.T.R.
   Schroeder Publishing and Consulting
   Kailua, Oahu, Hawaii

Shaw, Carol, M.S., O.T.R.
   Assistant Professor
   Occupational Therapy Program
   Kean College of New Jersey
   Union, New Jersey

Shoemyen, Clare, M.B.A.O.T., O.T.R.
   Psychiatric Staff Therapist
   Veterans Administration Medical Center
   Gainesville, Florida

Stowell, Mary Savage, M.S., O.T.R.
   San Diego, California

Trottier, Elizabeth Campbell, O.T.R.
   Supervisor of Adult Occupational Therapy
   Vista Hill Hospital
   Chula Vista, California

Williams, Susan, M.A., O.T.R., A.T.R.
   Former Staff Therapist at
      Langley Porter Psychiatric Institute
   University of California
   Current Director of ISIS
   San Francisco, California
   M.B.A. Student in Health Services Management
   Golden Gate University
   San Francisco, California

PART 1
INTRODUCTION

1
The Evaluative Process

Barbara J. Hemphill, M.S., O.T.R.

What and how does the occupational therapist evaluate? How does the occupational therapist know what is important, and that the results from the evaluation are valid? The answers to these questions and how they relate to the evaluative process are the subject of this chapter.

After searching the literature, it becomes apparent to the reader that other occupational therapists are attempting to answer these questions, yet few of them have completed all the necessary requirements for validation and standardization. Other occupational therapists do not go past the interview. From my recent survey I have found the results demonstrate that 47% of clinicians use the interview method as their only means of evaluation; thus, they never arrive at the answers to any of the above questions.

This is not to imply that the interview should not be used by occupational therapists. It is my belief that the interview should be conducted systematically and in conjunction with other appropriate evaluation procedures. This will be discussed further as the evaluative process is considered.

The Evaluative Process

The evaluative process is defined as using a specific method to measure essential behaviors in a sequential manner. Figure 1.1 illustrates the entire procedure that should be implemented for providing patient care. The evaluative process contains acquisition of the referral and data collection, which includes a chart review, interview, and testing procedures. The latter should be specifically designed to evaluate each client's level of functioning in four areas—psychological, behavioral, learning, and biological. Each of the need areas to be evaluated are influenced by the client's social environment and developmental level. These will be discussed in greater detail later in the chapter.

The results of the evaluative process if appropriately obtained, should enhance the determination of the needs areas, which in turn should indicate appropriate treatment. Re-evaluation should be an integral part of the treatment process to determine if the client's needs have been met. The same testing procedure which is used initially to identify the needs area should be used during re-evaluation in order to assure that the client's progress—or lack of progress—is measured with the same criteria. The results of the re-evaluation may indicate whether the client has progressed, not progressed, or has regressed. In the case of the first, the therapist may choose to continue or discontinue treatment. In the case of the latter two, re-

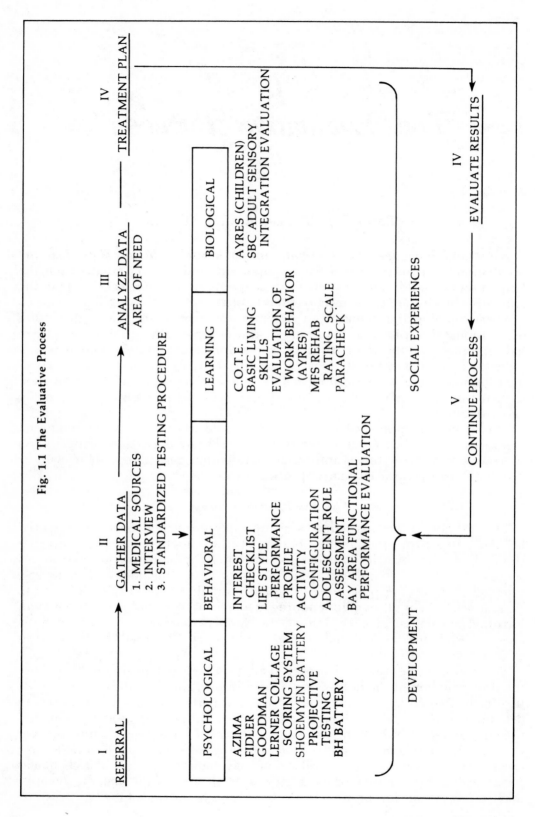

Fig. 1.1 The Evaluative Process

I	**II**	**III**	**IV**
REFERRAL	GATHER DATA	ANALYZE DATA	TREATMENT PLAN
	1. MEDICAL SOURCES	AREA OF NEED	
	2. INTERVIEW		
	3. STANDARDIZED TESTING PROCEDURE		

PSYCHOLOGICAL	BEHAVIORAL	LEARNING	BIOLOGICAL
AZIMA	INTEREST	C.O.T.E.	AYRES (CHILDREN)
FIDLER	CHECKLIST	BASIC LIVING	SBC ADULT SENSORY
GOODMAN	LIFE STYLE	SKILLS	INTEGRATION EVALUATION
LERNER COLLAGE	PERFORMANCE	EVALUATION OF	
SCORING SYSTEM	PROFILE	WORK BEHAVIOR	
SHOEMYEN BATTERY	ACTIVITY	(AYRES)	
PROJECTIVE	CONFIGURATION	MFS REHAB	
TESTING	ADOLESCENT ROLE	RATING SCALE	
BH BATTERY	ASSESSMENT	PARACHECK	
	BAY AREA FUNCTIONAL		
	PERFORMANCE EVALUATION		

DEVELOPMENT

SOCIAL EXPERIENCES

V CONTINUE PROCESS

IV EVALUATE RESULTS

4

Barbara J. Hemphill

evaluation indicates that more data must be collected through medical sources, interviews, and/or testing procedures. This would be necessary, because re-evaluation may indicate deficits in other areas of human function. Thus, the circle becomes complete, indicating the need to conduct the evaluative process again.

Referral

The evaluative process commences with the acquisition of the referral. It is recognized that many institutions operate under a variety of referral systems. The point is not to pass judgment on the referral mechanism, but to emphasize that the referral should provide a description of client behaviors rather than merely an indication of diagnosis, or lists of client psychological needs. The occupational therapist should then be able to direct his attention to the evaluation of those behaviors which require treatment. In other words, occupational therapists need not be concerned with diagnosis or client needs, since it is the behaviors that must be considered. That change of focus, from treating by diagnosis to treating by behaviors, came about when occupational therapy introduced the referral in place of the prescription.

Between the late 1950s and early 1960s, occupational therapists and physicians advocated the referral in place of the prescription. They believed that the prescription "fostered lack of initiative, provided little opportunity for increasing knowledge, and inhibited the development of a working relationship with the doctor."[1] It was also believed that the prescription constricted therapeutic benefits to the client—the occupational therapist treatment plan was too complex to be specifically prescribed. Consequently, when occupational therapy relinquished the prescription for the referral, occupational therapists had to assume the responsibility of transferring diagnostic judgment into occupational therapy goals and processess. Therapists are expected to have knowledge sufficient to make it possible to indicate the nature of appropriate treatment processes. Therefore, in order to be able to determine appropriate goals and treatment, the occupational therapist is obligated to evaluate the client's functioning. While the responsibility of the physician may be primarily diagnosis, delineation of pathology, and resultant treatment needs, it is the occupational therapist's primary responsibility to evaluate the client's behavior and provide treatment to change those behaviors that interfere with the client's maximum functioning.

On the other hand, in institutions which do not use a referral, therapists are obligated through their expertise to identify those clients needing therapy services. It is impossible for therapists to treat every client, nor is it likely that every client requires occupational therapy. Therefore, occupational therapists must have established criteria for screening, which must be developed according to: 1) the therapist's areas of expertise; 2) facilities available; 3) the manpower available; 4) the needs of the client; 5) the number of referral agencies; and 6) the type of treatment program. It is imperative that a systematic screening process be developed in order to ensure that those clients who would benefit from occupational therapy are serviced appropriately.

Data Gathering

Once the mechanism for obtaining clients, by referral and/or by screening has been conducted, the next step in the evaluative process is data gathering. Data gathering is broken down into three component parts: medical sources, interviewing, and testing procedures. These three facets are necessary in order to determine the needs area of each client.

Medical Sources. Occupational therapists must learn that much of the information they require about individual clients can be found in the medical chart. Many times therapists and other health care professionals seem to find it necessary to request information from the client which could either be found in the chart or culled from other colleagues in the health care delivery team. Oftentimes the client is asked the same questions by every member of the team, and it is no wonder that sometimes the client becomes anxious, passive, hostile, or indifferent. Therefore, the time spent looking in the medical chart at such items as the social history, admission summary, nurses' notes, summary of psychological testing, psychologist's report, physicians' reports, and other pertinent reports is well worth the time, and can save the client added aggravation. In order to enhance the data gathering a checklist of items would help when reading the chart. By drawing up a checklist in a carefully systematic manner, the therapist can gather information which will aid in carrying out the interview. *(face sheet)*

Interview. The interview should be an integral part of the data gathering process. The purpose of an interview is to obtain an understanding of the client's problems and to give the therapist direction for further evaluation. Therefore, the interview must be approached in a systematic manner. It is important that the occupational therapist know in advance the type of information that needs to be collected during the interview. The interview must be objective in nature, well-planned, and specifically concentrate on various areas of functioning.

It is not enough to use the interview for the purpose of developing rapport, relying on spontaneous emergence of information, and expect to receive valid and reliable data. Facts which are simply permitted to emerge without actively requesting them, result in conflicting, incomplete information, prolonged interviewing, and inaccurate documentation. It is not suggested that the therapist interrogate the client, but rather an attempt should be made to establish rapport and at the same time to systematically gain pertinent data. It is amazing how much time can be saved in the evaluative process if the interview is carried out in such a manner. A more detailed discussion of how an interview should be conducted is presented in Chapter 2.

The interview should provide a framework for obtaining specific information about the client's problems in four areas: psychological, behavioral, learning, and biological. The psychological area is the one area with which most occupational therapists are most familiar. It is the area that is concerned with the psychological functioning of the client in such areas as reality contact, social relationships, intrinsic gratification, body concept, defense mechanisms, impulse control, problem solving, and orientation. Information about these functions may be obtained through the interview. For example, the therapist may ask the question, "How do you feel about that?" or "How do you get along with your parents?" The client's answer may indicate information about intrinsic gratification and social relationships.

The second area is behavioral. Fidler maintains that the human organism is put together in such a way that action is innate to the organism. Additionally, anything that is alive is directed, and genetically programmed, to act. It is the action which enables an organism to survive in an environment. The transformation of random action into purposeful behavior involves action directed towards the environment through the process of reinforcement. Reinforcement enables an individual to

Barbara J. Hemphill

acquire a repertoire of behavior; when there is interaction between the environment and the organism that results in maladaptive behavior, the individual is in dysfunction.[2]* Function in the behavioral area includes such items as interest, adaptive behavior, and extrinisic gratification. To elicit information about adaptive behavior, the occupational therapist may ask an angry client a question such as: "What makes you angry, and what do you do about it?" The response may indicate that the client has been reinforced for maladaptive behavior.

The third area is learning. The theory related to this area is based on the acquisition of learned skills. It is those skills in which an individual becomes competent that allows him to become master of his environment. Such skills as activities of daily living, work, social, problem solving, decision making, and the like, are important to an individual's survival. Without the necessary skills the person is in dysfunction. Here, the occupational therapist might ask a female client if she is able to bake a cake for her child's birthday. The response to the question may indicate that the client is perfectly able to complete this activity.

The fourth area is biological. This area is developed from the knowledge that sensory integration plays a major role in assessing the individual's ability to benefit from purposeful action and to learn to cope and adapt to the environment. The individual's ability to organize, integrate, and interpret both internal and external stimuli is the nucleus of the perceptual process. "The functions of the brain in integrating and screening the sensory stimuli with which human beings are continuously bombarded are of monumental importance in determining human behavior. Thus, if the perceptual process is interrupted or if the neurological system is in some way dysfunctional, the resultant perceptual distortions may prevent normal interactions between the individual and the environment and make reality testing and the establishment of health, functional, cognitive, and motor abilities difficult."[3] The occupational therapist must be concerned with the integrating function of the nervous system while evaluating the client. Responses to questions about their physical behavior such as: "Do you consider yourself clumsy?" may indicate problems in this area.

In summary, the evaluative process is an organized and systematic way of determining client needs through a chart review, communication with other health professionals, interviews, and testing procedures. If the interview is to be effective in identifying problem areas, it must be pre-planned and contain questions pertinent to the four areas of human functioning: psychological, behavioral, learning, and biological. On the other hand, the establishment of rapport may be an important aspect of the interview if it is developed to meet that objective. The occupational therapist should then be able to follow the results of the interview up with appropriate evaluations in the areas in which the client indicates dysfunction. The interview itself should be limited to gathering information which cannot be obtained from other sources, and in many cases should require only a short period of time.

My experience is that approximately 80% of the information therapists felt was pertinent to know about clients could be found in the chart or from other health care professionals. It indicated to most of them that an interview for the purpose of obtaining information was unnecessary. On the other hand, they did not determine if the interview should be maintained for the purpose of establishing rapport. Each therapist must determine the emphasis that will be placed on the interview. Each

Taken from a presentation given by Gail Fidler at Cleveland State University, May, 1977.

therapist must decide if using the interview to aid in establishing rapport is necessary. If the decision is made that the interview is unnecessary for data gathering, perhaps another mechanism could be utilized for initiating the establishment of rapport. This process could be initiated during the time prior to orienting or preparing the client for the testing procedure.

While discussing these four specific areas of human functioning, examples of questions were given which might elicit information about the client's performance. The therapist should provide actual testing situations involving the client's functioning rather than, or in addition to, asking questions. Oftentimes, when the client reports that he can adequately function in a given situation, a demonstration proves otherwise. It is mandatory that the occupational therapist be knowledgeable of the variety of evaluation tools available, and to be able to select the appropriate instrument to assess the client's problem areas. The mark of a professional evaluator is one who uses specific techniques to evaluate patterns of behavior in a specific content area. In each of the four areas, there are specific tools presently available to occupational therapists.

Testing Procedure. In the psychological area, testing procedures have been proposed by Azima,[4] Fidler,[5] and other psychoanalytically oriented therapists. They proposed that occupational therapists use projective techniques as a testing procedure. What better way is there to evaluate such psychological functions as reality contact, intrinsic gratification, body concept, decision making, problem solving, defense mechanisms, and social relationships? The client is able to project his unconscious needs through symbolic projections. Originally, the focus of projective techniques was primarily analyzing symbolic content. Fidler suggests that the process by which an individual completed a task was the basis for personality assessment in occuational therapy. If the premise that human action as the epitomy of psychological makeup is accepted, then viewing the client in action is invaluable. Therefore, projective tests should be utilized by the therapist as a means for observing psychological behaviors. Many times occupational therapists become so involved in analyzing the content of the projective material, they miss the most significant symptoms of dysfunction because they did not observe the process. The projective techniques thus far developed include the Azima, Shoemyen,[6] and Fidler batteries. However, it must be noted that these testing procedures do not have standards through which actions can be rated through the projective material. Two other projective tests, the Goodman Battery and Carol Lerner's Collage Scoring System,[7] are also projective tests. Presently, these two are in the process of standardizing their rating scales.

Our body of knowledge about the behavioral area can be found in the theories proposed by Fidler, Mosey,[8] Shannon,[9] and Matsutsuyn.[10] In these, the therapist is concerned with the assessment of the acquisition of maladaptive behaviors. They involve an analysis of the client's ability to perform in work, play, and daily living activities within his environment. The occupational therapist has the expertise to evaluate these three areas. Testing procedures which have been developed in the behavioral area include: the Interest Check List, Life Style Performance Profile, Activity Configuration, and the Bay Area Functional Performance Evaluation.

The evaluation of the learning area involves a task that assimilates the actual skill to be performed. The learning area is concerned with the skill level performance of the client and the reason for the deficit. The occupational therapist must always bear in mind that an interview will not demonstrate skill; the therapist should be familiar with those testing procedures which evaluate skill. It was previously

Barbara J. Hemphill

suggested that in the learning area the therapist could ask a female client if she was able to bake a birthday cake for her child. How much more relevant it would have been if she was required to demonstrate that ability. Likewise, the therapist would have had a more accurate picture of the client's functioning level and would have been able to identify why the client was or was not able to perform the task adequately. Testing procedures which have been developed by occupational therapists to evaluate the learning area include the Comprehensive Occupational Therapy Evaluation,[11] Basic Living Skills,[12] Evaluation Work Behavior,[13] MFS Rehabilitation Rating Scale,[14] and the Paracheck Rating Scale.[15]

The biological area has been carefully researched by Lorna Jean King and Jean Ayres. The testing procedures in this area evaluate sensory integration functioning. While Ayres has researched this area in great detail, presently, The Southern California Battery has been standardized only for children. Therefore, at this point, it is inappropriate for psychiatric adults. On the other hand, King has published a great deal about the treatment of schizophrenic clients using sensory integrative principles.[16] Currently, she has not developed a formal evaluation of sensory integrative dysfunction; however, King does use the Person Drawing to assess body concept and spatial integration. This will be discussed in greater detail in Chapter 11. The one test which relates to the testing of the biological area is Schroeder's SBC Adult Sensory Integration Evaluation.

To summarize, therapists should be proficient in administering and interpreting those evaluative tools which are available to them. Likewise, the therapist should be able to determine which tools will best evaluate which behaviors. It would be futile for the occupational therapist to use all testing procedures on every client. On the other hand, since occupational therapists profess to treat the entire person, it would be just as futile for occupational therapists to operate and evaluate exclusively in one area. For example, many therapists are more familiar with the psychoanalytical approach to treatment, and devise their treatment based on Freudian concepts, often completely neglecting the evaluation of daily living skills, sensory integration, or work adjustment. In that way they neglect the client as a total human being. This may also be said for any therapist who is concerned exclusively with any of the other three areas of human functioning. However, it is apparent after examining each of the evaluations, that many of the aspects of human functioning overlap in the four areas that have been described. The therapist needs to use more than one testing procedure to evaluate a client's functioning. Until specific evaluative tools in each of the four areas of human functioning have been developed, the therapist will have to determine which evaluation will precisely identify specific problem areas of his client.

A survey I recently conducted clearly indicated that clinicians throughout the country were not using many of the testing procedures which have been developed by occupational therapists, and for the most part published in the American Journal of Occupational Therapy. Over 45 testing procedures were identified, and yet few clinicians reported that they were even familiar with them. If Occupational Therapy is to remain a viable health care profession in mental health, it is imperative that clinicians become knowledgeable and proficient in administering and interpreting all testing procedures which evaluate the four areas of human functioning.

It is clear from the previous discussion that therapists need to be more than just familiar with existing instruments in order to effectively use them in planning treatment. To determine if an evaluation is appropriate for specific use, occupational therapists should be proficient in research methodology used in developing assessment tools. Chapter 17 will deal with this matter in greater detail. However, regardless of whether the therapist is knowledgeable about research methodology or not, it is essential to develop the skill for choosing the appropriate tool. The following questions are designed to aid the therapist in this process:

1. Does the author give a viable and reasonable rationale for developing the instrument?
2. For what population is the instrument designed?
3. Are the behaviors defined in measurable terms?
4. Are there any studies reported regarding validity or reliability?
5. Is the procedure for administering the instrument clear?
6. What need area is the instrument designed to test—analytical, behavioral, learning, or biological?
7. Is normal behavior considered in the instrument?
8. Does the author explain how to interpret the results?
9. Under what circumstances would this instrument be used?

This guide for critiquing an evaluation must be considered when choosing an instrument. It also identifies the limitations of an evaluation and assists in determining areas of further research.

Problem Areas When Using Evaluations

Having completed the evaluative process, comments regarding the issues when employing evaluations need to be discussed. It is my opinion that knowing about and being proficient in administering evaluative tools also requires knowledge and understanding of the principles of standardization of procedures and norms. It should be obvious from previous remarks that while there are many evaluations available, few of them have been standardized. Regardless of what testing procedures are employed, each must be administered under uniform conditions with standard directions to a group of clients for whom the test is intended.

The research that has been missing for most of the existing evaluations is the determination of scores in the standardized group, or norm group. Frequently, the therapist is unable to interpret the results by comparing them to norms. Therefore, each therapist could undertake to develop norms in any one of the tests in order to have a more valuable instrument. If this seems like a formidable task, a group of therapists could undertake such a project. Then when occupational therapists use the evaluative tools, they would be able to interpret them with confidence. It is my opinion that because occupational therapists are unfamiliar with the existing evaluations, they spend a great deal of time and effort developing their own evaluation tools, rather than completing the necessary research to make the existing tools meaningful. Another reason for therapists not using existing tools is that they are unfamiliar with the process and essential factors involved in developing evaluation tools. If occupational therapists wish to develop an evaluation, there are several processes which should be kept in mind:

1. Determine what to evaluate—what attributes or abilities are to be evaluated.
2. Define what is being evaluated in measurable behavioral terms.

Barbara J. Hemphill

3. Select appropriate situations for eliciting those behaviors.
4. Devise a method for recording the behaviors.
5. Devise a method for scoring the behaviors.

These five essentials must be considered when developing any type of evaluation, regardless of its purpose or form; and once developed, the necessary research procedures must be incorporated. It must be made absolutely clear that whether the occupational therapist is using an established evaluation tool or developing his own, the tool must be administered to the population for which it was designed—unless the therapist establishes norms for a different population. A perfect example is that therapists are using various areas of The Southern California Battery to evaluate adult psychiatric clients. Therapists freely state they know that norms have not been developed for this population, yet they continue to use the test procedures. I ask, "How can they interpret their results when they do not know how normal adults would perform?" Are not occupational therapists wasting their time and effort as well as the clients' time and effort when they administer tests to populations for which norms have not been developed?

Another comment needs to be made about evaluations available to occupational therapists. This has to do with adapting existing instruments to meet the therapist's own objectives. Occupational therapists tend to adapt everything with which they come in contact, in order to treat clients. I have heard it said: "OTs do it better: We're adaptive." Occupational therapists talk about adapting equipment, adapting environments, and some therapists attempt to adapt evaluative tools for something other than what they were intended. Those therapists must be cognizant of the fact that when an instrument is adapted for a different population than what it was originally intended, reliable and valid results will not be obtained. For example, The Adolescent Role Assessment[17] was designed as an interview instrument to evaluate adolescents. The occupational therapist who uses that tool for a different population will have invalid results. On the other hand, some therapists pick and choose isolated items from an instrument to evaluate behaviors which are different from the intended purpose and then expect results to be meaningful. What has been done is to illegitimize the original evaluation and to produce a tool which does not yield reliable results. Furthermore, therapists frequently take one form of an evaluation tool, such as an observation scale, and use it for a different purpose, such as a daily record keeping form. In other words, they have not followed the procedure as outlined and have adapted the scale to meet their own needs. What is really unfortunate is that many times the clinician is not even aware that this is poor procedure. Since this has become common practice, many therapists with whom I am familiar have indicated their hesitancy in publishing their tools for fear that once published, they will never be able to recognize them again.

Finally, let me make a comment about borrowing evaluation tools. It is important that if one borrows an evaluative tool from a colleague or adopts a tool from a publication, that credit be given to the person who developed the tool. In the past few years, I have seen an entire published rating scale in a medical chart, without any credits being given to the author. After researching occupational therapy evaluation instruments, it is apparent that there are almost as many interest check lists as there are therapists. There are also a variety of object, work, and advocational histories. It is almost an impossible task to determine who originated each of them.

The Evaluative Process

Conclusion

By leading the reader through the evaluative process, this chapter has attempted to deal with questions regarding what and how occupational therapists evaluate psychiatric clients. The evaluative process starts with the referral, which could provide enough information to give the therapist direction in collecting data about the client, by means of the medical chart, and communication with other health professionals. Having gathered pertinent data, the evaluative process is continued by interviewing the client, and evaluating the client with specific testing procedures, thus answering the question regarding what is important in evaluating the client with psychiatric disorders.

A framework for evaluating mental health in four areas of human functioning—psychological, behavioral, learning, and biolgical—has been presented. It should be apparent that there is a need for specific assessments in mental health settings which should be based on the theoretical framework of occupational therapy.

Problems surrounding psychiatric assessments, such as standardization of evaluation tools and the inappropriate adaption of specific tools have been identified, thereby dealing with the question of how the occupational therapist knows that the results from the evaluation are valid. The need for assessment tools to be written in measurable behavioral terms has been discussed. In the end, our primary concern is to develop excellent tools which will be widely used to evaluate the behavior and performance of clients, in a way that is unique to occupational therapy.

References

1. Fidler G: The prescription in occupational therapy. A J Occu Ther 3:122, 1963.
2. Fidler G, Fidler J: Doing and becoming: Purposeful action and self-actualization. A J Occu Ther 32:305-310, 1978.
3. Hopkins H, Smith H (eds): Willard & Spackman's Occupational Therapy. New York, The Macmillan Co, 1973, p 287.
4. Azima H: Dynamic occupational therapy. Disease Nerv Syst 22:1-5, 1961.
5. Fidler G, Fidler J: Occupational Therapy: A Communicative Process. New York, The Macmillan Co, 1967, p 99-117.
6. Shoemyen C: Occupational therapy orientation and evaluation. A J Occu Ther 24:276-279, 1970.
7. Lerner C, Ross G: The magazine picture collage. A J Occu Ther 31:156-161, 1977.
8. Mosey A: Activities Therapy. New York, Raven Press, 1973, p 89-100.
9. Shannon P: The work-play model: A basis for occupational therapy programming in psychiatry. A J Occu Ther 24:215-218, 1970.
10. Matsutsuyn J: The interest checklist. A J Occu Ther 23:323-328, 1969.
11. Brayman S, Kirby T, Misenheimer A, et al: Comprehensive occupational therapy evaluation scale. A J Occu Ther 27:95-100, 1976.
12. Casanova J: Basic living skills. A J Occu Ther 30:101-105, 1976.
13. Ayres J: Form used to evaluate the work behavior of patients. A J Occu Ther 8:73-74, 1954.
14. Wolff R: A behavior rating scale. A J Occu Ther 15:13-16, 1961.
15. Parachek J: Paracheck Geriatric Rating Scale. Scottsdale, Greenroom Publications, 1976.
16. King L: A sensory integrative approach to schizophrenia. A J Occu Ther 28:529-536, 1974.
17. Black M: Adolescent role assessment. A J Occu Ther 30:73-79, 1976.

Barbara J. Hemphill

PART 2
INTERVIEWING PROCESS

2
The Interview Process

Carol Shaw, M.S., O.T.R.

In the helping professions, interviewing is the central and primary mode of communication. It is a fundamental technique which any helping person must acquire and perfect. Occupational therapists use interviewing for many different purposes in countless situations, and with a wide variety of persons.

Interviewing is a skilled technique which can be improved with practice. However, just practicing the technique will not perfect the therapist's skill in interviewing. Only by acquiring knowledge about the theory of human psychodynamics, the principles and concepts of interviewing, and conscious and constant examination of one's own interviewing, can one develop real interviewing skill.

This chapter will provide the reader with some basic information about the interviewing process. The interview will be defined and its purposes discussed, as it relates to the evaluation process in occupational therapy. The essential attitudes, components, and conditions necessary for a successful interview will also be presented. Additionally, information will be presented on how to conduct an interview, and some potential problems will be briefly touched upon.

Definition of an Interview
and its Purposes in the Occupational Therapy Process

Definition

An interview is defined by Harry S. Sullivan and others as a situation in which two or more people verbally communicate with each other around a particular subject matter (usually the client's patterns of living) for a specific purpose. The specific purpose is determined by the individuals involved and by the nature of the setting or facility in which the interview is taking place.[1] As Sullivan points out, the interviewer or therapist is the "expert" in the field of interpersonal relationships and behavior, as well as someone who is knowledgeable in the fields of psychopathology, and normal growth and development. As such, it is the interviewer's responsibility to identify the needs of the interviewee and how he will benefit from their interchange.

These last two concepts: 1) to discover what the needs of the client are, and 2) how best to help or benefit him, are key concepts to remember and focus on as one begins to conduct a professional interview. With these two ideas in mind, many of the pitfalls and anxiety-producing situations of the novice occupational therapist can be lessened. For example, a beginning occupational therapist might be more concerned and anxious about how she is perceived by a client, or if the "right" questions are being asked, rather than eliciting the necessary information to plan treatment, or establishing a comfortable interview situation in which the client will be more likely to trust and share his thoughts and concerns.

Purposes of the Interview

Why do occupational therapists bother to interview clients? Why not just put the clients into activity groups or give them something to do which might help them? Why bother to gather information? As a helping professional, the therapist must evaluate the client, his strengths, and limitations, before initiating treatment. It is the evaluation process and subsequent treatment plan that distinguishes a professional occupational therapist from an arts and crafts teacher or an activity worker. The interview is a primary technique in the process of evaluation and treatment.

Data Gathering. This is the first component in the evaluation process. The interview with the client serves as the primary source of data. Other sources include, but are not limited to, the client's family and significant others, the client's chart, and other helping professionals working with the client.

Information obtained during an interview will also help the occupational therapist to check the reliability and validity of previously gathered information. Clarification of data previously gathered may also take place for both the therapist and the client.

The amount and type of information gathered should be limited to the knowledge that is needed in order to help the client, not to satisfy the curiosity of the interviewer. The client must feel that each question is important and relevant to his problem or circumstance. If the purpose of the question is unclear, it is the responsibility of the therapist to explain why the question is being asked and for what purpose. Clarification can become a first step in the building of a trusting relationship, which is essential to the evaluation and the subsequent treatment process.

The interview should be focused on understanding the client, not in trying to find out what is wrong with him. The purpose of the interview should be known by both parties in order to lessen both the client's and the therapist's anxiety. If the client's anxieties are too great, important problems or issues may remain unclear and unrevealed. The occupational therapist's anxiety, if too great, may interfere with the ability to ask for and solicit the needed information. The purpose of the interview determines how an interview will be conducted and how the data obtained will be collected. If, for example, the purpose of the interview is to explore unconscious conflicts of the inteviewee, information will best be elicited by asking effective, open-ended questions, or by using projective materials and affective oriented tasks. On the other hand, if the purpose of the interview is to evaluate the activities of daily living skills of the client, then the nature of the questions and/or tasks will concentrate on this subject. The purpose of the interview somewhat determines the nature of the content and method of data collection. Also, if the evaluative procedure is standardized, then the interview must be conducted according to specific instructions, methods, or procedures, again influencing how the interview will be conducted.

The nature and amount of data sought is also influenced by the facility or agency in which the interview occurs. If the facility is acute, short-term, and community oriented, the data sought and evaluative procedures used will be very different from data collected in a long-term geriatric facility. For example, if an occupational therapist is working in an acute facility, she needs to know more about the client's

Carol Shaw

social support system, his ability to manage time, and his ADL acitivities rather than the client's capability of learning a new leisure-time skill.

Problem identification. Another important purpose of the interview is to identify problems, strengths, limitations, and resources of the client. An occupational therapist must understand the problems the person is experiencing and their possible causes. The nature of the difficulty must be clear to the interviewer—under what circumstances the problem manifests itself, or the client notices problems in living.

By mutually identifying in specific detail the nature and extent of the problems the interviewee experiences, both the therapist and client become actively involved in the beginning of a therapeutic alliance which will facilitate the treatment process and the attainment of treatment goals. The mutual identification process will convey to the client the therapist's interest, understanding, and concern. To be really listened to and perhaps to be understood is an experience few people enjoy. The actual process of being listened to and understood may, in and of itself, be of great benefit to the client, and can often be as important as finding solutions to his problems. Active listening by the occupational therapist will be discussed later in the chapter.

The clarification and delineation of the actual problems being experienced by the client often helps him to get a handle on his problems. The process of specifically outlining the difficulties serves to reduce the problem and makes it more accessible to solution. It is no longer an overwhelming mountain of difficulties but instead, has become a series of serious but certainly solvable issues. This realization oftentimes helps to motivate the client to actively attempt solutions which were previously not seen as present or possible.

If mutual problem identification does not occur, then both parties may find themselves working at odds with each other, or going in circles. This situation will eventually lead to frustration, anger, and probable termination of the interview, evaluation, or treatment process. Sometimes the client may feel that certain problems are more crucial and need to be discussed first, rather than those identified by the therapist. If this occurs, it is essential that the occupational therapist acknowledge them while suggesting alternative ways of viewing the client's problems. For example:

> A young woman comes to the pre-vocational program, stating that her problem is that she cannot type accurately or fast enough for employment. However, the occupational therapist soon realizes through observing both her behavior and her responses during the inteview, that the client is not able to concentrate on the subjects being discussed, and she is often tangential in her responses. Unless the discrepancies in the identified problems are worked out, the probability of a successful outcome for the client is very limited.

Problem-solving process. The accurate and precise identification of a problem is the first step in the problem solving process upon which the occupational therapy treatment process is based. After accomplishing this first step, the occupational therapist and client can begin to determine what additional information is needed, and where, how, or from whom to obtain it.

An intensive exploration of the identified and possible solutions may become the purpose for the interview. In the exploration of the problem, the occupational therapist learns how the client approaches problems, how he feels about his circumstances, and the characteristics of the social and economic system in which he is living. The therapist also learns the client's possibilities for change, the resources available to him, as well as his values, attitudes, strengths, and limitations. The occupational therapist may wish to encourage the expression of the client's fantasies and fears in order to understand what inhibits his attempts to solve or reduce his anxieties. This process of exploration is a continuous one which occurs throughout the helping relationship. It is one of the most challenging, difficult, and rewarding processes in the helping relationship, and can often be the therapeutic essence of it.[2]

Goal setting for treatment. Once the interviewee's problem has been identified, the purpose of the interview will change. The interview will then focus on the development of goals and objectives for the treatment plan and the therapeutic relationship. This again must be a mutual process in which both parties collaborate and agree upon the goals and objectives of treatment.

This type of interview can be done sytematically or informally. A systematic approach may be used when a client is manipulative or needs to have written, concrete goals because of poor recall or an inability to focus and proceed in a logical manner. With such clients, a formal contract should be drawn between the occupational therapist and the client, delineating the duties and responsibilities of both parties and the consequences of either fulfilling or breaking the contract. For example:

> Anna, a client in the day center, wanted to be part of the pre-vocational training group. However, she was often late in arriving at the center and was disruptive in the groups she attended. These two dysfunctional behaviors were identified and a contract was drawn. A contract was used with this particular client because of her inability to commit herself to a concrete step-wise plan, and her repeated accusations that the staff never kept their end of the bargain.

However, goal setting is usually done in a less formalized or concrete manner. Generally, no formal contract is written. Instead, the client and the occupational therapist will discuss the goals for treatment. A verbal agreement is made about the activities, groups, or actions needed to accomplish the stated goals.

Whatever the objectives of the therapeutic relationship are, it is also important to specify the priority of goals. This last concept of time-limited treatment is often left out of treatment planning. By including specific proposed time limits, the client is given an important message. He is told that the accomplishment of this goal is attainable in the near future. He is capable of reaching this goal and then moving on to the next one. But if he is unable to attain the goal within the alloted time period, then a re-evaluation can occur which may provide other alternatives, more information, or another goal.

Final interview. The final interview has several purposes. It can provide the therapist or client with an opportunity to get an overview of what has happened in the course of their relationship and work together. This overview can serve either as a reinforcement to the learning that has occurred or as an indication of what further intervention might be needed.

A final interview might focus on a review of the information obtained during the evaluation process in order to establish goals for treatment. At the end of treatment, an occupational therapist might wish to delineate potential problems or difficulties the client might experience in the near future, and discuss with him possible alternatives or solutions.

Carol Shaw

Content and Process of an Interview
Content of the Interview

The content of an interview is the factual information given by the interviewee to the interviewer. It is material which is readily accessible to the interviewee and can be generally validated by the occupational therapist. Content includes the client's thoughts, feelings, and experiences about the past, present life situations, and future life plans. This information has been labeled *introspective data* by MacKinnon and Michaels.[3] The introspective data provided by the client serves as a baseline of information regarding how the client sees his particular situation and what he sees as his problems, strengths, and limitations. It can also indicate to some degree his motivational level, ie, how much energy and resources he is willing and able to apply to his problems.

In addition to introspective data, the interview provides other information, called *inspective data.* This is the non-verbal behavior of the interviewer and interviewee.[3] In general, the client does not know or understand the important and significant messages or data which are being communicated on a non-verbal level. It is the occupational therapist's responsibility to know, analyze, and use this non-verbal data to help understand the client and what ails him.

Non-verbal communication is the more basic and primitive form of communication. It provides a continuous flow of messages without verbal accompaniment. Non-verbal communication can also be a vehicle for confusion and misinterpretations. For instance, someone may say verbally he is pleased to see you, while non-verbally conveying a very different message.

Non-verbal messages can be communicated in many different ways by a person in the interview setting. The person's physical appearance, dress, posture, body odor, body sounds, facial expression, gestures, tone of voice, and eye contact are all vehicles for non-verbal communication. Examples of some of these messages are:

1. *Tone of voice*—This can reveal a myriad of emotions, or an attempt to conceal emotions by using a non-committal tone of voice.
2. *Gestures and body movements*—These are commonly used as indicators of a person's anxiety, tension, attitudes, and ideas. Biting nails, shifting the feet, and restlessness are just a few examples.
3. *Dress and physical appearance*—How someone dresses and takes care of his physical appearance will definitely communicate something to the observer. This has to do with how the person feels about himself and what he wishes to tell the world about himself. For instance, society could label a man "crazy," if he wore a torn, dirty T-shirt with food stains on it and a pair of pants equally torn and dirty. If the same person wore a clean shirt, tie, and pressed trousers, he could then be seen as a "normal" and approachable person.
4. *Body posture*—This can often indicate if an individual is feeling depressed, tired, or energetic.
5. *Eye contact*—The degree of eye contact can often indicate an individual's ability to engage in interpersonal relationships in a meaningful way. Eye contact can also be an important factor in helping the interviewer to assess the interviewee's state of being or how he is feeling at a particular moment. However, it is particularly important to be aware of and sensitive to cultural norms and differences. In some cultures, eye contact is considered rude and often is seen as insulting and threatening.

As indicated previously, the non-verbal communication component of an interview may or may not agree with the verbal messages. The non-verbal language of the occupational therapist or client may, however, enhance, or clarify the often limited verbal language of the individual. In some cultures where the expression of emotions or needs is not allowed, a great deal of information and understanding can be conveyed to the listener by the speaker's non-verbal language. For example, in many cultures men are forbidden to show any emotions. The inteviewer, by being aware and sensitive to non-verbal communication, can observe and listen to the non-verbal messages being sent out on an unconscious or preconscious level, so as to ascertain the emotional state of the client.

These disguised messages require the interviewer to develop a third ear. Theodore Reik described listening with a third ear as the process in which the therapist begins to sense on a conscious level what the client is covertly communicating. This information is integrated with previous knowledge and emotions in the unconcious of the therapist and is then brought back to consciousness after it has been changed into a meaningful and useful interpretation of what the client has revealed. The therapist is, in essence, being sensitive to the hidden or concealed messages which the client is conveying.[4]

Process of the Interview

The process of an interview is an important source of information, as is the content of an interview. Process is defined as any change in the relationship of the interviewer and interviewee. The process can usually be noted when there is a change in the attitude of the interviewee or interviewer, which is usually reflected or mirrored back in the client's attitude. This latter change is often difficult for the interviewer to notice, and therefore requires a greater effort made during the interview. What is the importance of noticing, examining, and then, hopefully, understanding the process of an interview? The answer lies in the belief that the manner in which an individual interacts with another person is characteristic of and reflects his skills in interpersonal relationships.

The following questions are offered to help the reader begin the process of analyzing the process of an interview:

1. Did my comments include empathy and understanding?
2. Did I speak too rapidly, too professionally, or too glibly?
3. Did I help to refocus or redirect the course of the interview in a facilitating way?
4. Did I speak to him in words which were understandable and which showed my concern?
5. Were my questions leading, reassuring, or confusing?
6. Did my questions demonstrate understanding of the interviewee's thoughts and feelings?

The above questions are only a small example of the type of questioning and analysis which will help the interviewer learn from the process of the interview. A few other tools the beginning interviewer may use to analyze the interview as a whole will be described below.

Shifts in conversation. While it may not be immediately clear as to the reason(s) for the shift, it is usually possible to discover the reason through studying the process and the possible unconscious links between or among the subjects. Other times, the shift will indicate that the client is becoming anxious or tense about the topic. It may be too painful or too revealing for the client to express certain thoughts at that particular moment. Sometimes, shifts from one topic or another are not unrelated or disconnected. The topics have, for the client, a significant relationship. It behooves the occupational therapist to note these relationships and to explore with the client their nature and meaning. For example, a young mother may be discussing a minor illness in her husband. She then starts to talk about what she did over the past weekend. By exploring the events of that weekend, it becomes clear that she passed by her previous home where her mother's death occurred, and connected it with her husband's illness. How these two separate events are connected for this client will give the therapist a greater understanding of the woman's thoughts and feelings.

Repeated themes. The repeated themes or ideas which the client discusses are also of considerable importance. If the client discusses the same themes over and over again, if he states and restates the same ideas and feelings, the interviewer must begin to question in his own mind what the possible reasons are for this perseveration. If the interviewer feels that his repetition is hindering the collection of data and needed information, then he must try to intervene in the process and gently redirect, or probe with a question.

Gaps. If the client consistently repeats specific themes or ideas, the likelihood of there being gaps in the information becomes greater. These gaps are significant, especially when there is a pattern or similarity in the material being omitted. For example, if the client has discussed the reasons for his being fired from his last three jobs but fails to mention his relationship to any of his bosses, the interviewer should begin to explore the client's relationship with authority figures (ie, his bosses).

Inconsistencies. Another important factor to look for in the analysis of the interviewee is inconsistencies in the information given. Some examples are: 1) the client reports two different activities for the same period of time; 2) the client indicates finishing high school and then states the desire to get a high school equivalency diploma; and 3) a mother of two children gives conflicting reports of their ages, development, or current activities.

Hidden meaning. Finally, it is imperative for the therapist to listen with the third ear described earlier, for the hidden meanings which clients will inadvertently and invariably communicate. These hidden meanings provide clues about the client's problems which are difficult to verbalize, and about which he may be unaware.

Problems in Communication

Anxiety generally occurs when a person's self esteem or self-regard is in danger or is being threatened. A moderate amount of anxiety is often useful. This degree of anxiety may help to identify areas of difficulty a person is having and may motivate the person to change, or to seek help in order to change. Anxiety becomes unproductive when it overwhelms the person, and it can affect both the interviewer and interviewee. Neither is immune to the feeling of anxiety, nor to the effect too much anxiety will have on communication. Generally, too high a level of anxiety will hinder or block meaningful communication.

Behavior Resulting From Non-functional Anxiety

As the expert in interpersonal relationships, it is the therapist's responsibility to recognize the resultant behaviors of anxiety. Such behaviors include but are certainly not limited to irrational anger, misunderstandings of meanings, misinterpretations, lateness, pressured or rapid speech, confusion, authority acting, judgmental attitudes, talking up, down, or around an issue, using professional jargon, and using words or phrases with which the other person is unfamiliar. This list is endless and as the reader will note, includes behaviors of both the interviewer and interviewee. Both parties are susceptible to acting out their anxiety. It is, however, the occupational therapist's responsibility to avoid arousing unnecessary anxiety in the client. Sometimes a moderate amount of anxiety generated by the interview can be productive. However, the generation of anxiety should only be used when it is clearly in the best interest of the client. If the interviewer has any doubts about the efficacy of this therapeutic technique, it should be avoided. In most instances, the occupational therapist needs to act in such a way as to restrain the development of anxiety within the interviewee. It is helpful to reassure the client that some anxiety is natural, and it generally lessens as the interview proceeds.

Interviewee: "I'm feeling very confused and I'm not sure I'm making any sense."

Occupational Therapist: "I can understand how talking about this is difficult, and might make you somewhat anxious."

Anxiety may lead a beginning interviewer to create obstacles in communication. Therefore, it is helpful to be sensitive to the use of language. Is the therapist using a language similar to the interviewee's? Is the therapist using professionalism as a defense, by using words that a lay person would not understand? If the therapist is acting like an authority figure in order to ward off attacks or inquiry by the client, he needs to look at what ramification this stance is having on the communication flow.

Another indication of the possible presence of non-functional anxiety is allowing interruptions to occur during the interview. All too often, interruptions are viewed as a relief to the interviewer, especially during a difficult interview. By allowing interruptions to occur or by not ending them quickly and effectively, the interviewer is giving a clear, implicit message: "This interview situation is making me uncomfortable, because I'm anxious. . .bored. . .etc." Anxiety may also develop when the inteviewer interrupts the client as he is talking. If this occurs too frequently, the client will probably give up trying to talk. And why shouldn't the interviewee stop? It is clear from the inteviewer's behavior that he is not really listening to the client.

One last behavior resulting from anxiety, is judging the client's behavior or attitude. As an interviewer, the therapist might describe the client as uncooperative, a troublemaker, and/or eccentric. These judgments tend to limit the therapist's own self-reflection and evaluation of self behavior in the interview. It also tends to pigeon-hole the client into a certain category or classification. What will be missing is a real understanding of the client. All too often, a beginning therapist will also engage in self-judgment and in trying to be the ideal interviewer. This involvement in being the ideal interviewer, in asking all the right questions or in responding in just the right manner, can result in pulling away from the client, thus limiting or reducing the therapist's ability to communicate effectively. Since there is no ideal or perfect way to interview, this internal dialogue and preoccupation with self is both fruitless and unnecessary. What is most important to remember and to strive for at all times is an open, honest, and human interaction based on humanistic values.

Carol Shaw

Attitudes and Behavior of the Interviewer

An attitude is a reflection of the interviewer's mood or feeling about the interview, and about the client or topic of the interview. The attitudes and behavior which an occupational therapist demonstrates during the interview are crucial to the success or failure of the interview. For example, if attitudes are either judgmental or unempathetic, the client will most assuredly react either consciously or unconsciously and will be reluctant to share sensitive material. The interviewer's attitude and behavior reflect his basic philosophy of helping others.

Self-awareness and Self-acceptance

A beginning occupational therapist must become aware of his own attitudes and how they influence the behavior in the helping relationship—either positively or negatively. Some basic questions are offered below as a beginning to this process of self-examination.

1. How do I think and feel about myself?
2. How do I cope with and fulfill my own basic needs?
3. What is my value system and how does it influence my behavior and relationships with others?
4. What is my relationship to the society in which I live and work?
5. What is my lifestyle?
6. What is my basic philosophy of life and my work?

The more the therapist knows about himself, the more he will be able to evaluate, understand, and control his own behavior. Self-awareness leads to accepting oneself, including one's strengths and weaknesses. This honest self-acceptance and self-awareness will allow acceptance of the other person as an equal, deserving of respect as another human being who has his own values, beliefs, and attitudes.

With this self-awareness and understanding, the therapist is able to separate his needs, perceptions, and feelings from those of the interviewee. The interviewee will have the opportunity to know the therapist as another human being because the therapist will not have to hide behind a mask. This self-awareness and self-acceptance will also permit the therapist to attend to the client, and not to become preoccupied with himself and his own needs. Complete self-awareness is a difficult—if not an impossible—state to achieve. It should be something towards which occupational therapists strive but never really expect to achieve.

Humanness

Another essential attitude to have or develop is the idea of accepting the humanity of the interviewee. To respect the interviewee as another person, the therapist must first accept himself as a human being. The behavior that is demonstrated must not be robot-like. An interviewer is not an interrogator or a role model. The interviewer's behavior should convey sincerity, genuineness, and congruency. The interviewee must be able to trust that the therapist is really interested in helping him to understand and solve his problems. There must be respect for the client as a person capable of self-determination, and having worth as a fellow human being. The occupational therapist must demonstrate willingness to understand the client's background without any preconceived ideas or prejudices. The therapist must also understand and respect the concept that a person is both a part and a reflection of his culture, and that while the client may be geographically or physically removed from his culture, he is still emotionally and psychologically part of that culture.

Authenticity and Empathy

A professional attitude is not demonstrated by being a stiff, rigid, overly formal authority figure. A professional will demonstrate authenticity and warmth in his approach to the client. Authenticity implies a responsiveness on the therapist's part and willingness to understand the nature of the interviewee's experience and its meaning for him. This is empathetic understanding. Empathy is seeing the world from the position of someone else without losing sight of the self as a separate human being. One feels *with* the person rather than *for* him. The interviewer's empathetic understanding is communicated to the client by the verbal and non-verbal behavior of the interviewer. The client will know from the behavior that is shown if the interviewer is sincerely concerned and available to him.

With beginning occupational therapists, there is a tendency to confuse empathy with sympathy; however, there is a difference. Sympathy is the sharing of common interests and loyalties. As such, sympathy has no real place in the therapeutic relationship. Identification—the wish to be like another person—is also sometimes confused with empathy. Like sympathy, identification has no place in the therapeutic relationship. It is the empathetic understanding of the other person that underlies the helping relationship.

Objectivity

Another important attitude for which the inteviewer should strive is objectivity. This is essential to the evaluation process, and the interviewer must be as free of expectations as possible. It is important not to over-or under-estimate the other person, or to expect him to behave in a certain way. There is an old saying: "If you give a dog a bad name, he will bite you." This saying applies quite aptly to the preconceived ideas or expectations that a therapist may have about the client. To hear or see without imposing one's own ideas or feelings is a difficult task. It involves both control of attitudes, and self-discipline of emotional responses. This control, however, will allow the interviewer to use knowledge and skill most effectively and efficiently.

Objectivity can be lost through identification with the client or through projection of the therapist's own feelings upon the interviewer. For example, a young woman about 30 years old has recently lost her entire family in a car accident. The interviewer becomes completely immersed in her story of the accident, begins to become depressed, and loses his ability to conduct the rest of the interview.

Another example is a student who just had an argument with his clinical supervisor and feels unjustly treated. A young client then approaches the student to discuss a problem he is having with his teacher. The student finds himself siding with the client and getting angry at the teacher. At another time, the student would not have taken sides but would have handled the situation more objectively. The ability to be objective was lost in this incident because the student was both identifying with, and projecting his own feelings of being unjustly treated onto the client.

To reiterate: self-awareness, self-acceptance, humanism, authenticity, empathy, and objectivity are fundamental attitudes for a good interviewer to have and towards which to strive.

Types of Interviews

Structured-unstructured Continuum

There are a number of different methods of classifying or describing types of interviews. One method of classification states that the interviews occur along a continuum from structured to unstructured.

Structured interview. These are designated as standardized interviews. A standardized or structured interview has a specific area of concern or interest. In standardized interviews, similar and conflicting information about the client may be gathered from different people. This information can then be compared and classified. Similarities and differences in the answers given can be noted, and may reflect similarities and differences in the interviewee, not in the questions. A structured interview is one in which there are predetermined questions and fixed responses with which the interviewee may respond. There is little room to explore for further information or clarification.

Semi-structured interview. As in the structured, the semi-structured interview uses predetermined specific questions to gather information about an area of concern. However, in the semi-structured interview, the interviewer is free to ask other questions in order to clarify or probe for more information. There is generally a schedule of questions, or a general outline of the information being sought which assists the interviewer in this data collection.

Unstructured or unstandardized interview. In this type of interview, there are no predetermined questions. The occupational therapist explores whatever phenomena seem most crucial, useful, or pertinent to the interest of the interviewee. This type of interview requires great skill in and sensitivity to the client and the interview process, for it allows the occupational therapist to explore material or matters which are interesting, but relevant to the purpose of the interview.

Naturally, an interview may contain all these types of questions or formats. For instance, a structured section of an interview will ask for the name, address, date of birth, etc. Another segment of the same interview might center around an activity or work schedule, or an interest check list. This would be an example of a semi-structured interview. An unstructured segment of the interview would be the exploration of the interviewee's work relationship or past interests and/or activities.

Initial-terminal Continuum

Another classification system of interviews is one in which interviews are labeled as initial, on-going, or terminal.

Initial interview. As the name implies, this is the first interview. It is crucial to the establishment of rapport, since most people are often strongly influenced by first impressions. Unfortunately, first impressions, especially if they are negative, are hard to overcome. The initial interview provides a beginning basis for further exploration by establishing what needs to be evaluated in subsequent interviews. It is, however, the initial interview which sets the tone for the future.

On-going interviews. Again, as the name implies, on-going interviews occur over an extended period of time. They focus on single or specified issues which have been arrived at by mutual agreement. The interviews may be evaluative or therapeutic in nature. Naturally, the interviews are part of an on-going process, and where one leaves off is generally where the next one begins.

Terminal interviews. These occur at the conclusion of treatment. The focus of the termination interview is a review of the findings, and a general statement regarding the assessment of the interviewee's problems, strengths, or concerns. Treatment recommendations and plans are discussed and solidified. Anticipated difficulties are discussed and further recommendations or suggestions for other types of treatment might be made. At this time, issues of separation and loss are often crucial, and need to be addressed and discussed.

Consultations and Referrals

Consultations. Occupational therapists are usually asked to assess an individual's level of function within a particular area of occupational performance or to assess his potential for occupational therapy treatment. In the case of a consultation, the consulting therapist is rarely—if ever—the therapist who treats the client. However, the consultant will be asked to provide the treating therapist with information which will help to determine the nature of the treatment relationship, setting, or activities best suited to the client's needs. It is best to share the purpose and objectives of the consultation process. It is also important to share the assessment results with the interviewee so that he will be able to understand and use the information.

Referrals. These are made when it is clear that the occupational therapist or the facility cannot provide the services needed by the client. For instance, if a client needs to find a place to live, the therapist might refer him to a housing agent or a social worker, depending on the client's financial situation. The individual who does the referring generally makes initial contact with the person or facility for the client. Depending on the client's level of functioning, one of the following methods of referral may be used:

1. *Client contact*—After the client has been given information about the person or agency to whom he is being referred, the client makes all the necessary contacts.
2. *Therapist contact*—The therapist calls the agency and makes the appointment for the client, then gives the client the information.
3. *Joint contact*—The therapist goes with the client to the referred person or facility. This makes the transition and initial contact easier and less anxiety-provoking. This method also insures to some extent that the client gets to the facility.

Any of the methods described above may be adopted or modified to fit the client's needs and level of functioning.

It is important that the reasons for the referral and what the other person or facility has to offer be clearly explained to the client. Possible problems that the client might anticipate, and exploration of the client's concerns or fears might be discussed at this time. All too often, clients do not make a smooth transition from one facility to another, and do not avail themselves of the full benefit of that facility's services. This transition can be made smoother by helping the client understand the reasons for the referral and by helping him to become as comfortable as possible at the prospect of another helping person or environment.

Preparation for and Conduction of an Interview

Prior To Actual Interview

Before discussing what acutally takes place in an interview and how to prepare for it, there are certain things that need to be taken into account. The first consideration is how the interviewee comes for services. All these pathways will influence the interview process. Some of the pathways a client uses are:

1. *Referral for treatment*—Referral may come from a psychiatrist, psychotherapist, social worker, or any other health professional who recommends occupational therapy evaluation and possible treatment.
2. *Consultation*—This refers to a situation in which another occupational therapist or health professional wants an assessment of a person for a particular reason.
3. *Self-referral*—In this situation, the client feels that occupational therapy services might be beneficial to him.
4. *Self decision*—Self decision refers to the situations in which the occupational therapist initiates contact with the person because it is felt that the client would benefit from occupational therapy sessions.

Expectations

The expectations of the occupational therapist and the client about the interview situation will have an impact, at least initially, on the interview. Whether the client is arriving at the interview voluntarily, or under the direct or strong recommendation of his therapist (ie, somewhat involuntarily) he will experience apprehension which will influence his behavior. What has been heard or learned about the client's reasons for referral, life circumstances, or diagnosis will influence the therapist's preconceptions about the client. These circumstances may lead to different or hidden agendas. That is, each person may have different ideas as to the purpose, conduction, or possible outcome of the interview. For example, if the interviewer believes that an interview should be a collaborative effort, then how he conducts the interview will be in accordance to this belief. If, however, the client has different expectations, ie, he sees the interviewer as an authority figure or an advice-giver, then he may be disappointed, or confused by an interview conducted as a collaborative effort. For instance, the client is told by his psychiatrist he will be helped in getting a job, and therefore, he expects this from the occupational therapist. The therapist expects to evaluate the client's work habits and interests, and report the findings to the vocational counselor, psychiatrist, and client. Unless these different expectations are identified and resolved, the interview will probably be unsuccessful, in that neither party accomplished their expected goals.

Preparation for the Interview

The following list of responsibilities is offered as a guide in preparing for an interview:

1. *Physical setting*—Considerations regarding the physical setting are described later in the chapter, pp 37-38.
2. *Time considerations*—Schedule enough time to conduct the interview without being rushed or interrupted. Most interviews are scheduled to last between 45 minutes and an hour. Sometimes the interview may be as short as 10-15 minutes, whereas in crisis situations, they can last 2-3 hours. Usually, once an interview has lasted over an hour, fatigue for both parties tends to occur.
3. *Equipment and supplies*—Prior to the interview, so as not to waste time or present a negative impression, gather or arrange the equipment, supplies, and

evaluation forms which are going to be utilized.

4. *Background information*—Information regarding why and how the interviewee got to your clinic, ie, how he happened to need your services, is important to obtain. Usually some general historical or background information from the referring source is helpful. This information ought to be sent with the client's referral form.

5. *Purpose for interview*—A trained interviewer needs to have a clear idea as to what information is needed and for what purpose this information will be gathered.

6. *Essential attitudes*—Finally, the therapist needs to have acquired or to possess to some degree the attitudes basic to any helping relationship—self-awareness, humanness, objectivity, and empathy.

Stages of an' Interview

As with most events, the interview has a beginning, middle, and end. None of these stages are clearly delineated; rather, they evolve from one stage to the next.

The beginning or introductory stage. The focus of the this stage is the reason for which the occupational therapist and client are meeting. The stage ends when both parties understand and agree to what is going to be discussed. The reaching of this agreement may take five minutes, or considerably longer, if the two parties have different conceptions of the interview purpose. However, even before this agreement is reached, the interviewer meets and greets the client. As a general rule, social pleasantries have little place in an evaluative interview. However, this type of statement may be used to facilitate the initial transition from social interactions, which are usually more casual than the formal interview situation. Social pleasantries may also be used when the interviewee's anxiety level is obviously high. The use of these statements can help to relax the client to a point where he can participate fully in the interview.

A statement concerning the nature and purpose of the interview needs to be made by the interviewer. Especially in the evaluative interview, the purpose and outcome (ie, how the interviewee will benefit) are important to state. Further clarification is indicated if the client demonstrates some concern or distress with the interview situation. The introductory stage may also include either a statement or agreement about an initial definition of the interviewee's problems, and a delineation of the particular problems which will be addressed within this interview.

The development of rapport begins in the first stage. Even the therapist's manner of greeting the client may influence their rapport. For example, consider the following situation:

The client enters the office; you remain seated, non-verbally indicating where the client should sit. You then begin to question him about his work history.

Contrast this situation with the following set of circumstances:

The client is waiting in the clinic; the therapist approaches and introduces himself. The therapist invites the client into the office and suggests that he might be comfortable in a particular chair. The interview is formally opened with an explanatory statement regarding the purpose of the interview.

Undoubtedly, the potential for a successful interview is less likely in the first example than in the second one.

The middle or exploratory/development stage. The focus of this stage is the achievement of the agreed upon purposes or goals established in the beginning stage. This involves an indepth examination of the problems or areas of concern of the interviewee. This stage is the most difficult one to provide any specific guidelines to the beginning occupational therapist. However, the information presented later in this chapter, on pp 30-32 and 39-41, should help in conducting this particular stage of the interview.

The middle stage focuses on obtaining specific information. The focus, however, is of necessity dependent upon the nature of the information being sought, the problem being explored, or the stated purpose of the interview. See Table 2.1 for more information.

TABLE 2.1
INFORMATION OBTAINED IN THE EXPLORATORY STAGE

— Detailed inquiry of the problems and concerns of the client as directed by the interviewer.

— Client's own assessment and ideas about his problems.

— History/social, medical, psychological development of problems and related issues.

— Assets and limitations of the client and his available resources (physical, coping mechanism, social, and financial support system).

— Current level of functioning of client, or

— Future or potential level of functioning.

To assess the therapist's skills in conducting this second stage, the questions in Table 2.2 are offered to assist the feedback process.

The end or termination stage. The components of this stage are essentially the same as the introductory stage, except in reverse. The termination stage is equally important to the success of the interview as is the introductory stage. If it is handled poorly, it can be destructive to the entire interview.

Each person in the interview should be aware that the interview is ending, and accept this fact. Preparation for this aspect is usually done in the first stage. Usually, the therapist will have informed the client as to the expected length of the interview. If its purpose is accomplished prior to the end of its allotted time, then the interview is usually ended.

TABLE 2.2
QUESTIONS TO ENHANCE FEEDBACK PROCESS

— Did I enable the client to speak as freely as possible about himself without burdening him with my own values, biases, or concerns?

— Did the client gain some understanding of himself and his problems? Was he able to share with me how he felt and what he thought?

— Did I really listen to what his concerns were or did I try to program him to mine?

— Do I have a greater understanding of the person? Do I know what additional information I need in order to understand him better?

— Are the goals for treatment becoming more diffuse or more specific and clear? Are the goals my goals, the client's goals, or were the goals mutually arrived at?

— Did my questions and responses facilitate the client's discussion? Was I able to refocus the client's discussion when he strayed from the topic being discussed?

There should be a summary statement as to what has been accomplished. This statement needs to be kept simple and on a positive note. As summarization is a selective process, the therapist needs to ask the client if there are any questions or comments about the summary. Be sure to give enough time to answer the issues brought up by the interviewee. In summarizing, it is important not to discuss any new issues or concerns. Never give a diagnosis of the interviewee's problems. If the client asks for a diagnosis, explore why he is asking for one and what is the importance or significance of it to him. Sometimes the interviewee may be quite persistent, and will keep asking for one. In those instances, it is advisable to state that labels really have no bearing or effect on his problems or on the therapeutic relationship. This comment will usually close the discussion.

Arrangements for future interviews are generally made during this stage. If further evaluative interviews are not necessary, other action is usually recommended. These other actions might be referral to another facility, treatment, or no further contact.

Once these arrangements or recommendations are made and discussed, then the actual leave-taking occurs. This should be done with the same sensitivity as was illustrated in the introductory stage.

Basic Components of a Helping Interview

There are several basic components in a successful helping interview. These will be discussed briefly in the following sections. If greater detail is needed, check the books written on the interview, which are listed in the bibliography, p 42.

Listening

A fundamental operation of interviewing, listening is more than the physical sense of hearing. Listening entails both the mental and emotional functions of the person. It is truly a difficult process to learn; it requires constant effort. As a new occupational therapist, eagerness often gets in the way of precisely listening to the client. If the new therapist finds himself listening to less than two-thirds of the interview and talking more than one-third, he can be fairly sure he is the one being interviewed. Therefore, the therapist needs to look at what is happening, either in the client's situation or in himself, to account for this imbalance.

Be Ignorant

An excellent position to take as an interviewer is ignorance. The occupational therapist can then enter the interview situation without any preconceptions as to the client's problems. Poetically, the client is provided with a blank paper which he can fill with an unsmudged picture of himself. By making assumptions about what the client is like or what he might say, the therapist could find himself interrupting the client and perhaps finishing thoughts for him, often with disasterous, or at least non-productive consequences.

Active Process

Listening is an active process. The interviewer does not just sit back and let the interviewee talk. If this is done, a real opportunity to know the other person is lost. Knowing the other person means understanding how he thinks and feels about himself; how he thinks and feels about others in his world; how he sees others relating to him; what his goals, hopes, and plans for the future are; how he copes with problems, what defense mechanisms he uses; and what his belief system is.

Because listening is such an intense activity, there will be lapses in attention and in the listening process. Oftentimes, these lapses are caused by the interviewee repeating himself, or by the interviewer having an internal dialogue with himself. For example:

> A young man repeatedly discusses one particular event that happened to him over the weekend. Your attention lessens because you think you've heard this before. However, you later become aware that during this session he had described some crucial incidents which would have been useful to explore with him.

Internal Dialogue

Many times the client will be discussing a subject which will trigger an internal dialogue within the occupational therapist. For example: A woman is discussing her marital problems. The interviewer is reminded of her own argument with her husband earlier in the day. The therapist becomes lost in her own reverie. If these lapses in listening happen, and they surely will, it is best to be honest about them and say something like: "I'm sorry; could you repeat what you said? I missed some of it."

Selective Process

Good listening is a selective process. The good listener is actively attentive to general, recurrent, or major themes of the interviewee rather than to details. This selective effort requires that the occupational therapist know exactly why he is listening. This purpose or goal allows him to screen out what is not necessary information. For example, in trying to determine the reasons for the client's repeated suspensions from the sheltered workshop, the occupational therapist should pay close attention to the client's description of his relationship with co-workers and supervisors.

Languages

As a good listener, the therapist must also be sensitive to the subtleties of language and the different meanings of the same words to various cultural groups. For example, some people understand the word *horse* to mean an animal, while others understand it to also mean heroin. Certainly, this is an important distinction to know.

External Distractions

As listening involves hard work on the part of the occupational therapist, it is helpful to eliminate any external noise which may be distracting. It is also useful to look at the client. This will help to focus attention on what is being said, and to pick up additional non-verbal clues to assist in active listening.

Silences

During an interview, silences will occur. These lapses need to be listened to as actively as the verbal exchanges. Why is silence so difficult for the beginning occupational therapist and why does it create so much discomfort for both the participants? Silences are antithetical to this country's norm of self-expression, of speaking one's own mind. Silence is often seen as a rejection and an ostracism. Children are often punished by their peers by being given the "silent treatment." Silent people are often viewed with suspicion and fear—thus the phrase, "You need to look out for the quiet ones." Silence can be an effective means for achieving the purpose of the interview. An interviewer needs a certain amount of experience and security to allow silence to become productive. It may help the beginning interviewer to realize that there are many reasons, both positive and negative, for silences.

Collect and sort out thoughts. The client may be trying to gather himself internally in order to verbalize his thoughts and feelings. Interrupting him in this effort, by making some comment, may inhibit or thwart future attempts. This phenomenon may often be seen when the client pauses for a moment. A pause is defined here as a brief silence. The client may be searching for more to say and how to say it. It would be a mistake to rush in and make him lose his train of thought.

Natural termination of a topic. Silences may occur when the interviewee is finished talking about a subject. This may include the conclusion of a description of a particular incident or event. Or, the client may in fact choose not to discuss the subject further, but may or may not indicate this verbally. Oftentimes, the interviewee may also be waiting for a clue from the interviewer to know what to do next.

Resistance. Silences can and do occur as a reaction against or resistance to further probing by the interviewer. The interviewer may be viewed as an authority figure and therefore, may stimulate transference reactions. Silence can also be a result of anxiety on the part of the client. The interview situation or the material being discussed may generate sufficient anxiety to cause the interviewee to be unable to speak. In these last two instances, it is essential that the interviewer help the client work through these obstacles.

Observation

Active process. Observation is the active noticing or seeing which occurs continuously throughout the interview. Observation can be influenced by expectations or psychological set. In a recent study, students' observations of the same subject were reported to be significantly altered due to the information given to them prior to their observations.[5] Thus, as with listening, it is essential to be ignorant in an effort to reduce or eliminate, to as great a degree as possible, any biases and preconceptions. This is an important point and should be given serious consideration, as the new occupational therapist learns to interview.

Non-verbal communication. A great deal has been written about body language and non-verbal communication. The use of activities and other modes of non-verbal communication in the occupational therapy evaluation and treatment process makes it absolutely essential that the occupational therapist be knowledgeable about this form of communication. As non-verbal communication is more primitive, it is usually more reliable than verbal clues or messages. As with verbal messages, non-verbal communications must be validated. One cannot take a non-verbal message, such as lip biting, and label it a sign of anxiousness, or tongue movement, and say that it is a neurological symptom:

A client was observed to constantly lick the upper corner of her lip with her tongue. On the client's charts, a doctor had noted this movement and had written that the client had some neurological dysfunction based on his observation, and needed to be given a complete neurological examination. While talking to the client, a student asked her if she were aware of this repetitive movement and could she control it? The client exclaimed yes, and wished someone would help her cut off the long hair on her lip that had been annoying her so much!

As this example so beautifully illustrates, the interviewer must see non-verbal communication in the context of the situation. Be extremely careful not to draw firm conclusions without validating the meaning of the non-verbal communication with the interviewee. The interviewer must assess the situation and note the persistence, repetition, and quality of the behavior.

Non-verbal messages can often have as many different meanings as the number of people seeing the stimulus. For instance, if an activity group was using magazine pictures as a stimulus and focus for communication, each member of the group would see something different in the picture.

Self-observation. Not only must the interviewer observe the behavior of the interviewee, but he must also observe his own behavior and how it affects the client. If the interviewer is pressed for time and looks at his watch a number of times, or begins to look out the window instead of at the interviewee, he is sending out messages which will have a very definite effect on the interviewee. In the two above examples, the effect will probably be a negative one.

"How can I observe myself?" The answer is not an easy one. It will require the interviewer's developing an awareness of his own body language, and assessing himself throughout the interview. If the therapist is fortunate and can avail himself of a videotaping machine, this is an excellent way to observe both verbal and non-verbal communication, and to study their interrelationship.

The interviewer communicates non-verbal messages and information to the client as actively as he receives information back. It is imperative that the therapist be aware and sensitive to the impact he has on the interviewee. He needs to assess how age, sex, dress, and race will be viewed and reacted to by the interviewee.

Observing non-verbal messages allows the therapist to determine the nature of their relationship, and whether there is movement towards or away from the relationship. Non-verbal messages help to regulate communication through a feedback system. If the therapist watches the client's non-verbal behavior, he can learn whether or not the client is listening, bored, anxious, or wants to say something. The interviewer will also be able to assess covert messages.

Questions

Asking questions is another critical component in conducting an interview. How and when to ask questions are crucial issues for the beginning occupational therapist. If he asks too many questions, a pattern of interaction is established with the client which will be difficult to change. However, the therapist is also faced with the responsibility and need to elicit information from the interviewee.

When to ask questions. Questions should be asked when something the client said has been missed. The therapist simply asks, "I'm sorry. I missed the last part of what you were saying. Could you go over it once more?" Another use of questions might be to assess whether or not the client has actually understood. Additionally, the interviewer may also want to explore a particular area or issue more fully to clarify what the event actually meant. The client may also need to help in clarifying or exploring a thought or feeling, and may need a question to help refocus his thoughts. There are also occasions when the topic or feeling which the interviewee is discussing is a particularly difficult one for him to verbalize. A question asked with a supportive, understanding manner may encourage him, or help him to discuss it. For example: "It seems like a difficult topic. Is there something else you want to talk about now? Perhaps we could discuss that later."

Avoid asking too many questions. Questions must be asked in a facilitating way.

Too often, the beginning occupational therapist will ask too many questions at once. This barrage of questions probably has more to do with the therapist's own anxiety level than with the seeking of information. Many ill-timed questions can also effectively confuse the client by interrupting his concentration. Questions which force or impel the person to choose between two items or answers should also be avoided. For instance, asking someone, "Did you go to college or work at a job?" leaves him little opportunity to tell you what actually happened to him during that particular time period. Finally, avoid asking *why* too often. It is an extremely difficult question for most of us to answer—many people do not know why they behave or feel a certain way. The question also has a punitive connotation which might not facilitate a free flow of communication.

How to ask questions. Now that we have stated what not to do, we will discuss what kind of questions the therapist asks, and how he goes about doing it. If the therapist is seeking concrete information, direct, closed-ended questions are most useful. For example:

"What were the jobs you held over the last five years?"
"How many children do you have and what are their ages?"

For all other information, the open-ended type of question is the most facilitating:

"Could you tell me the circumstances surrounding your being fired?"
"How did you feel after your divorce?"

Questions should also be concerned with only one subject and be asked at a reasonable pace. The therapist will probably find that using an indirect question will dilute the impact or harshness of a direct question. For example:

"The group was pretty disruptive today. I noticed that you seemed quite upset and left the room."
"You've been attending the day center now for a week. There must be a lot you want to talk about."

Grammatically, these are not questions—there is no question mark. However, a definite, yet unstated question is being presented.

Listen to the answer. Once a question is asked, stop, wait, and listen for the answer—that is the ultimate reason for the question. All too often, interviewers race ahead in their thoughts to the next question, before the client has finished answering. If the client begins to answer the therapist's queries curtly and quickly, it behooves the therapist to look at himself to see if active listening is taking place.

Interviewer Responses

The verbal responses that are given during an interview will determine to a great extent, the client's comfort and willingness to share his thoughts and feelings. The responses will convey the attitude level of interest, concern, and understanding. It is hoped that verbal responses will help the interviewee understand himself and others more clearly, and clarify his feelings and thoughts about his life situation.

The kinds of possible verbal responses are practically limitless. Below is a listing of some of the responses most frequently used and described in the literature. The reader is referred once again to p 42 for more information on this subject.

Minimum verbal response. This response is the "uh-huh," "mm-mm," or "yes," utterances, or head nods of the occupational therapist which gives the client the sense that he is being listened to and understood. It also conveys the message that the client can proceed, since the occupational therapist is following his ideas. However, the information and emphasis of this response, if improperly used, sometimes denotes disapproval and criticism to what the interviewee is saying.

Paraphrasing. In this type of response, the interviewer uses most of the words used by the interviewee. The primary purposes are to reflect back to the client what he has said, to demonstrate to the client that the interviewer understands what is being said, or to stress one particular component or phrase of the client's statement. Example:

> **Client:** "I didn't do very well at work today."
> **Occupational therapist:** "Things didn't go well for you today at work?"

> **Client:** "It was very hard to tell her that I was angry at her."
> **Occupational therapist:** "It must have been very hard to say you were angry at her?"

> **Client:** "The boss yelled at me in front of all those guys. I really wanted to leave and never come back. I'm never going back."
> **Occupational therapist:** "Your boss yelled at you in front of all your co-workers?"

Reflecting. Reflection deals primarily with the unstated or implied feelings or concerns of the interviewee. It requires a great deal of sensitivity and empathy on the part of the occupational therapist, who must be able to accurately assess the feeling, tone, and attitude of the client, and to verbalize these feelings and attitudes in a clear and acceptable manner to the client. Examples of some reflecting statements are: "You really sound as if you want to cry," or "It sounds as though you were really very frightened by what happened."

Probing. To probe, the therapist generally uses an open-ended statement which attempts to gain more information about a particular subject, issue, or feeling. Statements which start, "Tell me more about..." "Let's talk about that for a moment longer..." or "I was wondering how that..." are some examples of probing responses.

Clarifying. Clarification of the information can occur for both parties in an interview. The occupational therapist's responses may be geared to help clarify something for the client or for himself. In the first instance, the occupational therapist might attempt to refocus or express something about which the interviewee is confused or is having difficulty expressing. In the latter instance, the occupational therapist needs to have something clarified for his own understanding of what is being discussed. An example of clarifying an issue for the interview would be:

> **Client:** "I just don't understand myself; I'm confused and anxious about every little thing."
> **Occupational therapist:** "It seems that even small things are making you anxious and unsure of youself."

> **Client:** "He really jammed me up; I didn't know where he was coming from."
> **Occupational therapist:** "I'm sorry. I don't really understand what you mean by jammed up."

Interpreting. Interpretation is the adding of something to what the interviewee is saying. It is a response which must be based on an honest understanding of the interviewee, his particular lifestyle, and internal frame of reference. If an interpretation is useful to the client, there will be a greater understanding on his part. If the interpretation is not correct or is not useful, then it will generally be rejected by the person.

> **Client:** "I can't seem to get myself to study for that course. It just doesn't interest me."
> **Occupational therapist:** "From what you told me earlier, you seem to resent the teacher's attitude toward you."

Confronting. Confrontation involves the occupational therapist giving honest feedback to the client about how he really sees what is happening to the client. Confronting must be done out of a genuine desire to help. If it is not done with this intent, confrontation can become a very destructive and hostile instrument. Confrontation responses are often best done by taking the *"I"* position. For example, "I feel that you are playing a game here," or "I wonder why you are so angry with me?" By sending *"I"* messages, the therapist is taking the responsibility for what is said and is openly sharing his thoughts or feelings with the client.

Informing. As the word denotes, informing is giving the interviewee information that is either factual or objective. This is quite different from advising. In giving advice, one is generally suggesting something which has a subjective aspect and may or may not have strings attached. Advice is generally to be avoided in the treatment process, and has no place in the evaluation interview or process.

General guidelines. The verbal responses described above are only a fraction of the kinds used in interviews. In these and other verbal responses, the therapist chooses to use certain guidelines or themes that are applicable. See Table 2.3 for more information.

Responding to personal inquiries. The occupational therapist is often confronted with the problem of having to deal with personal questions asked by the client. It is my opinion that personal comments have no place in the evaluation process as they may influence, inhibit, or in some way alter the interviewee's response or behavior. Personal comments or information may occasionally be used in the treatment to serve as an example. However, these examples or comments must be used sparingly and should be generalized and depersonalized. For instance, "Many students resent..." or "Many mothers have experienced the same thing."

If the interviewee asks a personal question of the interviewer, the interviewer needs to listen to the question with the third ear. If the therapist chooses to answer the interviewee's questions, it should be done honestly and with sensitivity as to the meaning of the question. For example, a client may ask if the therapist has children, what ages they are, and how they are disciplined. It is important to understand the motivation behind this type of questioning and what the client is saying about himself by asking such a personal question.

TABLE 2.3

GUIDELINES TO BE USED IN AN INTERVIEW

— Speak in the language of the interviewee; use his vocabulary.

— Speak slowly enough for the person to follow and understand what you are saying.

— Be concise; avoid verbosity.

— Talk directly to the interviewee; avoid talking about him as if her weren't there.

— Be aware of timing your responses to facilitate the communication.

— Make "I" statements when you are confronting or interpreting — "I" statements allow the interviewee to reject, accept, or change the message.

Carol Shaw

The interviewee may also ask questions about other people. As a helping professional, the therapist needs to respect the confidentiality of the person about whom the interviewee is inquiring. This may, in essence, reassure the interviewee of the interviewer's honesty and professional integrity. After reassuring him, the therapist needs to revert the focus of the interview back onto the client as soon as possible. Since all behavior is motivated, one can also assume that there is a reason for the interviewee's question about other people. The interviewer might want to explore the motives which stimulated the question at that time or later—whenever the timing is best.

The interviewee may also ask questions about himself. Again, the helping professional must understand the meaning of these questions and the motives behind them. If the therapist chooses to answer them he should understand the many ramifications of the response.

In order to arrive at a comfortable position with regard to answering personal questions, the following brief list is given. These are a few possible reasons or motives behind the interviewee's questions:

1. politeness
2. natural curiosity
3. an attempt to establish a relationship with the interviewer
4. an indication of an area of difficulty or conflict for the interviewee which is emotionally hot for him
5. the need for information

The interviewer must be sensitive to the concealed or latent meaning of these questions. Since all behavior is motivated, it has meaning and importance.

Additional Factors Which Influence an Interview

Besides attitudes, purpose, and components of an interview, there are other additional factors which influence the outcome of an interview and must be considered.

Physical Surroundings

The physical surroundings in which the interview takes place may influence the entire outcome of the interview. Some degree of privacy is essential. A client will most often be very reluctant to discuss private concerns if within earshot of others. Therefore, one of the preparations that needs to be made before interviewing is to make sure (or as sure as possible) that the interview will not be interrupted either by telephone calls, other staff members needing information, or other emergency interruptions.

A relaxed and comfortable atmosphere is also a crucial factor in the outcome of the interview. The room or office should be provided with comfortable seats and ventilation for the people involved in the interview. What the room or office should acutally look like is quite a difficult question to answer. Usually, a therapist's life space (the office) reflects in some part his personality. There is absolutely nothing wrong with this reflection. The therapist needs, however, to be sensitive to the impact the physical setting, content, and the atmosphere have on the interviewee, and what is being symbolically communicated to the client.

As occupational therapists begin to work more directly in the community, home visits or interviews conducted in the client's home will become a common practice. Whenever a therapist enters someone's home, it must be remembered that he is there generally at the invitation and with the permission of the client. Therefore, the therapist needs to understand and respect that the client is his host, and that he should arrive on time and accept the client's hospitality with respect and politeness. These homebound interviews can provide a wealth of information about the interviewee's life space, his values, beliefs, everyday living routines, and priorities which are absent from agency or institutional-based interviews. I strongly urge therapists to make use of this dormant information source and to realize its potential in helping the client within his actual living environment.

Whether the interview takes place in an office or elsewhere, the setting for the interview should provide quiet, privacy, and freedom from distractions.

Note-taking/Recording of Interview

The process of note-taking is an integral part of any interview. Notes are important as a means to refresh the memory, to remind us of plans which require action, to help us learn from the interview (ie, to see how we behaved, how we discussed, or failed to discuss certain conflict areas), and to indicate what other information needs to be obtained or explored further.

The question of how and when to take notes is generally of concern to the beginning interviewer. This is essentially a personal decision which is based on each therapist's own style and needs. For some people, a single word jotted down is sufficient. For others, more complete thoughts or phrases will be necessary. Whatever method is developed, some methods which should be avoided are presented below:

1. Do not use note-taking as a way to avoid making a real and meaningful contact with the client.
2. Do not become so involved with the process of note-taking that the real purpose of the interview is forgotten, ie, helping the client.
3. Do not keep the notes a secret from the interviewee. Be prepared to share the notes with him. Paranoid clients especially will be sensitive to note-taking and can often be reassured if the notes are shared willingly. Therefore, write down only factual information, not impressions and interpretations. These belong elsewhere, usually in the evaluation summary.

One last comment on notes and note-taking. The notes recorded during an interview require and deserve the same confidential status which are given the verbal communication of the interviewee. Notes should only be shared with the other staff members or supervisors working to help the interviewee.

Taping the interview either auditorially or audiovisually, provides the occupational therapist with an objective record of the interview and interview process. This objective record also gives the interviewer an excellent opportunity to learn how and what he is doing as an interviewer. Before using either method, the consent of the interviewee should be obtained. The client can also learn about his own behavior by listening and/or watching himself. Although initially, videotaping can be quite threatening to both the occupational therapist and client, it can be an invaluable tool for both parties by providing an objective record of the verbal and non-verbal messages.

Confidentiality

What the interviewee discusses and shares is to be respected and held in confidence. He has the right to know that this information will not be shared with people who are not directly involved with his treatment. The client also has the right to know with whom and for what purpose this information will be shared.

If the client gets a sense that the therapist respects his right to privacy and the confidential nature of the relationship, he will be able to begin to trust the interviewer.

It is also important to know and adhere to the facility's code of ethics regarding a client's right to privacy and confidentiality. It is the therapist's responsibility to become familiar with the guidelines and procedures of the facility.

Essential Information for the Occupational Therapist

The occupational therapist's primary focus is on the nature of the individual's relationship to the environment in which he lives or is expected to live, and on how he relates to society at large. In order to assess the individual's current level of functioning or potential for a functional and meaningful life, the occupational therapist needs to obtain specific information about the individual's occupational performance. Areas of focus and concern for the psychiatric occupational therapist are the individual's:

1. work or play history and current skills;
2. leisure time interests and pursuits;
3. daily living activities and time management;
4. mental status
5. social history

While the psychiatric occupational therapist is not responsible for obtaining a mental status examination or a complete and detailed social history, the occupational therapist must be familiar with the components of and information obtained from these interviews.

In the occupational therapy literature, a large number of evaluation procedures have been described and discussed. Numerous evaluation procedures have also been developed and presented at annual conferences, workshops, and in special interest groups on a state level. This section will present a number of previously published and unpublished evaluation procedures.

The various evalution procedures developed are reliable or valid. A beginning effort to develop reliability and validity for specific evaluation procedures has been initiated by American Occupational Therapy Association's Specialty Section for Mental Health. It is my hope that standardized evaluation procedures will be developed through this effort, and will thus provide the practicing occupational therapist with validated and reliable assessment tools for planning treatment.

Work History/Play History

While current work skills and behavior may be assessed through the use of task evaluations or simulated work situations, an individual's work history is best obtained through the use of an extensive semi-structured interview. Such an instrument has been developed by Linda Moorehead.[6] Correct use of this evaluation procedure is dependent upon the occupational therapist's knowledge of the occupational behavior frame of reference and skills in conducting a history-taking interview. These skills include the ability to ask questions that refocus the interviewee when necessary, and to elicit and clarify information pertinent to the areas under consideration or which are considered important.

In her article, Moorehead presents the theoretical basis and rationale for the development of this particular evaluation procedure. The author also suggests specific focuses with which to analyze the information obtained from the interview. Moorehead presents a case history as an example of the application to this evaluation procedure. This example beautifully illustrates how the information obtained through the interview was applied in the service of the client.

While an adult's work is generally his job or his primary occupation, a child's work is his play. Therefore, the occupational therapist working with children must be concerned with obtaining a complete play history. The book, *Play as Exploratory Learning,* offers an exciting and stimulating description of play and its place in the learning and socialization process. Included in the book is a chapter written by Nancy Takata in which she describes play history evaluation.[7,8]

The play history is an open-ended questionnaire which attempts to identify play experiences and play opportunities for the child. A detailed explanation of the information sought and how the information is then analyzed and applied is presented in Takata's chapter.

Leisure Time Interests and Pursuits

The occupational therapist uses a primary media for treatment which encompasses the interests and activities of the individual. In order to obtain information regarding the person's past, current, and potential interests, the occupational therapist often uses an interest check list. Such an instrument was developed by Janice Matsutsuyu.[9] Adaptions to this instrument have been made and are widely used by practitioners. Matsutsuyu defines six propositions upon which the interest check list and its subsequent analysis is based. It is important to mention that the check list is used in conjunction with a follow-up interview. This interview allows for further exploration, elaboration, and clarification of the information. Here again, the skills of the interviewer will determine, to some extent, the usefulness and completeness of the information obtained.

Daily Living Activities and Time Management

Occupational therapists are interested in how an individual occupies and manages his time. Occupational therapists also want to know the quality of the activity in which the individual is engaged. To obtain this information, the interview procedure developed by Sandra Watanabe is frequently used by occupational therapists. This interview method, the activities configuration, was developed from a theoretical concept first described by Watanabe in the article "Four Concepts Basic to the Occupational Therapist Process."[10] The interview form or schedule is presented in *Willard & Spackman's Occupational Therapy,* 5th Edition.[11] The activities configuration is of particular interest to the occupational therapist as it allows him to assess the specific activities in which the client engages, the function of these activities, their importance to the client, and degree of competency with which the client feels the activities are performed. This interview procedure can also provide the client with a concrete picture of how he spends his time, and what activities he does for himself or for others, either willingly or unwillingly. This kind of picture can sometimes be a starting point for treatment as it may become a barometer for change or a means of initiating self-reflection and self-evaluation in the client. The client and therapist may also use the tool to more accurately assess the client's current ability to manage his time, to problem solve, and to use time more satisfactorily in his work, play, and self activities.

Mental Status

A mental status examination is usually conducted by the psychiatrist at the time of the client's admission to the ward, day hospital, or other treatment program. The mental status examination is required by law in most states, and provides a current picture of the client's thought process, communication skills, and behavior.

Generally, the mental status exam helps in the detection and identification of psychopathology and may indicate causative factors. Most experienced interviewers will elicit the necessary information for a mental status exam without disrupting the flow of the interview. In general, the content of a formal mental status exam includes information about the following areas:[12]

1. Initial *appearance* and *behavior* refers to dress, posture, facial expression, motor activity, physical characteristics, mood, reactions, and the interviewee's specific mannerisms (ie, tics, repetitive gestures).

2. *Speech* refers to quality, quantity, and organization of speech (ie, tone, pressure, logic).

3. *Mood* refers to both the subjective determination by the interviewee, or the interviewer's objective determination or evaluation of the interviewee's thought; ie, whether the interviewee has obsessive-compulsive, ruminating, phobic, paranoid thoughts, or somatic preoccupations.

4. *Perception* refers to the presence or absence of illusions or hallucinations.

5. *Orientation* as to time, space, and person refers to the interviewee's level of awareness as to the date and place of the interview and who he is.

Social History

Social history information is generally obtained by the social worker on the mental health team. A detailed developmental history focuses on the individual's significant relationships and experiences during his development. Generally, each developmental stage is described, and the interviewer tries to get a picture from the interviewee of his strengths, weaknesses, values, attitudes, and basic characteristic patterns of coping behaviors and defense mechanisms. The interviewer usually wants to obtain a sense of the environmental factors which were influential in the person's development. These would include, but not be limited to, such things as social, economic, and cultural factors, as well as significant others. The social history is essentially an attempt to understand how and perhaps why the person seeking help got to that specific point.

Summary

This chapter has defined an interview and described its purposes, its essential components, and the stages of the interview. An attempt was also made to describe, however briefly, the attitudes and behaviors which are essential for a helping professional to have when conducting an interview. The chapter discussed the types of interviews which an occupational therapist might use, and the potential problems or pitfalls which are possible in any interview situation.

The importance of the helping interview cannot be overestimated. It is central to the helping process. The occupational therapist must strive to develop his knowledge, skills, attitudes, and techniques in the interviewing process if he is to be an effective helping professional. Interviewing is not an easy skill to develop and can sometimes be a difficult, anxiety-provoking, and unproductive situation. On the other hand, it is truly one of the most challenging, fascinating, and stimulating endeavors that can be attempted. This process of discovery, of trying to know and understand another human being can be a most challenging and rewarding journey. For one person to get to know and understand another human being takes an enormous amount of sensitivity, knowledge, and courage. The occupational therapist has the opportunity to engage in this thrilling process and to grow and develop both professionally and personally.

References

1. Sullivan HS: The Psychiatric Interview. New York, WW Norton & Co, Inc, 1954, p 4.
2. Okum F: Effective Helping: Interviewing and Counseling. North Scituate, Duxburg Press, 1976, p 81.
3. MacKinnon R, Michels R: The Psychiatric Interview in Clinical Practice. Philadelphia, WB Saunders, 1971, p 9.
4. Reik T: Listening with the Third Ear. New York, Grove Press, 1949, p 49.
5. Scott JE: Influencing students' observations. A J Occu Ther 29:143-5, 1975.
6. Moorehead LM: The occupational history. A J Occu Ther 23:329-34, 1969.
7. Takata N: Play as a prescription. In Reilly M (ed): Play as Exploratory Learning: Studies of Curiosity Behavior. Beverly Hills, Sage Publications, 1974, p 209.
8. Takata N: The play history. A J Occu Ther 23:314-8, 1969.
9. Matsutsuyu: The interest check list. A J Occu Ther 23:323-8, 1969.
10. Watanabe S: Four concepts basic to the occupational therapy process. A J Occu Ther 22:439-44, 1968.
11. Smith HD, Tiffany EG: Assessment and evaluation. In Hopkins HL, Smith HD (eds): Willard & Spackman's Occupational Therapy, 5th ed, Philadelphia, JB Lippincott Co, 1978, p 156.
12. Sands WS: Psychiatric history and mental status. In Freedman AM, Kaplan HI (eds) : Comprehensive Textbook of Psychiatry. Baltimore, Williams and Wilkins Co, 1967, p 508.

Bibliography

Argelander H: The Initial Interview in Psychotherapy. New York, Human Science Press, 1976.
Balinsky B, Burger R: The Executive Interview—A Bridge to People. New York, Harper and Brothers, 1959.
Benjamin A: The Helping Interview, 2nd ed, Boston, Houghton Mifflin Co, 1974.
Brill NI: Working With People: The Helping Process, 2nd ed. Philadelphia, JB Lippincott Co, 1978.
Davis JD: The Interview as Areana. Stanford, Stanford Univ Press, 1971.
DeSchweinitz EK: Interviewing in the Social Sciences. London, The National Council of Social Services, 1962.
Fenlason AF, Ferguson GB, Abrahamson AC: Essentials in Interviewing for the Interviewer Offering Professional Services. New York, Harper and Row, 1962.
Freedman A, Kaplan H: Comprehensive Textbook of Psychiatry. Baltimore, Williams and Wilkins Co, 1967.
Garrett A: Interviewing: Its Principles and Methods, 2nd ed. New York, Family Service Association of America, 1972.
Gordon R: Interviewing: Strategy, Techniques, and Tactics, Rev. Homewood, The Dorsey Press, 1975.
Kadushin A: The Social Work Interview. New York, Columbia Univ Press, 1972.
Matarazzo JD, Wiens AN: The Interview: Research on Its Anatomy and Structure. Chicago, Aldine Atherton, 1972.
Nemiah JC: Foundations of Psychopathology. New York, Oxford Univ Press, 1961.
Redlick FC, Freedman DX: The Theory and Practice of Psychiatry. New York, Basic Books, Inc, 1966.
Richardson SA, Dohrenliend BS, Klein D: Interviewing: Its Forms and Functions. New York, Basic Books, Inc, 1965.
Woody RH, Woody JD (eds): Clinical Assessment in Counseling and Psychotherapy. Englewood Cliffs, NJ, Prentice-Hall, Inc, 1972.

3
The Lifestyle Performance Profile: An Organizing Frame

Gail Fidler, F.A.O.T.A.

The design and use of evaluative or data gathering processes in occupational therapy has value to the degree that data being collected have discernable meaning and relevance to an overall frame of reference that defines the purpose and parameters of practice. The purpose of this chapter is to relate data gathering and assessment processes to a conceptual model that describes adaptive performance as the fundamental concern and focus for the practice of occupational therapy.

Definition

Human performance is viewed as the ability to undertake those roles and tasks of living that are essential to achieving social efficacy and personal satisfaction.[1,2] More explicitly, performance has been defined in an earlier work,[2] as comprising three critical skill clusters: 1) the ability to care for and maintain self at a level of greater independence than dependence; 2) the ability to engage in a variety of doing or action experiences that satisfy personal needs and provide intrinsic gratification; and 3) the ability to contribute to the needs and welfare of others.

This concept hypothesizes that achievement of a way of life that is health sustaining, is dependent upon the acquisition of such skills, and most especially on achieving and maintaining a life style that reflects an age specific, culturally relevant balance among self care activity, pursuit of personal need gratification, and those activities that contribute to the welfare of others. What may be described for any one individual, at any point in time as adequate skill or skill level, and an appropriate balance among the skill clusters, depends upon age, cultural norms, and biological endowment. Performance skill and life style expectations change with different stages of life and vary in accordance with cultural and social norms.[2]

Performance skill acquisition is influenced by factors in the external environment and by internal neuropsychological process or systems. The components or sub-systems of performance include such human and non-human factors in the external environment as culture, economics, family constellation, social class, housing, geography, and architectural structures. Those components of performance that comprise the internal processes are the sensory, motor, cognitive, and psychological systems. Maturational/developmental delays or deficits caused by trauma, impact performance skill behaviors. Likewise, factors in the external environment can inhibit or support skill development. Age appropriate social skills are essential to the achievement of satisfactory performance. Social behavior learning and development is made possible, or is impaired, by both internal and external factors or systems. Social skill development is a critical component of performance.

When viewed from these constructs, occupational therapy practice is basically concerned with skill development and achievement of a satisfying, health sustaining life style. Thus, delineation of existing strengths and skill deficiencies, description of the developmental lags and deficits in performance components, and identification of external barriers or resources, comprise the basis for planning intervention. Data gathering and assessment processes are thus directed toward these elements.

Behaviors Assessed

Impaired performance is frequently related to dysfunctions in one or more of the internal components of performance and in social skill development. If performance skill learning and remediation of deficits is to occur, intervention will need to address the nature of dysfunction in these components, and the system's readiness to respond and cope with stimuli and learning expectations. The components of performance that may require assessment can be described as including, at age and developmentally appropriate levels, the following:

1. Sensory/motor functions such as:

    Balance and equilibrium
    Ocular control and visual perception
    Tactile discrimination
    Bilateral motor coordination
    Visual-motor integration
    Visual-spatial awareness
    Language and auditory skills
    Gross motor coordination, mobility
    Fine motor coordination and dexterity
    Muscle strength and endurance
    Work tolerance

2. Cognitive functions such as:

    Temporal adaptation
    Retention and recall
    Sustaining focus-goal directedness
    Perceiving cause and effect relationships
    Coping with a variety of circumstances simultaneously

    Ability to:

    Interrupt attention without loss of task goal
    Use past experiences as resources
    Make deductions
    Discriminate, see similarities and differences
    Perceive parts in relation to the whole
    Abstract, generalize
    Coordinate, follow through in logical sequence and order
    Reason, use common sense logic
    Assess realistically
    Perceive various alternatives
    Evaluate and assess alternatives

Make choices
Organize and plan on basis of choice
Implement decision or plan
Inhibit extraneous stimuli
Establish and sustain appropriate priorities

3. Psychological functions such as the ability to:

Manage, cope with time pressures
Cope with ambiguity
Use inner control in the absence of external ones
Tolerate risk, accept, cope with elements of chance
Sublimate—channel drives
Master feelings—exercise appropriate expression and control
Modify behavior—have available varying responses
Postpone gratification
Compromise without loss of self values
Seek and experience intrinsic gratification—pleasure
Invest, make commitment to external objects, persons, task, events
Assess own skills, competence, limitations
Cope with external control, limits
Differentiate self from others
Set realistic goals and expectations
Cope with success, criticism, failure, competition
Balance structure and flexibility
Feel sense of self-competence, efficacy, and self respect
Have self reliance, internal motivation
Have a sense of autonomy
View self as agent
Frustration tolerance

4. Dyadic and group skills such as:

Relationship to peers
Relationship to authority, coping with subordinate role
Engagement in reciprocal peer relationships
Ability to give, receive, share
Capacity for trust
Responsiveness to needs and feelings of others
Ability to demonstrate warmth, respect for others
Appropriateness of expectations about others
Collaborative, interdependent relationship skills
Leadership skills
Group member role skills
Ability to elicit positive response in others

Administration

A first priority should be to obtain information that will make it possible to describe an individual's performance skills, deficits, and characteristic life style as well as the external resources and/or barriers that influence performance. Figure 3.1 outlines the critical areas that need to be addressed.

Information relative to each of the areas identified in this schema is necessary in order to be able to describe the kind and level of a person's existing performance

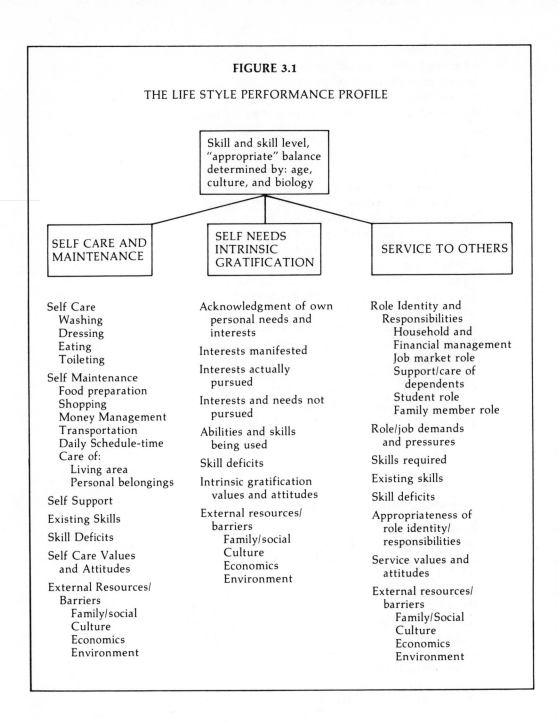

FIGURE 3.1

THE LIFE STYLE PERFORMANCE PROFILE

Skill and skill level, "appropriate" balance determined by: age, culture, and biology

SELF CARE AND MAINTENANCE

SELF NEEDS INTRINSIC GRATIFICATION

SERVICE TO OTHERS

Self Care
  Washing
  Dressing
  Eating
  Toileting

Self Maintenance
  Food preparation
  Shopping
  Money Management
  Transportation
  Daily Schedule-time
  Care of:
    Living area
    Personal belongings

Self Support

Existing Skills

Skill Deficits

Self Care Values
  and Attitudes

External Resources/
  Barriers
    Family/social
    Culture
    Economics
    Environment

Acknowledgment of own
  personal needs and
  interests

Interests manifested

Interests actually
  pursued

Interests and needs not
  pursued

Abilities and skills
  being used

Skill deficits

Intrinsic gratification
  values and attitudes

External resources/
  barriers
    Family/social
    Culture
    Economics
    Environment

Role Identity and
  Responsibilities
    Household and
    Financial management
    Job market role
    Support/care of
      dependents
    Student role
    Family member role

Role/job demands
  and pressures

Skills required

Existing skills

Skill deficits

Appropriateness of
  role identity/
  responsibilities

Service values and
  attitudes

External resources/
  barriers
    Family/Social
    Culture
    Economics
    Environment

skill capacities and deficits, as well as the individual's value orientation regarding performance and the ways in which the family, the culture, and the environment support or hinder performance skill development and maintenance.

Necessary data can be gathered from specific evaluations that test self care skills, and from leisure-time interest check lists. Most of the data, however, is best obtained by means of an interview, and supplemented by information contained in the social

Gail Fidler

history that is compiled by other professionals. Interviews must be planned and structured, and the Life Style Performance Profile provides a structure and organization for guiding the interview process.

A performance profile would be incomplete without a history of performance that makes it possible to describe and understand an individual's historic pattern of activity, characteristic interests and experiences, and family patterns that shape performance development, attitudes, and values. Plans and processes for intervention will have relevance and meaning to the degree that such information is the basis of formulations.

Various outlines and forms have been used in occupational therapy for obtaining activity history data. The one developed and used by Diasio and Jones[3] is perhaps the most thorough, reflecting a perspective of the interrelationship of many factors that shape and influence vocational choice and performance. The "Occupational History" represents an adaptation of some of their material in the interest of reducing data gathering time and broadening the history to include a wider client population and interest inventory (see Appendix A).

Conclusion

The Life Style Performance Profile presents a structure for organizing and identifying performance skills and deficits within the context of an individual's social-cultural norms and characteristic patterns of responding to and managing life tasks. It offers a focus for describing those social-cultural and environmental factors that can be tapped as resources to support skill development, and for delineating those external forces that interfere with learning and require intervention. Since impaired performance is related to neuro-psychological factors and interpersonal components as well as social-cultural ones, the evaluative process will need to include assessment of these components. Collection of such data should make it possible to describe:

1. The level and kind of skill deficits and strengths relative to self care, self needs, and service to others.
2. The social-cultural expectations for performance in each of these areas in terms of self and significant others.
3. The life style performance balance/imbalance within the context of age and culture.
4. The nature of family, social, cultural, economic, and environmental resources or barriers.
5. The sensory-motor, cognitive, psychological, and social skill strengths/ deficits impacting development.
6. Individual characteristics and interests that shape response.

Comprehensive, relevant interventions can then be planned, and appropriate priorities established.

References

1. A Curriculum Guide for Occupational Therapy Educators. Rockville, MD, American Occupational Therapy Association, Inc, 1974.
2. Fidler GS, Fidler JW: Doing and becoming: Purposeful action and self actualization. A J Occu Ther 32:305-310, 1978.
3. Diasio KB, Jones MS: The Role of Pre-Vocational Services in the Rehabilitation of Young Adult Psychiatric Patients. In Proceedings of the Fourth International Congress, World Federation of Occupational Therapists, London, 1966, pp 122-136.

4
The Adolescent Role Assessment

Maureen Black, Ph.D., O.T.R.

Literature Review

Much of the credit for the concept of adolescence in industrialized societies goes to G. Stanley Hall's *Adolescence*, published in 1905.[1] Hall was a maturationist who wrote that adolescents' lives are dominated by the inevitable conflicts, which include hyperactivity versus inertia, independence versus dependence, submission versus dominance, and responsibility versus self-absorbtion, and often result in inconsistent, and sometimes rebellious, behavior. Hall argued that, for successful passage from childhood to adulthood, adolescents be permitted to resolve these conflicts, and their behavioral inconsistencies be tolerated. Hall's work forms a baseline of thinking on adolescence in America and indeed, adolescents are afforded a freedom of expression unavailable either to children or to adults. Society expects adolescents to display occasional bouts of crazy behavior, and they comply.

In spite of the emphasis on the stress and strain of adolescence, most of the time adolescents are not in the throes of turmoil or rebellion, but are busy with school, family, and friends.[2] Most adolescents successfully pass through this stage of development to become competent adults. However, many adults with adjustment problems do have a history of adolescent misbehavior. It is difficult to discriminate between the expected turmoil of adolescence and the early signs of pathology, particularly because the boundaries of acceptable adolescent behavior are so flexible. Thus, very little is known about normal adolescent development or the effect of stress on adolescent adjustment.[3]

Even less is known about the adolescents seen by occupational therapists—those with physical or emotional disabilities.[4,5] The problems of these adolescents go beyond the expected conflicts of maturation. Not only are they in the midst of a change of roles from childhood to adulthood, but they have been identified either through their physical or behavioral abnormalities and may be denied many of the experiences of adolescence. For example, physically handicapped adolescents may not be permitted the independence and responsibilities periodically demanded by most adolescents, or schizophrenic adolescents may be unable to recognize the changing role playing expected of them. These adolescents may require additional support and guidance in successfully coping with the conflicts of adolescence.

Although the discordance of adolescence has been widely publicized both through professional and popular literature, attention should also focus on the consistencies of development. Such a perspective has emerged from a framework of occupational behavior, and enables questions to be raised about the acquisition and transfer of skills from one stage to another. In this way it may be possible to earmark the developmental strengths and weaknesses of adolescents seen by occupational therapists, rather than ignoring problems of adjustment, or automatically attributing them either to maturation or to pathology.

Occupational Choice

The theory of occupational choice, described by Ginzberg and others,[6,7] fits well within the framework of occupational therapy, because it outlines a progression of decision making stages from childhood to adulthood. The occupational choice process is conceptualized in three stages, characterized by specific evolutionary tasks. The first stage begins in childhood play and includes fantasy and exploration. Through play, children learn to organize rules for games, to win and to lose, and to receive spontaneous feedback from peers. Feedback enables children to distinguish acceptable social behavior from unacceptable behavior.

Through role models and experience, children build references for their fantasies. The stick becomes a director's baton, the parked car drives to the store, and the hat transforms the child into a fire fighter. Children daydream and explore make-believe alternatives as they increase the scope of their reality. From their dreams and fantasies, they develop interests and hobbies to guide further exploration.

The second or tentative choice stage emerges when the interests built in childhood are related to personal capabilities, values, and goals. Since adolescents are no longer licensed to actively fantasize by pretending to be fire fighters, they require more subtle outlets for their exploration. Childhood play is replaced by adolescent leisure activities, especially social interaction and interest development.

Adolescents are expected to assume responsibilities within the family, neighborhood, and school. They receive feedback from their performance and become increasingly accountable for their actions. This feedback assists adolescents in judging their own capabilities and forming values and goals. As values and goals are compared with interests, the search for possible occupational role alternatives continues.

By late adolescence, the alternatives narrow and adolescents enter the realistic stage or final phase of occupational choice. This stage is characterized by thoughts crystalizing on one choice and the development of skills and habits within that choice. To achieve satisfaction and competence in an occupational role, the role expectations must be consistent with adolescents' values, and within their skill level.

This theory, which originated as an explanation of the decision making process leading to the selection and preparation of an occupational role, and the feedback system inherent within the progression, makes it useful for working with adolescents, regardless of their presenting problems. The Adolescent Role Assessment (Appendix B) is an interview tool which is constructed from the stages in the occupational choice process.

Assessment

Administration

The Adolescent Role Assessment is administered as a semistructured interview through casual dialogue. The questions are phrased in the vernacular, and the therapist must be familiar with the purpose of the questions and the rating criteria. Specific rating criteria are included with each question in the assessment, and are

Maureen Black

designed to reduce value judgements and subjectivity as much as possible. For example, a question entitled *Goals* asks about future plans, and is rated by the adolescent's ability to mention goals and preparation, regardless of the actual goals. The ratings are based on normative adolescent behavior,[3] and are summarized on the Scoring Sheet (Appendix C): plus (+) indicates appropriate behavior, zero (0) indicates marginal or borderline behavior, and minus (−) indicates inappropriate behavior. For example, a positive response which addresses the question would receive a plus, a noncommital response of, "I don't know," would receive a zero, and a negative response such as, "I have no interests or friends," would receive a minus. A predominance of plus scores suggests appropriate role behavior, a predominance of zero scores suggests apathy and an unwillingness to respond, and a predominance of minus scores suggests serious doubt about appropriate role behavior. Intervention should be designed using the content from the interview as a guide for specific treatment planning.

Behaviors Assessed

The Adolescent Role Assessment is divided into six sections, representing various stages of development in the choice process. The first section includes questions about childhood play. During that period, children typically learn a variety of play activities and can identify friends, heroes, games with rules, make-believe games, and the development of interests. Adolescents who cannot identify these aspects of their childhood play may need remedial activities to help them to use role models or to fantasize.

By separating adolescents' primary sphere of influence into family, school, and peers, the next three sections of the assessment are used to investigate performance in a variety of concurrent roles. The items in the family section focus on the role as a responsible family member in terms of interactions, chores, and money. Through these items it is possible to determine if adolescents view themselves as passive victims or as active participants within the family.

School occupies a major segment of adolescents' time and energy, particularly in industrialized societies where education often extends into the mid-20s or beyond. The developmental tasks associated with school include an increasing recognition of the adolescent's own abilities and limitations within an institutional setting. In many ways school performance (ability to get along, rather than grades per se), serves as an index to subsequent vocational performance.

The peer group often acts as a shelter in which adolescents try out and practice various behaviors before entering adulthood and the larger society. The questions in the peer section address the variety of experiences available to the adolescent.

The final two sections involve occupational choice and work. The former section looks at work attitudes and concrete plans, while the latter section looks at the adolescent's ability to fantasize about long range ideas and goals.

The Adolescent Role Assessment outlines topics that should be considered in working with adolescents. In problem areas, the therapist should explore further to identify specific situations that could be incorporated into program planning.

Research

The Adolescent Role Assessment was administered to 12 inpatients at the Neuropsychiatric Institute of the University of California at Los Angeles. The subjects ranged in age from 13-17 years with diagnoses that included adjustment reaction, anorexia nervosa, school phobia, and depression. Subsequently it was administered to 28 normal adolescents aged 13-16 from schools in a suburban metropolitan area. Not only were the hospitalized adolescents more likely to give marginal and inappropriate responses, $t(38)=2.19$, $p<.05$, but the range in their responses was wider. The largest difference between the two groups occurred in the sections on family and school socialization. The hospitalized adolescents were less likely to mention themselves as accountable for their own actions, $X^2=3.92$, $p<.05$.

In order to verify the adolescents' responses, a battery of assessments including participatory observation, Rosenberg's Self-Esteem Scale, Bills' Index of Adjustment and Values, Interest Check List, Rotter's Generalized Expectations for Internal Versus External Control, and Buhler's Life Goals was given to the hospitalized group. The analysis suggested that weaknesses identified through the Adolescent Role Assessment also appeared through the other assessments.

Reliability was checked by administering the questionnaire twice to a small subset of the sample. Based on the rating criteria, the adolescents' responses are highly reliable, r = .91. However, the content obtained during the second interview was more copious and specific than initially obtained, probably reflecting the importance of a positive relationship between the adolescents and the therapist.

Critique and Suggested Research

The value of any interview depends on the respondent's willingness to cooperate in a truthful manner. Often this willingness may be influenced by the setting and by the therapist's interviewing skills. Thus, interviews taken by different interviewers may yield slightly different results. Furthermore, there may be discrepancies between what adolescents say and what they actually do. Whenever possible, results should be verified through observing, administering other assessments, or interviewing parents, teachers, or siblings.

The possibilities of future research are endless. Although this discussion has centered on adolescents in a psychiatric setting, the Adolescent Role Assessment could be used with any group of adolescents, regardless of their problem— physically handicapped, learning disabled, juvenile delinquent, etc. The assessment could be administered to various groups of handicapped and nonhandicapped adolescents in order to identify areas of greatest difference where intervention may be effective. For example, in my study, it was found that hospitalized adolescents were less likely than nonhospitalized adolescents to accept responsbility for their actions. This discrepancy could be incorporated into treatment planning, and a follow-up assessment could be administered to determine the adolescents' response pattern after treatment.

Either on an individual or on a group basis, the Adolescent Role Assessment may be used to evaluate behavior changes in response to specific treatment programs. These evaluations yield an index both on the adolescents' progress and on the effectiveness of the treatment.

Theoretically, those adolescents with the least adjustment problems should have the most success in their movement toward adulthood and adaptive occupational roles and, conversely, those with more adolescent adjustment problems should have less adult success. This prediction could be tested by dividing adolescents into groups on the basis of their scores, following them over several years, and then obtaining a measurement of their competence as adults. Outcome could include tabulations of the number of people in each group who live independently, have not had legal problems, work regularly, assume some responsibility for others, and other measures of general competence. The design of such a longitudal project could enable researchers to begin to identify and document adaptive paths from adolescence to adulthood that may be available to handicapped individuals.

Conclusion

Adolescents seen by occupational therapists frequently have two problems—in addition to a physical or emotional disability, they are experiencing the expected conflicts of adolescence. The Adolescent Role Assessment is based on an occupational behavior model, and enables therapists to focus on past, present, and future role adjustment through the decision-making stages of occupational choice. It serves as a guide for treatment planning and evaluation, rather than as a diagnostic tool. Nevertheless, it does discriminate between normal and hospitalized adolescents in the present sample. Moreover, the casual dialogue seems to facilitate the formation of a relationship in which adolescents are able to respond.

Although some behavioral inconsistencies are expected during the transition from childhood to adulthood, it is too easy to attribute all adolescent adjustment problems to maturational strains, particularly when other disabilities may be present. The Adolescent Role Assessment enables therapists to focus on past, present, and future role adjustment through the decision making stages of occupational choice. By incorporating data from the Adolescent Role Assessment, the occupational therapist can plan an intervention program relevant to specific adolescents, as illustrated in a recent case study.[8] Occupational therapists are in a unique position to provide opportunities for adolescents to explore, to search for alternatives, and to evaluate feedback. With an understanding of the Adolescent Role Assessment and the tools of occupational therapy, therapists may design and implement treatment programs to facilitate the transition through adolescence.

References

1. Hall GS: Adolescence. New York, D Appleton and Co, 1905.
2. Kett JF: Rites of Passage. New York, Basic Books, Inc, 1977.
3. Coleman JS: Youth in Transition. Berkeley, Univ California Press, 1968
4. Shannon PD: The work-play model: A basis for occupational therapy programming in psychiatry. A J Occu Ther 24:215, 1970.
5. Pezzuti L: An exploration of adolescent feminine and occupational therapy behavioral development. A J Occu Ther 33:84, 1979.
6. Ginzberg E, Ginzberg SW, Axelrad S, Herman JL: Occupational Choice: An Approach to a General Theory. New York, Columbia Press, 1956.
7. Ginzberg E: Toward a theory of occupational choice: A restatement. Vocational Guidance 20:169, 1972.
8. Black MM: Adolescent role assessment. A J Occu Ther 30:73, 1976.

PART 3
PROJECTIVE INSTRUMENTS

5
The Azima Battery: An Overview

Fern J. Cramer Azima, Ph.D.

Historical Development

Towards the end of the 1950s, I was involved in an assessment of psychiatric occupational therapy in Canada,[1] and the published findings caused shock, dismay, and marked criticism here and in the United States. Very quickly, I was invited by the American Occupational Therapy Society and later the American Psychiatric Task Force to present the findings, to report on a new test procedure, and a basically new philosophy and dynamic orientation for the field.[2-5] To review what transpired is now history, and yet the puzzle remains why the battery and the dynamic concepts advocated in four or five articles for psychiatric occupational therapists have survived the test of time.

The impetus for the battery was the department's simultaneous involvement in Analytic Group Art Therapy—renamed Projective Group Therapy[6,7]—and studies in the treatment of schizophrenia, and later, on prolonged sleep and sensory deprivation studies. The central pivot, in many ways, was the concern about understanding and clarifying distorted object relations, the regressive phenomena that occur in severe psychopathological, drug, or marked states of stress.

In those days, psychiatric occupational therapy was concerned almost exclusively with traditional occupational and recreational functions, and minimally with evaluation and "therapeutic functions". As I worked with occupational therapists, it became increasingly clear, especially while working with schizophrenics, that they were in many ways the primary therapists to evoke for the client a meaningful relationship to reality. I am convinced that the key concept proposed for dynamic occupational therapy is the central position of the object. As was stated, "It is contended that the presence of objects (ready made, offered, or created) and the dynamics of object relations as referable to an available external medium, is, and should be, taken as the distinguishing mark of occupational therapy from individual or group psychotherapies. Evidently, the dynamics of individual and group psychotherapy are applicable in the occupational therapy setting, but the presence of non-structured objects which can be structured according to the emergence of internal happenings marks the point of emphasis and of distinction of on-going processes in the occupational therapy setting."[2] In psychotherapy the individual is in a situation requiring verbalization, but not *doing;* and there is no unstructured object (taken in its physical sense) to which to relate, while in occupational therapy the setting allows both verbalization and doing.

Administration

With this starting point I devised a simple battery that would encourage the *free creation of objects,* utilizing three media and subsequent *free association and inquiry phases.* The patient is asked: 1) to do a free drawing with a pencil; 2) to draw a whole person and then a person of the opposite sex; 3) to make anything with clay; 4) to do a finger painting. The second part of the test procedure is to gain free associations to each production. The battery is usually administered individually with the occupational therapist and the client seated side by side before a small table on which there are the finger paints arranged in a standard order (yellow, red, green, blue, brown, and black) and a container of water on the right; the clay is kept moistened in a plastic container on the left hand side. Paper towels are provided, but no other objects such as a ruler or tools used in ceramics are allowed. The preferred order of presentation is pencil, clay, and finger painting, since the latter medium usually requires the hands to be washed before continuing with the *association phase.*

The occupational therapist asks the client's age, education, marital, and occupational status. After gaining some rapport, the therapist gives some orienting instructions such as:

> "As part of the evaluation routine of our hospital, I would like to carry out a battery of tests with you. I am going to ask you to make some different things with the various materials on this table. This is another investigation to help assess your mode of functioning and some of the problem areas that are not always visible on the surface, or even that you may be aware of. I may repeat the procedure at various intervals and at discharge to assess your progress."

After giving the instructions, the therapist moves slightly behind the client so as to be out of line of vision, and begins to record both time for each of the productions, as well as the total test time. The occupational therapist keeps note of the client's behavior, of the drawing, clay, and finger painting sequence, the verbalizations, and the total technique employed. During the *creation phase,* the occupational therapist refrains from talking, and responds minimally to allow the client maximum concentration and externalization. It is preferable to commence the *inquiry stage* after all the productions are finished. Exceptions to this rule are certain active children, organics, or memory damaged individuals where the inquiry for association is made as each product is finished. As with other projective techniques, associations are gained by such statements as:

> "Please tell me now what you have made; describe to me what you see and what you had in mind, and what comes to you now."

The therapist must be cautious not to project his own associations or directly suggest meanings, but to show positive interest, a need for elaboration, and understanding of the productions.

The client's motivation, behavior, and rapport to the test situation and examiner should be noted. For each part of the battery, the phases reaction and total time of: 1) preparation, 2) production, and 3) completion are recorded. For the interpretation of the battery an evaluation scale has been published. Briefly, the scale is divided into: 1) the organization of mood; 2) the organization of drives; 3) the organization of ego; and 4) the organization of object relations. For completeness the original scale is reproduced (Appendix D).

Fern J. Cramer Azima

Behaviors Assessed

Aside from the decoding of free associations, dreams, hypnosis, and the psychological projective tests of drawing and especially the Rorschach, few avenues are open to the exploration of an individual's inner world. The battery is a method that allows externalization of fantasy into a visible, tangible, physical object, and directs the association to it. Analysis is therefore possible of both the structure of the object and its corresponding verbal associations. The client, as it were, creates his own visible dream or Rorschach. The three media of the battery allow the projection on both two and three dimensional space. The battery evokes tactile, spatial, visual, auditory, and often olfactory sensory modalities. The change in media from dry to wet, from flat to thick, and into three dimensional objects again extends to externalization processes for the testee, and immeasurably widens the parameters of observation and understanding on the part of the tester. What has been described previously as object hierarchy and its development, and the object-situation or object field, are further concepts that allow the therapist to actually perceive how the client represents his object world, at what level of maturity, and with what degree of relatedness to others. The therapist can assess not only the primitive or primary thinking, but also primitive object development and its corresponding symbolic proximity—for example, why the over-sophisticated, verbally defensive client feels more comfortable with the pencil, while another allows himself to enjoy the manipulation and indulgence of smearing. The historical correlation of the present object with the early primary object needs is of special importance in psychotic states, and the concept of "gratification of basic needs" in the real or fantasized object is explored at some length in studies of schizophrenia.

Assessing the specific determinants of the battery is beyond the scope of this presentation, but the importance of evaluating reality contact, mood, level of functioning, and the quality of the object relations should be stressed. Structural, sequence, and content analysis are blended with the verbal analysis. Line, form, organization of space, interrelationship of parts, and the total gestalt are primary determinants, and act as the fulcrum of the scale. Movement, color, texture, and perspective add the dimensions of fantasy, spontaneity, sensitivity, and intelligence.

Phenomenological evaluations are preferred over symbolic interpretations, unless clear associations are given by the client. The dynamics of the object as a whole system are defined by its radiating and integrating subsystems, and they vary markedly from syndrome to syndrome, from psychosis to neurosis and organic features, including deterioration in form, distortion of perspective, lack of angulation, line tremor, and retracing. Motor organization and orientation to space may be traced over a number of weeks, months or years. Poor contact with reality is evidenced by bizarre, eccentric, or original representations or poor form, color, and content, as well as the presence of psychotic language and reasoning.

Reports should be clear and factual; a brief *Behavioral Analysis* of the client during the testing procedure should precede the *Examination Analysis,* where each part of the battery is briefly detailed and interpreted. The *Summary* should present the salient findings to be included in the client's chart, and should cover the following six areas:

1. Contact with reality
2. Degree of relatedness to others

3. Quality of mood expressiveness
4. Degree of ego control and coping
5. Degree of activity
6. Degree of clarity of communications as compared to defensiveness.

Differential diagnosis, treatment planning, and prognosis should be attempted.

Uses of the Battery

Further research in addition to the evaluation—diagnostic aid of the battery, its use for change detection, prognosis, therapy, and rehabilitation—are added dimensions. Since the testing procedure is a simple, uncomplicated one, it may be repeated several times to follow the affects of drug administration and clinical experimental procedures. It would seem that the procedure would be useful to track behavioral modules, such as desensitization, conditioning, implosion, and feedback. The muscular tonus is well demonstrated in toxic states, in studies of alcoholism, and anorexia nervosa (unpublished clinical studies).

An area that has been relatively unexplored is the battery's prognostic use for psychotherapeutic intervention. From the level of organization, integration, and freedom of expression, and the degree of primitive versus sophisticated productions and associations, one has a way of assessing the client's ability to comply with the test procedure and to show sufficient spontaneity, creativity, and easy association. It would be of interest to carry out test-retest with clients in psychotherapy or psychoanalysis, and to determine the change in free association and the created objects.

An adjuvant method for employing the battery is to instruct the patient to draw out his phobia, dream, past traumatic episode, a future goal, etc. This technique allows further specific evaluation and therapeutic planning. A snake, spider, or a scene of feared compulsion presents a physical presence of more acute intensity than only verbal suggestion or implosion. Verbalizations are often denied or suppressed, whereas the created objects are a "reality" that can be shared by both, re-shown, and re-discussed. A series may be presented as a group of photographs. Changes in size, line pressure, shading, repetition of theme, or regression-progression sequences give an independent assessment for the clinical changes.

At the same time that the battery has been used for diagnosis and change detection, there is significant usefulness for its adjuvant use in individual and group therapy with adults,[3,6-8] adolescents, and children. In a therapeutic day setting for emotionally disturbed children, its application by a multidisciplinarian team has been invaluable.[8] As in play therapy, the symbolic meanings of the material are quickly decoded. The group of children and staff create a world of objects—animate and inanimate. The added use of the television camera allows a playback dimension that creates a reappearance of the object, the child, and his peers, and then allows a subsequent restructuring, ie, a second chance to change, modify, and cope differently. The camera as a projective instrument brings alive to the group pieces of the object world the client had not seen before. In previous days, it was the fairy stories, songs, poems, myths, painting, and sculpture that was the method of preserving the past and communicating to the future. Projective batteries and others in this text are ways to render the person's hidden past into a visual identifiable form which gradually the ego recognizes and codes into language.

With the proliferation of family therapy, a family battery has been experimented with, as well as a comparison of batteries done independently by mother and child,

Fern J. Cramer Azima

by twins, siblings, etc. At times the parent has been asked to "interpret" the battery that his child has done, and this is very often highly revealing of hidden reciprocal family conflicts.

Conclusion

The Azima Battery introduced in 1960 originally as an evaluation diagnostic procedure was expanded as a therapeutic adjuvant and as a research instrument. This projective technique was based on *free creation* in three media—drawing, sculpture, and finger painting, and their subsequent free associations. Psychoanalytic and psychodynamic theories were the frames of reference for *object relations theory*, which was used to describe the central role of the object in psychiatric occupational therapy.

References

1. Azima H, Wittkower ED: A partial field survey of Occupational Therapy. A J Occu Ther 11:1-7, 1957.
2. Azima H, Azima F: Outline of a dynamic theory of Occupational Therapy. A J Occu Ther 13:1-7, 1959.
3. Azima H, Azima F: Projective group therapy: A systematic application of true creativity in analytic groups. Intern Mental Research Newsletter 2:9-10, 1960.
4. Azima H: Dynamic occupational therapy. Diseas Nervous System, Monograph Supplement 22, 1961.
5. Azima F: A dynamic theory of Occupational Therapy. In Crow LD (ed): Psychology of Human Adjustment. New York, A Knopf, 1967, p 561.
6. Azima H, Cramer F, Wittkower ED: Analytic group art therapy. Intern J Group Psychotherap 3:234-260, 1959.
7. Azima H, Azima F: Projective group therapy. Intern J Group Psychotherap 10:176-183, 1959.
8. Azima F: Group therapy for latency children. Canad Psychiatr Assoc J 21:210-212, 1977.

6
The Shoemyen Battery

Clare W. Shoemyen, M.B.A.O.T., O.T.R.

"The Shoemyen Battery" is a recently adopted name for the orientation and evaluation procedure used in the Occupational Therapy Department, Shands Teaching Hospital at the University of Florida (STHUF). The battery employs four expressive activities common to occupational therapy: mosaic tile, finger painting, sculpture, and clay modeling. The mosaic tile is a highly structured activity which requires no tools, and permits a wide choice of colors. Finger painting is a creative activity and provides a potentially sensual experience. Sculpture is both a destructive and constructive activity which requires the use of tools in three dimensional expression. Clay modeling is a constructive three dimensional activity in which the client is requested to create a human form.

Historical Development

The procedure was developed in response to the challenging leadership of Alice Jantzen, (then Chairman of the Occupational Therapy curriculum and Director of Services), and to the specific needs encountered by two of the psychiatric occupational therapy staff.

In 1963, Karen Rusnak, O.T.R., and I were responsible for planning and implementing the occupational therapy and recreation program on the 30-bed adult inpatient psychiatric unit of the hospital. Assistance was available from other staff, especially the nurses, but initiative fell to us. The clients were predominantly from an upper socio-economic level, encompassing a wide range of diagnoses, ages, and conditions. They were slow to admit enthusiasm for arts and crafts, were frequently negative in their initial responses, and disliked being scheduled; yet they were not willing to take responsibility for themselves. This difficult and demanding client group, combined with a pleasant and well-equipped setting, a generous initial budget, and many campus and community resources, presented a challenge unique to our experience. I began to see the need for a systematic orientation procedure.

Alice Jantzen's probing questions concerning how the psychiatric staff would assess functional levels, determine treatment goals, and know which activities to use with differing clients was the other major factor providing impetus to the development of the battery. Stimulated by Jantzen's interest and support, the two of us began thinking more critically of our practice. We tried to identify the clues which influenced treatment, and to examine the theoretical basis of our work.

Sharing reactions and experiences, we realized that we both relied heavily on observing and listening to clients' responses on, or soon after, the initial contact. Neither of us was comfortable with a formal information-gathering interview, which could duplicate much of the Admission Conference data. The Admission Conference was the initial discussion involving patient and spouse or parents, and representatives of each discipline.

The search began for a different initial approach that would provide information needed by the therapist, while promoting a natural relationship with the patient, and lead to collaborative patient-therapist treatment planning. Various combinations of skills and activities were tried. Some of those rejected were water color painting, which was seen by most patients as too difficult, and checker playing in an observation room, which proved impractical in terms of scheduling.

Sharing ideas with Nedra Gillette at the Occupational Therapy Conference in Denver in 1963, did much to clarify my thinking. We had many experiences in common. Our discussion of sculpture media led to the University of Florida's use of a sculpture block which was easily made in the clinic. After Karen Rusnak left Gainesville, other occupational therapists and interns became interested in the evolving process. One psychiatrist in particular, Dr. Deborah Coggins, expressed interest and suggested that a human form be included. None of the other orientation activities required a specific subject.

By the end of 1964 the process was developed, allowing for samples to be collected and compared with reasonable consistency. The next step was to develop an adequate recording system. Stimulation came from the Clinical Supervisors' Workshop in New York City, which I attended in January, 1966. Participants observed and experienced projective and task oriented techniques. Gail Fidler and others discussed the Azima Battery, its modifications, and related techniques. Material presented at the Workshop reinforced confidence in the value of what was being used on the STHUF psychiatric unit. The Workshop revealed deficiencies in communication, especially in recording, and inspired my first literature search.

Following the New York Workshop, I shared information and insights with colleagues, and made several attempts to incorporate what I had learned into the orientation and evaluation process and recording system. This proved an educational and soul searching experience for me and other therapists involved, but ultimately had little tangible effect on the procedure. Dynamic terminology and interpretation were incompatible with the philosophy and approach of the psychiatric team with whom we shared information. With time, the focus became more firmly established as observable behavior and performance. Symbolism was recognized by therapists and often by clients. Interpretation was only recorded when volunteered by or discussed with clients.

In October 1967, a report on what is now known as The Shoemyen Battery was presented at the Occupational Therapy Conference in Boston. It aroused interest and requests for detailed information and permission for its use. Since then, the process or modified versions of it have been fairly widely used, but inconsistently reported.

The procedure described in Boston is still used by Occupational Therapy staff working in the psychiatric unit of STHUF. Changes and variations have been made in recording format and in therapeutic use of the information gained. Because The Shoemyen Battery evolved in response to problems and questions encountered in the practice of occupational therapy rather than in exploration or validation of any specific theory or concept, there is no obvious frame of reference. In response to questions about this, I have attempted to retrace and identify

Clare W. Shoemyen

professional influences. It has been both interesting and overwhelming. There is the 16 year span from the battery's inception and development to its current use and modifications. There is also—more subtle and difficult to untangle—the influence of the previous 16 years which built my philosophy and practice of occupational therapy. In excavating my professional past, stored in memory and the pages of yellowed notebooks, I found a copy of what had been described to a new colleague as my *Principles and Guidelines for Psychiatric Occupational Therapy*. These must have been written in 1957, in an attempt to clarify my thinking, after pioneering experiences as the first and only occupational therapist in a newly opened psychiatric unit:

1. Occupational therapy is goal oriented, meaningful activity—a collaborative treatment which for goal setting requires mutual understanding and sufficient knowledge of the client's taste, interests, and experience to determine what is meaningful.
2. The occupational therapist attempts to identify the client's strengths and weaknesses. Treatment is usually built on strengths.
3. As a member of the treatment team, the therapist should be flexible in approach, and responsive to the client's obvious needs.
4. *Occupation* can be any activity through which therapeutic goals are achieved, ie, gardening, cooking, arts and crafts, dancing, writing, studying.
5. The occupational therapist should understand and accept herself well enough to be a positive example and, when needed, a substitute significant person.
6. The occupational therapist should expect the most rather than the least of a client, once a tentative ability level is determined, remembering that each client is a unique individual from whom we may expect to learn.
7. The occupational therapist should not bluff her way through an unfamiliar activity requested by the client. If a substitute is not available, she should try to find instructions or an instructor and learn with the client.

Though general and limited, this synthesis of training, experience, and reading covered my view of occupational therapy prior to Alice Jantzen's questions, and the challenge of the STHUF psychiatric unit. *Evaluation* and *orientation* were not mentioned as such, but were inherent in the treatment process. These seven points, which might be considered the foundation upon which The Shoemyen Battery grew, were not original, but neither can they be identified with or credited to any one lecturer or book. They were my eclectic frame of reference.

Administration

The procedure involves the therapist and one to four new clients, depending on the admission rate. Each new client is introduced to the four activities that he is expected to attempt. Further explanation is given only if requested, and is kept as direct and honest as possible, emphasizing future program planning and a mutual learning experience. The maximum time allowed for each activity is 45 minutes. The order in which they are attempted is left to the client, and is considered to have possible significance.

When the client completes all four projects, he is offered the opportunity to look at his work with the therapist. He is encouraged to express his feelings about each project. Questions from the client are stongly encouraged, as well as spontaneous interpretation. The client's questions are answered directly and honestly, with emphasis placed on his specific therapy. Interpretations, observations, and conclusions reached with the client are reported to the rest of the medical team.

The four activities and an analysis of behaviors assessed are as follows.[1]

Mosaic Tile

Materials and procedure. A piece of 6 x 6 inch plywood and a choice of ten colors in a square ⅜ inch tile are provided. The client is instructed to arrange and glue the tiles on the board as a sample of a tray or trivet.

Inherent qualities. The size of the product and its components are highly structured. The choice lies in selection and arrangement of two to ten colors.

Response variables. The client's common sense and self-confidence tend to show up in relation to method, timing, and spacing. Dexterity, precision and color are easily observed.

Finger Painting

Materials and procedure. The client is presented with three jars of primary colors in finger paint with a tongue depressor in each, and a sheet of 16 x 22 inch finger painting paper, a sponge, and a bowl of water. He is instructed to wet the paper and paint whatever he wishes.

Inherent qualities. Those offered by the activity are free aesthetic and motoric expression employing color as a major factor; and a sensual, especially tactile, experience that may be employed regressively or creatively.

Response variables. This often demonstrates artistic ability, suggestibility, concern for detail and design, perseveration, and guardedness. Another variable is previous exposure to this medium in kindergarten or through his own children.

Sculpture

Materials and procedure. The client is given a block (cast of three parts vermiculite to two of plaster) that is approximately a 4 inch cube. Tools are a skiving knife and metal modeling tool. The client is instructed to carve the block into any shape that is satisfying to him.

Inherent qualities. This activity requires ability to conceptualize in the round. It is a destructive rather than a constructive activity that involves the use of tools. The soft, crumbly material negates attempts at detailed fragile sculpture, or should, if the client has any sense of appropriate use of the medium.

Response variables. It is for most clients the least familiar of these activities, and as such, demonstrates most clearly the client's problem solving potential and his susceptibility to multi-dimensional form. Dexterity, and fine and gross motor skills are obvious variables.

Clay Figure Modeling

Materials and procedure. The client is given a ball of moist, well-worked clay about the size of a large orange, a slab on which to work, and a pencil as the only tool, if specifically requested. The client is instructed to model a human figure.

Inherent qualities. A highly expressive plastic medium is used. The process is primarily constructive in contrast to the sculpture. The sensual characteristics of the medium often evoke strong emotional reactions. The specified subject, the human figure, encourages portrayal of self-concept or significant other person.

Response variables. Variables include concern for detail, technique, and dexterity, as well as positioning.

Many people have asked how The Shoemyen Battery handles contaminated response and less opportunity for observation when more than one client is oriented at a time. The answer is that the situation is accepted as one with more variables. I feel that though purity is lost, the opportunity to observe suggestibility and dependence on others is enhanced. It does require the therapist to have competent observation skills and a good memory.

Recording Assessed Behaviors

Rereading reviewers' comments and correspondence concerning The Shoemyen Battery since 1967, I have found universal interest in the recording mechanism and the means of arriving at conclusions. Unfortunately, these are the battery's least developed aspects, ones for which help and feedback have been consistently requested with disappointing results. Copies of most versions of recording forms used in the STHUF psychiatric occupational therapy practice since 1964 are available, but would be too space-consuming to include. The forms have progressed from a short, simple format to a longer, more specific, and more objective format.

The earlier form used in 1964 and 1965 fitted on one page and had a simple evaluation key. Soon after adoption of the clay figure as a fourth project, a second two-page form was devised. The summary for inclusion in the chart was based on a recording outline designed by Alice Jantzen. Later in 1965, the Regional Research Institute of the University of Florida was consulted. Several of the staff were interested and enthusiastic about the orientation-evaluation concept and possibilities, but felt the forms too simple and subjective for useful information collection. With their help, a four-page form was designed which did not include the summary and goals for chart and department files. The second page of the previous form seemed adequate for this purpose.

New forms with several check list modifications followed. Some therapists used these comfortably and consistently, while others found them too general to be very satisfactory.

The 1978 version is the most recent of those designed for and used in the psychiatric unit program. Since the objective of this chapter is the evolution and description of The Shoemyen Battery, the latest of these forms is included for readers' examination. It includes a portion of a form that Sally Bendroth and Marti Southam, in collaboration with me, devised for recording the arrangement and use of the tile. The STHUF form is designed to be a complete occupational therapy information summary. The first page includes information gained from the Admission Conference or chart, and is kept in the occupational therapy departmental files. Pages two and four are intended for both occupational therapy files and the client's chart. Page three is kept in the occupational therapy files for reference. The form is designed for use with its own key and guidelines. The form and key are included in Appendixes E, F and G.

Over time, different therapists used these recording forms with varied perceptions and points of view. There were changes in referral systems, and several charting changes. Except for legal purposes, the most effective communication remained verbal: in rounds, conferences, and one-to-one reporting. Most therapists using The Shoemyen Battery while associated with the University of Florida program agree that there are problems with subjective assessment of results and subjective definitions; yet they feel that the communication potential compensates.

The Battery provides a framework where materials, instruction, and time frame are consistent, while client response is varied. The procedure usually forms an excellent basis for discussion, planning, and goal setting. In the occupational therapy program of STHUF there have been, as case materials will demonstrate, different uses for the information derived. It is made clear to the client that results will be shared with the other members of the treatment team. A client's products are stored in the occupational therapy office until a physician requests a view or the client is the subject of a teaching conference. Clients' work is always kept as long as they are in the hospital. Many sets were photographed before being destroyed. The tile is recycled since the type used is no longer available.

Case Studies

During an Audio-Visual Workshop for Health Related Programs in 1971, a group of occupational therapy faculty at the University of Florida decided to use The Shoemyen Battery for their project. I gave permission for a slide series to be made, showing the use of the process and photographing examples of clients' work. I was asked to select three examples demonstrating different problems and responses to the Battery which were not of too recent production, and to create and narrate a script to accompany them. History and personal information which might identify clients were omitted for obvious reasons. Excerpts from this script will be included in the case examples that follow. The Workshop and project material were funded by the Center for Allied Health Instructional Personnel and the Kellogg Foundation.

Case Example 1

The first case was a male college student, who though shy, was friendly and cooperative when introduced to the occupational therapy orientation procedure. He commented that he was slowed down from his medication, but would do his best. He chose to start with the carving. He carved with apparent enthusiasm and considerable skill for the 30 minutes available, discussing archaeology with another client who was working in the same area. Whether his somewhat primitive, but artistically carved head precipitated the discussion or vice versa, is uncertain.

In his next session the client chose to do finger painting, and though he was courteous and somewhat friendly to the other patients sitting around the table, he seemed completely absorbed in what he was doing. He appeared preoccupied with the possibilities of mixing colors and the use of his fingers as well as in portraying his thoughts.

On the third session he spent the first part of the time smoothing a long block of clay. When reminded of the therapist's instructions to form a human figure, he became visibly anxious, said nothing, and proceeded to tear at the oblong piece of clay and form a crude figure with relatively long legs and a small head. The initial figure had no arms. He then worked carefully on the feet and the shaped legs, which he covered with scratch-type marks, until he reached the pelvic area. The client continued to work on the thighs and the diaphragm, and formed flipper-like arms out of what had been shoulders. He then formed a simple suggestion of a face in profile, scratched some hair, rather violently forced a hole to represent the umbilicus, and made a smaller hole in the side of the head (Fig 6.1). While doing this, he seemed oblivious of other people sitting at the table, and proceeded to his final touch. Using a modeling tool picked up from another patient, he jabbed the genital area of the figure at least 30 times. Having done this, he got up abruptly and left the room.

At his final session in occupational therapy the client worked for about 40

Clare W. Shoemyen

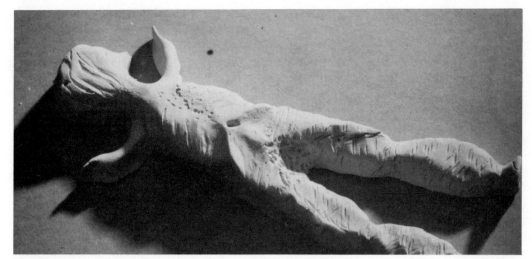

Fig 6.1: Case 1.

minutes on the tile. Again, he seemed upset and preoccupied while working. He appeared irritated with the other clients at the table, but did not verbalize his feelings. He arranged and rearranged the tiles several times, choosing the back of many of the tiles, and adding several in apparently random formation on top. When the client indicated that it was complete, no attempt was made to discuss the project with him, since he appeared very agitated and hostile. Unfortunately, there was no opportunity during the next few days to talk with him about his work, as he had to be restrained in his room. Just prior to his transfer to another hospital, the therapist spoke to him briefly about these projects. He discussed them as follows:

The carving pleased him, although it was incomplete. It apparently demonstrated his ability to express some tension through physical activity when appropriately goal-oriented. He spoke of enjoying doing it, and being pleased with the result. The finger painting apparently frightened him, as he said he remembered the scary faces, serpent, and strange beasts that were threatening him at the time. The tile he described as, "simply the way I wanted it that day; good and bad, right and wrong, all colors, all shapes, all sizes." The figure he would only describe as part human and helpless. He appeared quite shaken at seeing his figure.

Though it was not possible to carry out treatment with this patient, the set will always be remembered as a vivid example of tortured thinking and violence expressed through art media.

Case Example 2

This case, a man in his early 40s, was an extremely quiet, gentle individual whose depression had resulted in extreme weight loss and withdrawal from his family and work situation.

The client began with finger painting and spent the full 45 minutes on this activity. He used the three colors presented in approximately equal amounts, very neatly and carefully, with no overlapping or mixing, one line of each color and three circles, each demonstrating a concentric color sequence. He was most careful to get no paint on the table, to wipe his fingers after each time he touched the page, and to keep perfect balance. He even timed the painting to be complete in 45 minutes.

On the second day he spent about 30 minutes forming a human figure with realistic proportions, but in a smooth, stylized effect with absolutely no detail or facial features (Fig 6.2).

This client's third attempt was carving, which in the end took slightly longer than 45 minutes, as there were interruptions. The carving is skillfully and stiffly representative of a horse's head mounted on a plaque. He appeared completely absorbed in this, and spoke to no one while carving.

The client left the tile project to the last and did this in slightly less than the appointed time. The tile design is balanced rather than symmetrical, and features a subtle color combination. It may represent his ability to work more freely with the most structured of the four activities. Perhaps he was simply more comfortable by the last session.

If this client had not been discharged for financial reasons, it would have been a pleasure to work with him and help him to use his considerable technical ability and precision in more creative and experimental ways. He expressed pleasure in the evaluation procedure and had looked forward to becoming involved in the program.

In summary, the two sets described, Cases One and Two, have some interesting similarities and many differences. Time spent in the process was similar for both of them—above average—but their motivation appeared to be different.

Case One expressed much of his fantasy life and problems during the process. The physical activity involved in the carving, the project chosen first, may have accounted for less apparent anxiety during that session than in the others. His later three productions appeared to the therapist very clear indications of his disorganized thinking and frightening fantasy life. The asexual, only half-human type figure which he proceeded to attack was an extremely direct message.

Although Case One's products were bizarre, they showed dexterity and some artistic talent that would have been interesting to channel had the opportunity arisen.

Case Two may have taken a long time on his projects because of his perfectionistic tendencies and the satisfaction derived from performing in this area

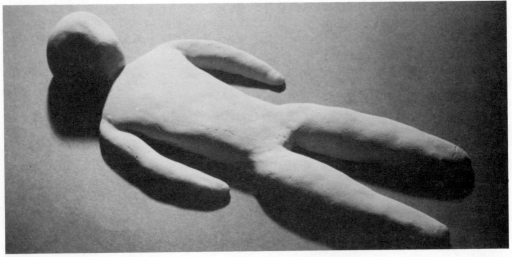

Fig 6.2: Case 2.

Clare W. Shoemyen

rather than being under pressure to communicate verbally. The whole set suggests concern with control, smoothness, and balance. The client used colors subtly rather than boldly. His human figure was beautifully formed in terms of smoothness and proportion, but in terms of detail, posture, or any other expressive characteristic, remained strikingly non-committal.

In this series the selection of cases was based on contrasting products and response to the situation rather than on value as diagnostic material and a step in treatment planning. The following case example has been chosen to show a more complete picture of this procedure leading to treatment.

Case Example 3

This case was a 17 year old, single female with a preliminary diagnosis of adolescent adjustment reaction. She complained of severe headaches and feeling depressed and burdened. The client spoke of contemplating suicide several times in the past three to four years, but had not been able to communicate these feelings to her parents. She felt that she was living under heavy pressure. Her parents were separated and she and her younger brother and sister lived with her mother. Though the mother denied assigning responsibility for the siblings and household tasks to the client, she felt that she had to assume these responsbilities. At the time of admission she was tremulous and crying, biting her lips and scratching herself. She stated that she felt guilty, specifically in reference to her parents' marital problems.

The occupational therapy evaluation procedure was started three days after admission. Forty-five minutes were spent on each project, with much of the time used in planning. The finger painting was the first project and the client described it as symbolizing her feelings of fear and guilt, represented by the blue and yellow, and of new blood, represented by the red, flowing in to make things better.

The carving was identified by the client as something peaceful. She expressed great concern over not being able to complete this project to her satisfaction.

The third project was the clay figure and was identified as "a Renaissance Madonna" in which concern was expressed about detail and about the body showing through the clothing (Fig 6.3).

The last project, the tile, was identified as a "Spanish tile," prompted by the client's desire to go to school in Mexico.

While the client was working, the therapist observed a high degree of creativity and organization, concern for detail, a good attention span, but noticeable signs of tension such as biting her lips and scratching herself. Upon completion of the four projects (Fig 6.4) the therapist discussed with the client her feelings and reactions. The client said that structured activities did not allow enough creativity for her, and that she had thus put off the tile project until last. She also spoke of having feelings and emotions that she did not know how to handle, and that she tended to put herself into situations of pressure by setting high goals for herself. In discussing the clay figure, she expressed concern and some confusion about her sexuality, and made several references to religion and time spent reading the Bible.

On the basis of her performance and the discussion of the projects, the therapist felt that the client needed to learn to acknowledge her feelings, and to express these outwardly instead of directing them inward; that she needed an opportunity to pursue her creativity in a non-pressured setting; and that she needed to develop an understanding of her sexual identity.

Treatment in occupational therapy started one week after admission. As she had felt frustrated by not being able to complete the carving project in the evaluation,

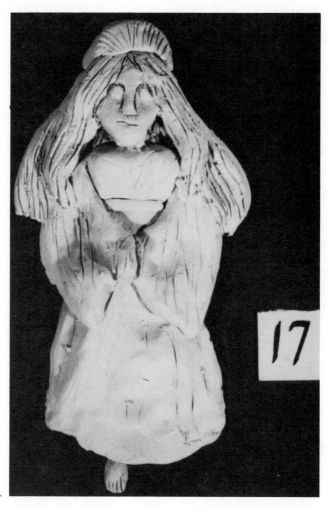

Fig 6.3: Case 3.

and was interested in attempting something similar, this was chosen as an initial project. She carved on a 10 inch block, stating that she wished to make a pawn, as in chess, since she felt that she was the pawn in the family game between her mother and father. She worked for several days on this project and expressed satisfaction with the release of tension and anger she felt the carving provided. On completion of the carving she expressed interest in learning a craft with which she had no previous experience, and decided to attempt a leather project. A stamped belt for herself was suggested, and the client was soon involved in the creation of the design. Release of tension was again noted in very heavy stamping.

During her hospitalization, *Case Three* was also involved in the group art therapy sessions conducted by the occupational therapist. These sessions were held twice weekly, and provided varied experiences for the clients, in an attempt to stimulate awareness of themselves and their feelings. Expressions of these feelings were encouraged initially on a non-verbal level, working towards a goal of verbal expression. During the initial session, *Case Three* was asked to depict herself at the time of admission, at the present time, and in the future (Fig 6.5). At the time of admission she showed herself as, "tearful and distraught", at the present time as,

Clare W. Shoemyen

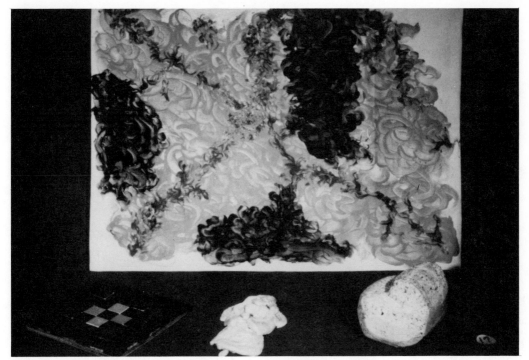

Fig 6.4: Case 3—total set.

"shaky and tense", and for the future she identified herself as, "peaceful". During another session she was asked to depict her world. She chose a black background, and used white string, wound tightly in a coil, but gradually loosening (Fig 6.6). The client said she was becoming less uptight and tense. For the third session, she was asked to make a mask for herself for the future (Fig 6.7). This mask she desribed as having quizzical eyes and a half-sad, half-smiling mouth. She spoke of it as showing a general feeling of doubtfulness, but with some hope for a better future.

Other treatment during hospitalization included group therapy and family therapy in which the client was encouraged to acknowledge and express her feelings, particularly in relation to her parents. She was discharged one month after admission, with plans for follow-up family therapy and continued private psychiatric treatment in her hometown. Her future plans included attending a university in Mexico in order to be, "as far away from home as possible." Subsequently, the client was reported as doing well.

Case Examples 4 and 5

These cases were a husband and wife, admitted together as inpatients. Prior to their year of stormy married life, they had been graduate students in the same program.

The husband described himself as depressed and confused. His wife had wanted private outpatient care during her husband's hospitalization, but was encouraged to become an inpatient also. Since both expressed concern over their marriage at their admission conference, it was recommended that they become involved in family therapy on a daily basis, with emphasis on sharing responsibility for treatment plans and decisions.

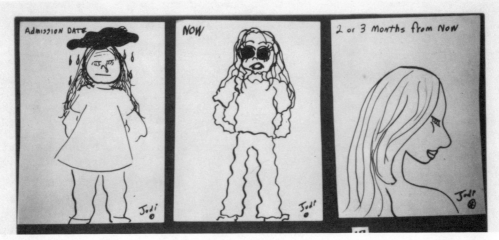

Fig 6.5: Case 3.

The couple was scheduled to start occupational therapy orientation and evaluation the morning following the admission conference. During their first session, two other clients were concluding their orientation and evaluation. The husband and wife became part of a small group at once. Both were cooperative and very courteous, and expressed their interest in the process and in trying anything that the staff recommended. The wife tended to talk for both, helping her husband get settled, telling the therapist that he was artistic and she was not. Her first choice was to work on the tile mosaic; and while working on this she continued to talk and to remain part of the group.

Her husband chose finger painting and sat as much removed from the group as possible. He became very much involved in his painting and spent the full 45

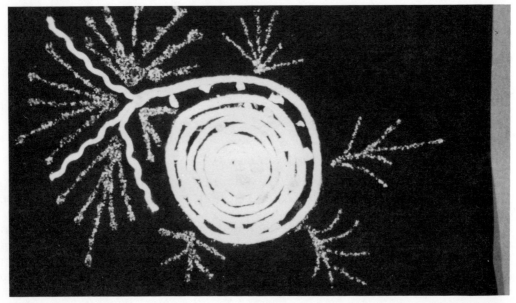

Fig 6.6: Case 3

Clare W. Shoemyen

minutes allotted to this task. His wife wished to comment on his work, but was told this should wait until each of the four projects was completed.

In the second session the wife chose finger painting and hesitated about starting until another patient near her took the lead. When her very similar painting was completed she left the area.

The husband chose clay, and again worked independently and with apparent concern for slightly more than 45 minutes.

In the third session the wife chose clay and worked hard on a figure for the full time. The husband worked with tile. When the mosaic was almost complete he was interrupted and told to report for X-ray. At his request he was permitted to take the tile mosaic to his room to finish.

In the last session both husband and wife carved. Each appeared to enjoy the destructive quality of this activity. They both talked freely to those around them, and their conversation was less superficial.

Both clients and their social worker and psychiatrist expressed interest in the evaluation of their products. After the brief individual sessions arranged by the occupational therapist, they combined, together with their products, for a joint

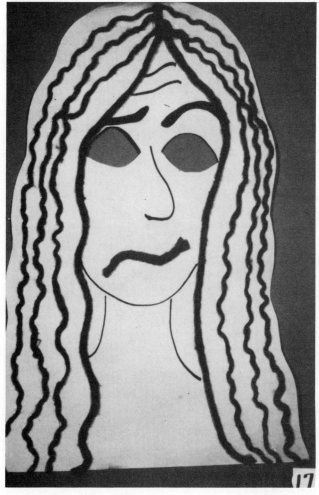

Fig 6.7: Case 3.

session where these were used for discussion and program planning.

In their initial approach to evaluation, both clients were similar in that they expressed interest and were very cooperative. Differences became apparent as they worked. The wife was concerned about fulfilling the requirements, always remaining in control of the situation, and avoiding failure and risk. On the other hand, the husband became very much involved in each activity and seemed unaware of those about him. Both wife and husband had qualities that were assets and liabilities. The primary ones, considering the problems recognized at the time of their admission, seemed to be as follows:

The wife's assets were seen as perseverence, recognition, and to a large extent, acceptance of her limitations, a good sense of design, and security within a structure. Her liabilities were seen as her extreme suggestibility, dependence, and lack of originality.

The husband's assests were seen as dexterity, care and precision, originality, ingenuity, and a sense of humor. His liabilities were seen in his guardedness and intellectualization used in an isolating and confusing manner, both toward the client and his associates.

Comparisons of these primary assets and liabilities were discussed at some length in the initial group session and used in treatment planning. Some of the conclusions reached will be shown through descriptions of each project.

The husband's ambivalence and need to control is suggested in his use of finger painting, which is the least structured of the media, and was his first choice. His painting was anxiously experimental and overworked. It covered every scrap of paper, and used several approaches—hand printing, drawing, and smearing (Fig 6.8).

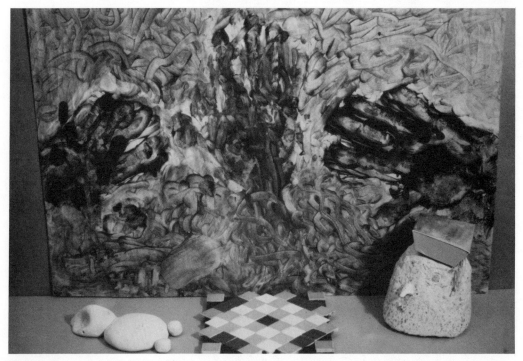

Fig 6.8: Case 4 (husband)—total set.

Clare W. Shoemyen

In the mosaic tile he produced a highly structured and symmetrical design at variance with the instructions given to him, as if to assert his originality, and maintain the last word in a confrontation (Fig 6.9). His final independent touch was to use his wife's eye liner to paint in the spaces he had left bare on the board.

His clay figure is full of symbolic messages (Fig 6.10), including perhaps his

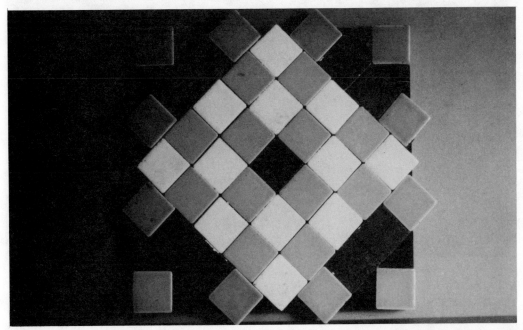

Fig 6.9: Case 4 (husband).

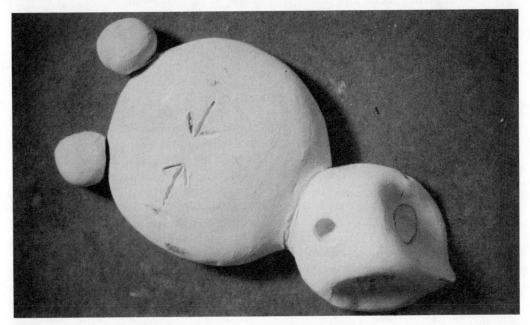

Fig 6.10: Case 4 (husband).

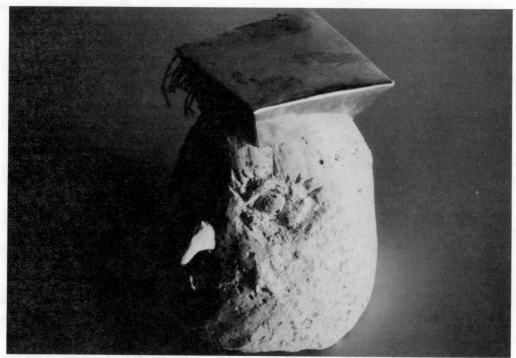

Fig 6.11: Case 4 (husband).

concept of himself as having a pointed head. Arrows accentuating the lack of umbilicus suggest strong feelings about family ties and dependency. The inhuman, insect-like form probably represents two levels of awareness: denial and guardedness with peers, and low self-concept.

His carving of a one-eyed owl (Fig. 6.11) with an ash-tray perched like a mortar board, probably represents both guilt and paranoid feelings in relation to his unfinished course work, and is another example of humor used defensively.

The wife's rigid, Victorian positioned and dressed clay figure may well imply conflict in sexual roles in a very dependent individual. The free-standing position also suggests her concern over dependence (Fig 6.12).

The subject of her finger painting was influenced by another client in the room.

In discussion, it became obvious that the house she carved was both an easy subject and a conflictual area. She dreamed of decorating her own home, but up to the time of hospitalization, she had either lived in her husband's "bachelor pad", or had travelled. She lacked the confidence to assert herself as a wife and homemaker (Fig 6.13).

Occupational therapy goals for the wife were focused on building up her own self-image and self-esteem. Opportunities were provided through the occupational therapy clinic and the recreation program for success in feminine, homemaking activities and entertaining, as well as for developing new interests and hobbies for herself. Since one of the early problems noted in therapy was the wife's dependence on approval from her husband and a tendency to cling, fuss, or be provocative, it seemed helpful to encourage independent projects and interests which could be considered separately.

In daily occupational therapy sessions, the husband worked by himself, steadily

Clare W. Shoemyen

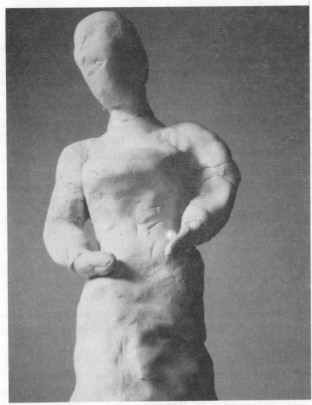

Fig 6.12: Case 5 (wife).

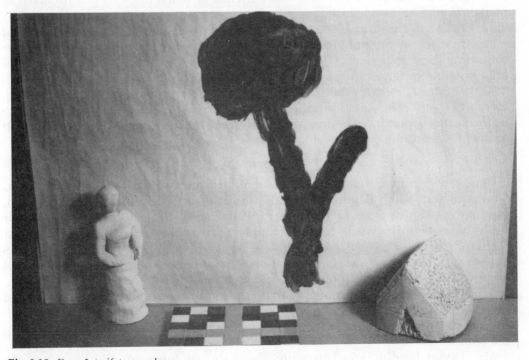

Fig 6.13: Case 5 (wife)—total set.

The Shoemyen Battery

79

and skillfully, on designing and building an elaborate box, which was much admired by patients and staff who had been unaware of his talents.

The wife, meanwhile, chose to work in another area of the clinic, and strengthened her self-esteem somewhat through indepth learning of the ceramics and the copper enameling processes, and in helping other patients at the occupational therapist's request.

Though she did not use occupational therapy to develop free, less rigid expression as was hoped, she did broaden her interests, and experimented considerably in the area of ceramics. She also learned several methods of artificial flower-making, and spent time with the occupational therapist in the garden project in the care and arrangement of flowers.

The individual goals in occupational therapy, within the total treatment program of each of these individuals, were obviously different in most instances. However, because the goals concerned the behavioral patterns and reactions which affected the other, they were interrelated and dependent.

Intellectualization and guardedness diminished as they experienced real success, in both creative activities and social situations. Opportunities for even more direct expression of feelings through art therapy were provided, as were opportunities to express frustration and hostility in acceptable physical ways. In place of the provocative games and mixed messages, more honest communication developed between husband and wife. Attempts were made to ascertain real feelings about their education and to help them face reality in this area.

Throughout their stay, both clients spent more than average time in the occupational therapy clinic. Insights and conclusions reported there, as well as the clients' total response to treatment, derived from the program as a whole. Due to their daily family therapy sessions, their time in occupational therapy usually coincided with the physically disabled patients, or when the staff was involved in preparation. This seemed undesirable, but in the long run the arrangement may have worked to the couple's advantage. Both developed more independence and self-sufficiency in the hobbies of their choice, and more meaningful one-to-one communication experiences with the occupational therapists than would have been possible in larger groups.

At the time of discharge, both clients appeared more spontaneous and sensitive to each other and to be functioning on a firmer basis of reality. Their plans were to furnish a newly purchased mountain cabin and to make a garden around it, hopeful forms of continuing occupational therapy.

Research

I know of two investigations of the orientation and evaluation procedure. Marti Southam and Sally Bendroth,[2] while students at the University of Florida, conducted a study entitled, "Objective Evaluation of Projective Material." Their study focused only on tile mosaic, which was the most structured of the four evaluation activities. Devising objective criteria and techniques for scoring the 149 patient projects was an awesome and time-consuming job, requiring a great deal of effort, cooperation, and professional and technical assistance.

The other attempt was initiated at about the same time at Chapel Hill. Since I had been sent a detailed description of the very elaborate (six month grant funded) project during its first month, Mary Lyn Taylor was contacted for follow-up information.

Ms. Taylor kindly agreed to write about the situation for the benefit of the

Clare W. Shoemyen

occupational therapists attempting research. Most of what she wrote is as follows:

The research effort conducted in the psychiatric occupational therapy department at the North Carolina Memorial in 1971-1972 was nobly thought out and designed, but produced data almost impossible to interpret. The value of recording a research project failure lies in the enormous quantity of hindsight and wisdom acquired that can be shared with others embarking on a similar adventure.

The goal of the effort was to investigate the possible relationships between clients' working diagnosis and their task performance in occupational therapy. The task performance was recorded through an evaluation battery modeled after the one used at that time at Shands Teaching Hospital in Gainesville, Florida. The client evaluation section consisted of 54 statements concerned with the clients' abilities and responses to the task. The project evaluation was made up of eight to 13 statements concerned with the clients' work methods and the physical details of the project.

Forms and protocols were developed for each aspect of the battery. Due to treatment time constraints, each client was asked to select and do two of the four tasks. Two forms were completed by the occupational therapist on each project done by a client. The forms were then filed, put on coding sheets, and keypunched. At the end of the project, several computer runs were made. It became apparent that the data spread was so diffuse that meaningful correlations could not be derived.

The obvious glaring error of this project was its broad scope and incredible number of variables. This effort should have been broken down into several components and pursued individually. The notion that, "while we are into it this far, let us learn all that we can" proved erroneous and unproductive.

Another major problem of the project was the reliance of the data collected upon the working diagnosis of the client. The clients were administered the battery soon after admission and there was often considerable lag time before a working diagnosis was established by the physician. This often affected accurate and complete data recording, as well as having the study rely on undescribed and undefined diagnostic criteria and methods.

The final and greatest lesson learned, aside from project size, was the absolute necessity of having experienced research and statistical resource persons available during the entirety of the project. This study suffered in that a great deal of research consultation was available at the planning and beginning phases, but persons unfamiliar with the project had to be sought at its conclusion. This resulted in many remedial hours, unanswerable questions, and unbelievable frustration.

Despite the study's lack of results and conclusive findings, a great deal of knowledge was acquired by all who participated in the study.

Obviously, it would have been good to hear of more positive and conclusive results. This situation reminds me that though information gained from the Battery often substantiates a diagnosis under consideration by the treatment team, diagnosis was never a major purpose of the Battery.

Students ask, why collect this information if it does not have definite predictable use? In my opinion the Battery administered under appropriate conditions is the first step in occupational therapy—the jumping off place for collaboration and mutual goal setting.

Suggested Research

I feel that there is potential for research based on The Shoemyen Battery if, as Taylor emphasized, the questions or elements of concern are broken down into separate components and addressed individually. This will only happen if there is interest, and if occupational therapists using The Shoemyen Battery in several settings agree on a question and are willing and able to be consistent in administering the Battery and in collecting data from a predetermined number of samples. A coordinator or project director experienced in methodology with access to computer facilities would be essential.

Since 1970, one of the questions of interest to me is whether there is in fact correlation between dependence (or defense against it) and the free standing clay figures created by some clients. Other simple questions relating to use of color in both finger painting and tile, or order of project choice might be possible to address simultaneously if the proposal is designed correctly.

Conclusion

History of The Shoemyen Battery from 1963 to the present would not be complete without mentioning that time constraints have reportedly kept a good many therapists from using the Battery in spite of their interest and expressed need for a routine initial procedure. Recently, some shorter forms were tried, with my knowledge, in private hospitals and the Veterans Administration system.

The Veterans Administration and Medical Center in Gainesville, Florida has just started using a modification of The Shoemyen Battery designed for completion within an hour. The staff, of which I am a member, would be willing to share the forms with interested therapists. Broader use will help to determine whether it is beneficial. Again, I request feedback, so that all may learn.

References

1. Shoemyen C: Occupational therapy orientation and evaluation: A study of procedure and media. A J Occu Ther 24:276-279, 1970.
2. Bendroth S, Southam M: Objective evaluation of projective material. A J Occu Ther 27:78-80, 1973.

Bibliography

Azima H, Azima FJ: An outline of a dynamic theory of occupational therapy. A J Occu Ther Sept/Oct, 1959.

Berne F: Games People Play. New York, Grove Press, 1967.

Beccle H: Psychiatry for Nurses. London, 1953.

Dunton W, Licht S: Occupational Therapy Principles and Practice. Springfield, IL, Charles C Thomas, 1957.

Fagan J, Sheperd L: Gestalt Therapy Now. New York, Harper and Row, 1971.

Fidler G, Fidler J: Occupational Therapy—A Communication Process in Psychiatry. New York, MacMillin Publishing Co, 1963.

Gillette N: Standardizing Observation Techniques Through Available Occupational Therapy Media. Proceedings of Psychiatric Subcommittee, October, 1964.

Glasser W: Reality Therapy. New York, Harper and Row, 1965.

Jones M: Social Psychiatry in Practice. London, Penguin Books, 1968.

Linn LS, Weinroth LA, Shamah R: Occupational Therapy in Dynamic Psychiatry. Washington DC, American Psychiatric Assoc, 1962.

Llorens L: Facilitating growth and development: The promise of occupational therapy. Eleanor Clarke Slagle Lecture, 1969. A J Occu Ther 24, 1970.

Macdonald EM: Occupational Therapy in Rehabilitation. London, Balliere, Tindally, and Cox, 1960.

Machover K: Personality Projection in the Human Figure. Springfield, IL, Charles C Thomas, 1948.

Willard H, Spackman C (eds): Occupational Therapy, 4th ed. Philadelphia, JB Lippincott Co, 1971.

Acknowledgments

All Occupational Therapy staff, students, and faculty associated with the Shands Teaching Hospital psychiatric unit and Occupational Therapy Curriculum,

Clare W. Shoemyen

University of Florida, have participated to some extent in the development of The Shoemyen Battery.

In addition to those mentioned in the text, the following individuals have been particularly helpful and influential:

Ethel Alford, COTA
George Barnard, MD
Jean Deitz, MEd, OTR
Kathleen Fowler, OTR
Ken Grantham, OTR
Holly Howard, OTR
Lela Llorens, PhD, OTR, FAOTA
Ferol Menks, MS, OTR

Mary McCaulley, PhD
Rene Moyer, OTR
Nancy Nashiro, MS, OTR
Mary Robertson, PhD
Jane Slaymaker, MA, OTR, FAOTA
Florence Stattel, MA, OTR, FAOTA
Grace Straw, OTR

Without cooperative clients, nothing would have been developed to describe.

Case Number Three was evaluated, treated, and described by Kathleen Fowler, OTR when on STHUF Occupational Therapy staff.

Material from the slide series was produced in an Audio-Visual Workshop sponsored by the Center for Allied Health Instructional Personnel and the Kellogg Foundation.

Photography of client productions was by Nancy Nashiro and Nicholas Fowler. These were reproduced in black and white by the Medical Media Production Service of the Veterans Administration Medical Center in Gainesville, Florida.

Thank you all.

Clare W. Shoemyen, MBAOT, OTR

7
The Goodman Battery

Marsha Goodman Evaskus, O.T.R.

The Goodman Battery evaluates the ego assets and deficits directly affecting an individual's ability to function. The tasks in the Goodman Battery are administered in a progression of decreasing structure, from copying a specific mosaic design to the spontaneous drawing and figure drawing, and finally, the clay task. In each, an assessment is made of the client's ability to conceptualize the task, organize, and plan procedures that will enable him to carry through and achieve a meaningful, integrated whole. The client's responses to the various tasks reflect the strength and integrity of his ego boundaries. The strengths and weaknesses of the ego, emerging needs and conflicts, and defenses utilized are assessed within the framework of the ability to function within varying degrees of structure.

Development

The work by the Azimas,[1] which promoted the use of occupational therapy materials for assessment, the development of the Azima Battery[2] and its later modification, and the Diagnostic Battery Scoring and Summary[3] developed by Fidler, formed the basis for the development of the Goodman Battery in 1967. The diagnostic battery described by Androes[4] influenced the decision to include structured media in the Goodman Battery. The media used in both the Azima and Fidler batteries represent decreasing degrees of control through the progression from drawing to finger painting, and then to clay media. According to Azima, this progression allows for "an increasing degree of projection of primary process modes of object-relations."[2] The diagnostic battery described by Androes includes five tasks (drawing, ceramics, painting, woodwork, and leather work), administered in a developmental progression of increasing complexity. Structured tasks are included so as to assess the individual's ability to follow directions, his cognitive processes, and planning ability.[4] While the activities included by Androes provide a range of complexity and structure within which to assess the client's responses, the battery is time-consuming and expensive to administer. The tasks in the Goodman Battery provide a range of structure and stimuli that elicit information regarding the client's level of cognitive and affective ego-functioning, while offering the advantages of a comparatively brief administration time, and materials that are readily accessible, portable, and inexpensive.

Theoretical Base

When assessing ego functioning, it is useful to consider the two categories of ego functions described in the literature:[5] 1) the executive *conflict-free* portion which consists of the biological capacities or skills, including thought, perception, intention, comprehension of objects, and motor development; and 2) the synthetic *conflict-born* portion which deals with emerging conflicts and issues of drive and impulse control. The relationship between the individual's level of ego functioning and his action potential is emphasized. As discussed by Polansky,[6] the presence of a strong conflict-free ego increases the ability of the individual to function efficiently in relation to the environment—to deal with new situations, demonstrate good concentration, attention, and to problem solve. These ego-functions become less effective when the individual's energy is consumed by conflicts and defenses. Therefore, an interdependent relationship exists between the two functions of the ego, with weakness in one area of function affecting the proper development and emergence of the other function.

The strength of ego boundaries also affects the individual's ability for thought and action. Federn describes ego boundaries as providing the "sense of self as separate from the world...without which action cannot proceed effectively."[5] According to Polansky, a loosening of ego boundaries affects performance on tasks, as seen in a higher incidence of distraction, greater disorganization, and the inability to follow through and complete.[6] There may be an emergence of ideas and images from the unconscious, as seen in bizarre responses to tasks, and illogical and disconnected thinking and associations. Looseness of ego boundaries also affects the ability to "sustain structure," demonstrated by poor impulse control and the need for immediate gratification.

If firm inner boundaries have not been established through the internalization of external structures and controls, impairment of ego functions may be seen in situations providing little external structure. Likewise, situations providing too much structure may overwhelm, by placing too much demand on the ego.

In the Goodman Battery, the mosaic task provides the greatest structure and limits in its fixity of materials, and predetermined design. Observation of executive ego functioning in response to a specific task is facilitated, and can be interrelated with boundary and control issues. A less structured, more ambiguous stimuli situation, as in the drawing and clay tasks, allows for more varied range of responses,[7] with the potential for evoking responses of a more projective nature.[8] In the spontaneous drawing, the content or end-product is subject to the client's control, and as such, has the potential for revealing conflicts, needs, and drives, as well as the ability to organize and present concepts. Though the figure drawing offers more structure in that the client is told what to draw, it is administered after the spontaneous drawing, so as not to influence the content of the free drawing. The figure drawing is included to more directly gain information regarding the client's concept of self and/or others. While the drawings offer the structure provided by the limits of the size and form of the paper, and the control allowed by the properties of the pencil, the inclusion of the clay task provides information regarding the client's response to a changeable, messy form. Boundary and control issues are evoked because of the amorphous quality of the clay. The added dimension of the client's tactile response and the opportunity for manipulation of the media can elicit regressive and/or aggressive responses more graphically than in the other tasks.

Literature Review
Mosaic Tile

The use of mosaic pieces for the study of personality was introduced in 1929, by Margaret Lowenfeld of London.[9] In the Mosaic Test, an analysis is made of the

Marsha Goodman Evaskus

spontaneous productions of clients using a set of 465 small wooden pieces in varied colors and shapes. The Mosaic Test was later adapted by Wertham, and in a study done by Wertham and Golden, a method of analyzing and interpreting mosaic designs based on a diagnostic correlation between characteristics of designs produced, and specific clinical entities or reaction types, was described.[10] While specific diagnostic correlations are not emphasized in the interpretation of results from the Goodman Battery, certain findings described by Wertham[11] have been seen in the mosaic task. The level of organization present in the pattern produced is important to Wertham's description of characteristic responses of the different diagnostic categories. For example, Wertham found a very low level of organization in the designs produced by deteriorated schizophrenics, while in depressive psychosis there is an inability to initiate organization. In addition to organization, Wertham's characteristics of coherence or incoherence of design, completeness or incompleteness of design, and distinctness of configuration (or Gestalt), are findings also emphasized in the mosaic task of the Goodman Battery. Other characteristics of designs described by Wertham are less comparable to the findings on this mosaic task, because they pertain to spontaneous creations rather than to the copying of a specific design.

Other studies have also demonstrated the value of using mosaics to assess disturbances in personality structure.[12] In an extensive study by Diamond and Schmale,[13] the grading of mosaic performance was based on the achievement of a satisfactory and well-organized Gestalt. The researchers concluded that the ability to produce a recognizable Gestalt or pattern within the limits of the test materials reflected basic personality integration. The severest disturbances in the mosaic Gestalt were revealed in schizophrenia, psychopathic personality, and severe organic brain syndromes, while conditions in which the personality structure is less disordered showed less abnormality in the Gestalt produced.

The Goodman also emphasizes the importance of producing an organized form configuration, but to more clearly demonstrate the processes of conceptualization and organization, the client is asked to copy a specific mosaic design. Because the Mosaic Test and related occupational therapy test batteries[14] utilize a form of spontaneous or free production with mosaics, certain psychological tests in which the client is required to copy a specific design were surveyed.

In both the mosaic tile task of the Goodman Battery and the Bender Visual-Motor Gestalt Test, the client is required to copy a specific design with emphasis on the abililty to reproduce the configuration, as seen in both the process utilized and the end-product produced. An understanding of basic Gestalt principles is useful when assessing the client's performance in both tests. The visual-motor function is described by Woltmann as the ability to "perceive, interpret, integrate, and organize stimuli,"[15] mastered through successive stages of maturation. The inclusion of the advanced diamond form in the center of the Goodman mosaic design is based on the developmental progression of the visually perceived form observed by Bender: from the circle, to the square, the triangle, and finally the diamond.[15] Therefore, the level of visual perception of form can be assessed, eg, is the client able to perceive and copy the diamond form as well as the simpler square form?

From the Bender Gestalt test performance, an evaluation can be made of how the individual approaches and organizes a specific task, the capacity to reproduce perceptions, and the level of visual motor coordination.[16] Similarly, the ability to integrate the parts of the figure to the whole so as to reproduce the total configuration is assessed in the performance of the Goodman mosaic tile task.

Disturbances in the perception of the configuration, or Gestalt, can be detected in the sequence followed by the client in placing the tiles.

The inclusion of restrictions in a test situation reveals the client's reaction to and way of handling limitations and the subsequent frustrations added to the task. For example, in the Bender Gestalt test, the limitation of using one sheet of paper and the subsequent manner of organizing the nine figures on the same sheet reveals qualitative differences in the client responses.[15] Lerner states that defined boundaries, such as those of the paper "evoke ego functions which reflect reality testing judgment, boundary awareness, and respect," or they may "reflect cognitive capacities: the ability to anticipate, organize, plan for, and execute a task under the terms set."[17] Specific manifestations of disturbance seen in response to the Bender Gestalt are described by Halpern, and include fragmentation, elaboration, perseveration, displacement, compulsivity, crowding or overlapping of figures, and the "too-perfect performance".[16] Similar responses may also occur in response to the limitations inherent in the Goodman mosaic task. The reader is referred to *Behaviors Assessed,* pp 101-105, for a discussion of the specific findings on this mosaic task.

Comparisons may be drawn between the functions assessed in the Similarities and Block-Design subtests of the Wechsler Adult Intelligence Scale (WAIS),[18,19] and the functions assessed with the Goodman Battery. In the Similarities subtest, described by Matarazzo as a test of abstraction or concept formation,[19] the client is asked in what way two items are alike.[18] Mayman[20] and Rapaport[21] define verbal concept formation as the ability to see similarities and differences, and to identify ideas or objects as belonging together. In the Goodman Battery, the client is asked to think of a use for the mosaic tile product and to see similarities in his productions and manner of working on the tasks. As in the Similarities subtest of the WAIS, responses may indicate concrete or abstract levels of concept formation. The ability to sum up the essential common characteristics of objects would demonstrate the ability for abstract conceptualization. The flexibility and appropriateness of the client's thinking is also revealed.

The Block-Design subtest of the WAIS, is described in the literature as measuring visual organization and visual-motor coordination, dealing with the relationship of perceptual and motor processes.[19-22] In both the Block-Design subtest and the Goodman mosaic task, the client is asked to reproduce a specific design from parts, with the pattern kept in view, measuring the ability to conceptualize the pattern as a whole, break it down into its component parts, and then reproduce it. While Goldstein emphasizes the function of abstract ability in any sorting task, Rapaport considers these tests of concept formation.[21] The process of reproduction involves analysis and synthesis, in which "the complex design must be broken down by the subject into units equivalent to faces of the block . . . [involving] a steady interaction between presented pattern and available blocks."[20] In the same way, the ability to see the relationship of the parts to the whole, to achieve differentiation of the design, and a synthesis leading to reproduction of the pattern, is assessed with the mosaic task of the Goodman Battery.

Rapaport describes an efficient performance on the Block-Design subtest as involving an appropriate amount of regard for the pattern, for the parts already constructed, and for the remaining spaces and blocks.[21] Various steps may be taken in the performance of the Block-Design, with implications for the level of visual organization utilized. Rapaport finds that intially, the client inspects the design. Through this inspection: 1) the pattern may be immediately differentiated into its

Marsha Goodman Evaskus

parts, with a firm concept of how the pattern is to be reproduced, 2) only a vague idea of the pattern as a whole is achieved, with only an idea of the starting point, or 3) no ideas of either whole or parts is achieved, with the client turning to the blocks for an indication of the pattern. Performance by "pattern coherence", described by Goldstein and Scheerer as, "the concrete matching of patterns without abstract conception of the design construction,"[21] refers to the use of motor trial-and-error attempts when visual organization is impaired. Rapaport characterizes this approach as one in which the pattern is reproduced piece by piece without an organized picture of other than isolated parts of the pattern. The pattern is not experienced as a whole, and the approach is not guided by "organization, image, meaning, or plan".[21] This piecemeal approach can be compared to the fragmented, segmental sequence followed by some clients in placing the tiles for the Goodman mosaic task.

Spontaneous Drawing and Human Figure Drawing

The literature on the use of drawings for assessment of the personality is extensive. Machover's findings,[23,24] based on the clinical use of figure drawings, provides the theoretical concepts and rationale for many of the studies that followed. The reader is referred to literature on the projective use of drawings for a thorough study of the subject, and specifically to the writings by Buck,[25] Hammer,[26] and Levy[27] on interpretation of figure drawings, and to the studies by Anastasi and Foley[28,29] on the interpretation of spontaneous drawings. The findings from the literature which are used in the interpretation of the drawings in the Goodman Battery are summarized in the section, *Behaviors Assessed,* pp 105-109. While much of the literature is empirically derived from clincial studies, and emphasizes qualitative findings, Buck also emphasizes quantitative findings and the use of the House-Tree-Person Test (H-T-P) as a measure of intellectual function.[25] An extensive and detailed description of Buck's quantitative and qualitative methods for scoring the H-T-P, as well as illustrative cases, can be found in the H-T-P manual.

While the clinical value of using human figure drawings for personality assessment has been supported in the literature, discrepancies have been described between the results of research studies and clinical experience. Swensen has extensively reviewed the human figure drawing research literature.[30,31] In the first review, Swensen found little evidence to support Machover's hypotheses concerning figure drawings. He concluded that the figure drawing may be valuable as one part of a diagnostic battery, but that in itself, does not provide sufficient diagnostic evidence.[30] Swensen recommended further research into the validity and reliability of human figure drawings. Hammer disagrees with many of Swensen's criticisms, emphasizing the clinical importance of signs even though they may appear infrequently, and the importance of considering the extremes on a continuum.[32] These signs should not be cancelled out by only comparing the means, as often is the case in research studies. Hammer states that it is the deviation in either direction from the mean that is important clinically, and recommends the use of a research design that employs a "3-point (or 5-point) rating scale: 1) overemphasis, 2) normal emphasis, and 3) underemphasis or absence"[32]

In Swensen's study of research literature from 1957-1966,[31] increased empirical support was found for the use of human figure drawings as a clinical tool and specifically, as a diagnostic instrument. The studies suggest that the validity of a particular aspect of the drawing is directly related to the reliability of that aspect of the drawing. Global ratings, which encompass the total drawing, have the highest reliability and validity. This measure of the overall quality of the drawing is found to be a useful screening device for gross maladjustment. Contradictory results regarding the reliability of structural and formal aspects of drawings (eg, size, placement, and the line quality), are still reported. However, Swensen also found an increase in the number of significant results reported, particularly regarding the structural aspects of size (reflecting self-esteem) and stance (reflecting stability and security), with omissions and distortions found to be especially reliable indicators of severe disturbance. Individual signs (eg, rendering of particular detail or body part) are found to be the least reliable and least valid, with findings being either conflicting or negative. While the sex of the first figure drawn has been related significantly to self-concept, it still remains a complex area of study. The evidence presented by Swensen reinforces the importance of analyzing patterns of signs, rather than an individual sign. However, findings on the Goodman Battery also support Hammer's comments regarding the clinical importance of extreme deviations in signs.

Clay

Although the use of clay for personality assessment has not been documented extensively in the literature, psychodynamic and developmental frameworks for understanding responses to clay medium have been found in the fields of psychology, occupational therapy, art therapy, and education. Implications for the use of these frames of reference in interpreting response to the Goodman clay task will be noted and discussed further in the section, *Behaviors Assessed*, pp 109-111.

In considering the expressive potential and psychodynamic value of clay, the properties of the clay medium, and the responses that may be elicited, should be understood. In the literature, the unstructured, plastic nature of clay is contrasted with the properties of more structured media. According to Frank,[8] the amorphous quality of clay allows a cathartic expression of affect, and an opportunity for symbolic release of hostility. Robbins and Sibley[33] also described the increased expressive aspects elicited by the changeability of the clay material, as contrasted with the safer, repetitive quality of more easily controlled materials. The reversible quality of clay, allowing for flexibility in making changes, is also described. This plastic nature of clay that permits the form to be easily altered, may present difficulty for the individual with distortions in perception of reality. Fidler emphasizes the importance of clear delineation of form and procedures in providing support for the individual with poor reality testing skills.[34] Her "Outline for Activity Analysis"[34] provides an excellent framework for understanding the basic psychodynamic characteristics of a given activity, and specifically, for considering the implications for the meaning of clay.

Using a psycho-analytical framework, clay can be considered a primitive anal medium.[2] The use of clay to provide opportunity for expression and actual or symbolic gratification of primitive needs has been described by Bender and Woltmann,[35] Azima,[2] Fidler,[34] and others.[36] Fidler discusses the value of clay in eliciting unconscious material, the expression of hostility, and in exploring self-concept.[34]

Considering both the psychodynamic and developmental aspects, Bender and Woltmann[35] discuss the use of plastic material (plasticene) in treating children with behavior problems, correlating maturational aspects of the responses to plasticene, and drawings with the personality development of the child. The authors describe the initial response of the child as initiated by the drive for motility expression and the reaction to sensory and tactile stimulation. During this stage of nonspecific treatments as in the scribbling stage in drawing, there is no intention to copy or create form. Accidentally made forms are given a name and function. In the next stage, more integrated rhythmic rolling leads to the first attempts in object representation. The suggestibility of the child in response to the clay form is described: "Every touch or pressure upon the material will produce changes in form which might lead to a different interpretation by the child. . . a child will start out with one intention and change it a number of times before the creation is completed."[35] Emotional values now enter into the creative activities, permitting expression of fantasy life and resolution of problems. According to Bender and Woltmann, the plastic medium lends itself to the "repetitive-aggressive-destructive type behavior,"[35] characteristic of children, and the unconscious gratification of regressive needs.

Lowenfeld uses a cognitive developmental framework, describing the first stage of a child's interaction with clay as a primarily kinesthetic experience, involving beating and pounding of the clay with no visible purpose, comparable to the "scribbling stage" in drawing (age 2-4).[37,38] This early kinesthetic response is comparable to the overinvolvement in the process seen at times in the Goodman clay task. Lowenfeld observed that the child, with a need for more controlled activity, begins to break the clay with or without order, and may form coils and balls without attempting any specific object, parallel to the "controlled scribbling stage". These early forms still lack a definite purpose or meaning. The readiness to establish a relationship between his representation and the things he wants to represent is indicated when the child begins to name the forms, parallel to "naming of scribbling", marking a change from kinesthetic thinking to imaginative thinking. In the "pre-schematic stage", Lowenfeld describes the beginning use of form seen in the first representational attempts.[37] A variety of forms may be used to represent the same object, developing into a representative pattern or schema by age 7, when "achievement of a form concept" occurs. Lowenfeld describes two modes of thinking that are reflected in the method utilized in working with clay: 1) the *analytic method*, having a concept of the total from which details will be developed, involves pulling out the single details from the whole; and 2) the *synthetic method*, building up a synthesis out of partial impressions, involves putting single parts together to form the whole.[37] These two methods have implications for the assessment of concept formation in the Goodman Battery.

Hartley and Goldenson describe a similar developmental progression from the smearing, tactile experience (including feeling, smelling, squeezing, etc), to experimenting with taking apart and putting together, leading to the creation of form (eg, cakes, balls, snakes, snowmen, dishes).[39] The child at age five builds forms out of parts, and by age seven displays a readiness to form out of one piece. From age seven, there is an increase in forms used and subject matter represented. According to Hartley and Goldenson, tools can be used as an extension of the self to increase and vary the effects produced by the hands alone. This use of tools to achieve form with greater control represents a progression in development from the earlier, primitive pleasure in the feel of clay.

Golomb described the results of a study of the development of representational forms, and specifically, the human form, in the drawing and clay productions of children ages two through seven.[40] Concerned with the relation of form to cognitive development, Golomb did not deal with the psychodynamic aspects of representation. The researcher described a progression from motor action with no representational intent (eg, holding the clay passively, turning it aimlessly, hitting the table with it) to an increased range of actions that lead to the rolling motion and formation of the snake form. Other early forms, based on the use of the circle and verticality, include the flattened pancake, rounded ball, and standing column. The child progresses from "action-imitation", in which the interpretation of form is based on the function of the object (eg, bouncing a ball form) with no attempt at perceptual likeness, to "verbal designation", in which the form is made to conform to the original intention despite the lack of visual similarity. Golomb found that continued exploration and development of form leads to the first representations of the human figure: the upright standing column, the ball or slab with facial features, and the array of separate parts (two-dimensional graphic models).

These developmental studies have implications for the interpretation of responses seen on the Goodman Battery clay task, especially regarding the degree of involvement in process, the ability to maintain intention and constancy of form versus the degree of suggestibility, and the level of form representation achieved.

Administration

General Considerations

The Goodman Battery has been developed for use with individuals with psychiatric disturbances, including psychotic, psychoneurotic, and character disorders. It is not intended for use with retarded individuals, though it has been administered to clients with low intellectual functioning (eg, IQ 70+). The battery has been used in both inpatient psychiatric hospitals and psychiatric day care centers, administered to clients ranging in age from 12 years through adulthood.

Ideally, the client is seen for evaluation soon after admission and before entering the occupational therapy treatment program. Before testing, an assessment should be made of the client's ability to tolerate the testing situation. Contraindications for evaluation include clients who are heavily medicated, too disoriented to understand the instructions or attend to the tasks, or agitated clients.

Prior to the testing (two or three days), the client is contacted and told the day and time of the evaluation. It is explained that the evaluation will consist of several tasks involving mosaic tiles, drawing, and clay media. When indicated, to minimize anxiety or confusion, the client should be told of the schedule for testing the day prior to, or the morning of, the scheduled evaluation.

When preparing to administer the Goodman Battery, the following time considerations should be noted: 1) the administration of the battery generally takes one hour; however, because some clients may require more time, a leeway of one half hour should be allowed when scheduling the time; 2) sufficient time should be allowed for setting up the battery materials; 3) test materials should be prepared ahead of time (eg, the bases pre-cut, clay pliable, tiles available in needed colors); and 4) the Goodman Battery is administered in one sitting.

Materials

Mosaic Tile Task:
1. one masonite or wood base, 2¼ x 2¾ x ¼ inches
2. one completed model of the tile design to be reproduced (Fig. 7.1)

Marsha Goodman Evaskus

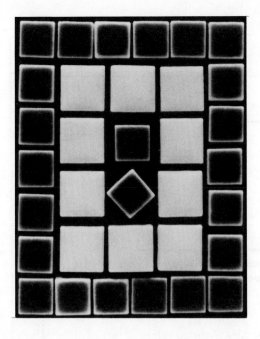

Fig 7.1: Mosaic tile model
(actual size 2¼ x 2¾ x ¼ inches).

*3. one container two thirds filled with ⅜ inch square mosaic tiles in assorted colors

*4. one container two thirds filled with 5/16 inch square mosaic tiles in assorted colors

5. white glue in a small bowl

6. several paper towels

7. one tongue depressor blade

Drawing Task:

1. one sheet of white drawing paper, 12 x 18 inches

2. one #2 pencil with eraser

Clay Task:

1. one 2 pound ball of white Amaco art clay on plaster bat

2. assortment of three clay tools, including one serrated edge, one pointed end, one rounded end, and one wire end tool

3. sponge and water in a bowl

Procedure

   The room used for testing should contain minimal stimuli. The client should be seated at a table where materials have been arranged according to the diagram (Fig. 7.2A). The examiner should sit to the left and slightly behind the client, so as to view the client and his work inobtrusively. The client is told that notes will be taken throughout the procedure. The approach to the tasks, verbal and motor behavior,

---

*The containers are opaque; 46 fluid ounce juice cans covered with blue yarn are used.

Source for tiles: S & S Arts and Crafts, Colchester, CT 06415

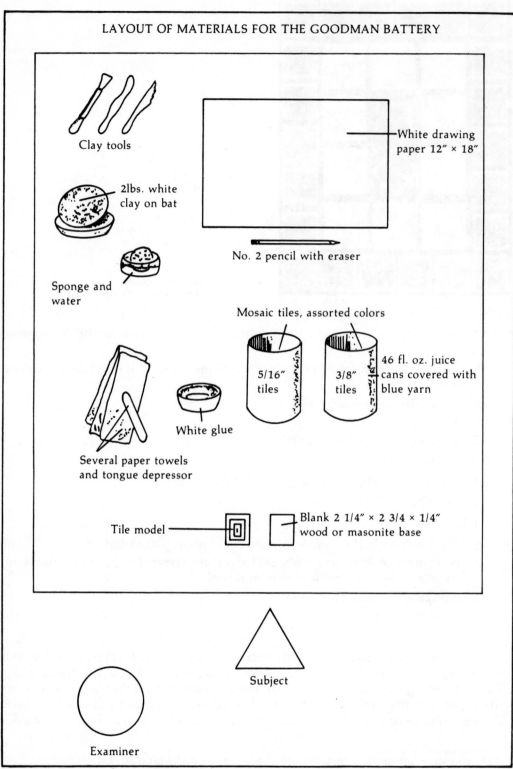

LAYOUT OF MATERIALS FOR THE GOODMAN BATTERY

Clay tools

2lbs. white clay on bat

White drawing paper 12" × 18"

No. 2 pencil with eraser

Sponge and water

Mosaic tiles, assorted colors

5/16" tiles

3/8" tiles

46 fl. oz. juice cans covered with blue yarn

White glue

Several paper towels and tongue depressor

Tile model

Blank 2 1/4" × 2 3/4 × 1/4" wood or masonite base

Subject

Examiner

Fig. 7.2.A. Diagram showing layout of materials for the Goodman Battery.

Marsha Goodman Evaskus

and work processes, should be recorded by the examiner. The examiner's responses and questions should also be recorded.

The Goodman Battery is administered to clients on an individual basis. Other individuals should not have access to the testing area during administration. Any interruptions that do occur should be noted in relation to the effect on the client's test performance, including requests made by the client (eg, smoking, bathroom). Projects from the evaluation battery are to be kept by the examiner for assessment purposes, and not given to the client.

Introduction. The examiner says to the client, "I will be asking you to do something with mosaic tiles, something with paper and pencil, and something with clay. This evaluation usually takes about one hour, but some people take more time, some less. There is no time limit. I will be taking notes as you work. Do you have any questions?"

Mosaic Tile. The examiner then says, "Using the materials available, make a mosaic tile just like this one. The tiles are in the cans, the glue is on the table." Often the client will ask if he is to make it the same, use the same colors, etc. The examiner should only repeat or rephrase the directions, but not be more specific.

When the client states or otherwise indicates he has finished, the examiner says, "What were you thinking about as you were working?" After recording the client's response, the examiner says, "Compare your tile to the model—how is it the same? Are there any differences?" Finally, the client is asked, "What are some possible uses for the tiles?"

The client is then asked to put the leftover tiles back in the cans, if he has not already done so.

Spontaneous Drawing. The paper and pencil are placed in the cleared area in front of the client, with the paper in a horizontal position. The examiner says, "Do something with the paper and pencil." Often, the client will state that he is not a good artist. The examiner then says, "This is not a test of how well you draw." If the client says that he does not know what to draw, the examiner should repeat or rephrase the initial directions, but not be more specific. The client can be told, "Do whatever you want with the paper and pencil; it is up to you."

When the client indicates he has finished, the examiner says, "What were you thinking about as you were working?" Next, the examiner asks the client, "Tell me about what you did." *After* the client has volunteered information about his drawing, he may be asked to further discuss some aspect of it about which the examiner is unclear. Be sure to record which comments were solicited and which were not.

Figure Drawing. The client is then told, "Turn the paper over and draw a person." If he protests about his inabilities, say, "This is not a test of how well you draw." If he asks if he should draw the whole person, or what kind of person, etc, he should be told that it is up to him. The examiner should not be more specific.

When the client indicates he has finished the task, he is again asked, "What were you thinking about as you were drawing?" Next, the examiner says, "Tell me about what you did." If the client offers little information in response to the non-directive questions, the examiner can become more directive (eg, "Tell me about the person you drew; make up a story about this person."); however, these responses should be clearly designated in the recording as solicited by direct questions.

Clay. The examiner places the clay in the cleared area in front of the client, and says, "Do something with the clay. The clay tools and water are available."

When the client indicates that he is finished, he is asked, "What were you thinking about as you were working?" The examiner then asks him, "Tell me about what you did."

Comparison of productions. After completing and discussing all the tasks, the client is asked, "Look at all your productions. Do you see any similarities in what you did? In the way you worked? "He is then asked, "Which did you like the most? Why? The least? Why?"

Problems with Administration

The trend towards briefer periods for psychiatric hospitalization and high client turnover presents realistic time problems for the therapist in providing necessary assessment of client functioning. Goal-directed treatment based on the results of appropriate assessment of the client's level of ego functioning is essential to the practice of psychiatric occupational therapy. In settings where clients remain for only brief periods, the occupational therapy assessment of ego functioning is especially important in the diagnostic process and in after-care planning, including recommendations for outpatient treatment, day care settings, and/or community support systems. Evaluation must be seen as a vital part of the psychiatric occupational therapy program and as such, should be allotted adequate time so that ideally, all clients can be seen for evaluation. In settings where turnover is great, the occupational therapist should be involved in determining criteria for client referral to occupational therapy, and the service to be provided. In some cases, the provision of assessment only is indicated. The use of group assessment techniques, when appropriate, is helpful in maximizing the use of limited time; however, individual assessments for greater depth of evaluation should still be used when indicated.

Evaluator versus therapist? The right to evaluate. The need of some therapists to be supportive and/or an agent of change may confuse the purpose of evaluation with that of treatment. When administering the evaluation, the therapist's role is to observe and record, not to intervene and treat. Although the therapist may feel discomfort in the role of the non-directive examiner, as Gillette emphasizes, the process of assessment must be seen as integral to the concept of the professional occupational therapist, not as an intrusion into the client's privacy.[41]

On being non-directive. Consistency in the examiner's affect, and wording of directions and responses are essential for standardization of test administration and results. Variables must be kept to a minimum so as not to influence the client's responses. The therapist's anxiety may translate into the need to respond more directly to the client's questions and concerns. While directions may be repeated and encouragement offered, the protocol should be followed to avoid projection of the examiner's anxiety onto the client. It is also important that the examiner not interfere during the production phase. The examiner can, however, ask questions regarding any unusual response during the association phase.

Indications for direct intervention. Professional judgment must still be used in the framework of the non-directive approach. A determination of when to intervene requires assessment of the degree to which the client is capable of controlling his responses to the testing situation. Issues such as fear of exposure, sexual stimulation, or loss of ego-boundaries may cause increasing anxiety and agitation, with the potential for loss of impulse control or immobilization. In such cases, direct intervention, such as verbal reassurance, moving to the next task, or stopping the evaluation, may be necessary. Rescheduling of the evaluation may be indicated.

Marsha Goodman Evaskus

Direct intervention in the form of time limits may be needed for the compulsive individual taking excessive time for task completion. Verbal limits and directions to focus on the task may be necessary with the client who tries to engage the examiner in discussions not directly related to the test process, or who tries to reverse the role of client and examiner.

Taking notes. Accurate recording of responses to the evaluation battery is vital to correct interpretation of test results. Most clients accept this need, and note-taking is not usually an issue. In some cases, however, the suspicious client may make frequent glances towards the examiner, hide his work from view, and/or may ask to see what is written. The client may be told that the results of the evaluation can be discussed with him at a later time. If refusal to participate occurs, the examiner should be aware of the issues of power and control raised, and assess whether to continue with the evaluation.

Refusal. The client may refuse all or some tasks in the battery. This refusal in itself is an important response and should be recorded. If possible, the reason for the refusal should be ascertained and the client encouraged to participate. If he persists in his refusal, move to the next task. If indicated, the evaluation can be rescheduled if the client refuses the entire battery.

Knowing when the client is finished. The examiner should not influence the client's time of completion by asking prematurely if he is finished. Generally, the client will indicate his completion of the task through verbal or non-verbal means. Typical responses include stating he is finished, saying, "There," putting the pencil down and looking at the examiner, just stopping and staring, or pushing the project away. If the examiner is not certain that the client has completed the task, he may then ask for verbal confirmation.

Sharing information with the client. The examiner should exercise good judgment, and use discretion in selecting material for discussion with the client. Test material should be presented at a level useful to the client, and in keeping with the treatment approach.

Response of drawing a person for the spontaneous drawing task. Even if the client draws a person in response to the spontaneous drawing task, the figure drawing task should still be administered.

Test materials. Although the test materials are standardized, a premade kit is not currently available, allowing for possible human error in the assembly of materials.

Behaviors Assessed

The client's responses to each task, as observed in the approach, process utilized, end-product achieved, comments, and associations, are assessed for level of ego-functioning, expression of needs and defenses, and repeated behavioral patterns. The following *Outline for Analysis of the Goodman Battery* is provided as a framework or guide for the observation and interpretation of responses to each task. As the functions assessed are interrelated, the items listed in the outline may overlap. Following the outline, the discussion of each task further clarifies the interpretation process. Four rating scales have been developed, placing the responses to the Goodman Battery into continuums of function (Appendixes H, I, J, K). Because further refinement of the scales is needed, they are presented and discussed in *Suggestions for Research,* pp 121-123.

This interpretation of responses to the Goodman Battery is based on findings from the literature, and empirically derived clinical evidence. The reader is advised that additional variations in response may be seen, and the meaning of the responses are not fixed and inflexible.

Outline for Analysis of the Goodman Battery

A. General Considerations

    1. Approach to task and to examiner—some descriptive terms:

      a) cooperative

      b) guarded

      c) suspicious

      d) talkative

      e) silent

      f) compliant

      g) self-depreciatory

      h) grandiose

      i) hostile

      j) seductive

      k) confused

      l) attentive

      m) distractible

      n) hesitant

      o) impulsive

      p) indecisive

      q) methodical

      r) rigid

    2. Length of time to complete each task and total evaluation:

      a) slow

      b) appropriate

      c) fast

    3. Response to structured vs. non-structured media:

      a) level of functioning

      b) preference

B. Mosaic Tile Task

    1. Level of organization

      a) sorting and selection procedure

      b) sequence of tile placement

      c) application of glue

      d) work space

    2. Level of concept formation

      a) ability to reproduce pattern

      b) complete or incomplete

Marsha Goodman Evaskus

3. Ability to perceive size and space relationships

4. Problem solving ability

a) flexibility in making changes

b) ability to recognize errors

c) ability to follow through and complete

5. Level of impulse control and frustration tolerance—ability to delay gratification

6. Independency-dependency needs: response to authority

7. Ability for abstract thinking

C. Spontaneous Drawing and Figure Drawing Tasks (process analysis)

1. Level of organization

a) latency period

b) sequence followed in drawing details

c) complexity—amount of detail included

2. Size and space relationships

3. Graphics—types of lines used

a) pressure—faint, heavy

b) continuity—sketchy, broken, flowing, jagged

4. Differential treatments

a) omissions, distortions, erasures

b) reinforcements, excessive shading

c) overworking of a particular detail

5. Verbalizations and associations

a) appropriate, related, or loose, unrelated to content

b) amount—excessive, appropriate, or minimal

D. Spontaneous Drawing Task (content/end-product analysis)

1. Level of concept formation—integrity of completed whole

a) related theme vs. unrelated objects

b) complete or incomplete

2. Nature of content

a) realistic vs. symbolic

b) animate vs. inanimate

c) comprehensible vs. idiosyncratic

3. Relatedness of content and form—reality testing

a) size and space relationships

b) presence of bizarre relationships, idiosyncratic symbolism, schematic or stylized drawings

4. Feeling tone and attitudes conveyed through content and associations

a) empty, happy, sad, controlled

b) inner drives, needs and responses—view of world, others, his role in it

E. Figure Drawing Task (content/end-product analysis)

1. Level of concept formation
   a) complete or incomplete
   b) details related to whole
   c) amount of differentiation
2. Strength and integrity of ego boundaries—note graphics
3. Identity issues
   a) same or opposite sex
   b) self or other drawing
   c) body image
4. Amount of differentiation
   a) organization—primitive or sophisticated, (eg, stick figure or more complex)
   b) amount of detail—sexually differentiated, clothing, etc
   c) cartoon, stereotype, etc
5. Feeling tone
   a) facial expression
   b) perspective—full face, profile, rear view
   c) stance and degree of movement—rigid, relaxed, action-oriented
6. Relatedness of content and form—reality testing
   a) presence of bizarre relationships (eg, three eyes, disconnected parts)
   b) transparency (eg, internal organs drawn)
   c) labeling
   d) idiosyncratic symbolism, stylized drawing
   e) mechanical-looking figure
7. Associations
   a) information regarding self concept, interpersonal relationships
   b) self-esteem: degree of satisfaction with self

F. Clay Task

1. Level of organization and concept formation
   a) latency period
   b) process vs. end-product orientation
   c) working from whole or building up form from parts of clay
   d) ability to achieve integrated end-product
   e) level of object representation achieved
      1) primitive vs. complex form
      2) abstract, realistic, or symbolic content
2. Level of impulse control and strength of ego boundaries—presence of

aggressive and/or regressive responses
   a) nature of contact with media
      1) use of hands and/or tools
      2) smoothing, stroking, patting, etc
      3) cutting, pounding, jabbing, etc
   b) degree of involvement in process
   c) ability to control media
      1) degree of suggestibility
      2) presence of compulsive defenses
   d) number of changes made
      1) destructive or constructive
      2) issue of permanency
3. Associations—related, appropriate

Discussion of Mosiac Tile Task

The client is presented with the task of reproducing a specific mosaic tile design (Fig 7.2B). To do so, the client must select, sort, and arrange the mosaic tiles into the particular design configuration—the conceptualized whole.[8] This sorting and

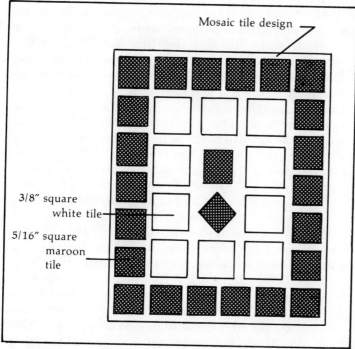

Mosaic tile design

3/8" square
white tile

5/16" square
maroon
tile

Fig 7.2B: Detail of the Mosaic tile design used in the Battery.

selection process requires the abilities of concept formation, organization, and perception of color, size, and space relationships. The ability to cope with multiple stimuli, to exert control, and not be overwhelmed during this process is assessed.[41]

Is the client able to see the relationship between the parts and the whole? Are the correct color and size tiles readily perceived and selected? Use of incorrect size tiles

The Goodman Battery

will affect the spacing. If this occurs, is the client able to identify the source of the problem and make corrections? Asking the client to compare his product to the tile model regarding similarities and differences is important in differentiating between perceptual problems and other causes. For example, if the client is able to identify differences but states, "My design is better," or "I wanted it different so that I could tell which one was mine," the presence of issues of defiance of authority or the need to include differences to maintain individuality and boundaries could be indicated. In some cases, variations could be the result of low energy level, poor frustration tolerance, or a passive-aggressive response. If colors and/or sizes of the tiles are mixed, reversed from the design, or if the center diamond shape tile is not included and the client is not able to point out or correct these differences, problems in perceptual functioning should be suspected. More extensive assessment of perceptual functioning may then be conducted at a future time.

How does the client approach and organize the process of getting the tiles out of the cans? Responses range from pouring all the tiles out at once—an impulsive, less controlled approach, to peering into the can to pick tiles out one at a time—a more cautious, guarded and/or compulsive approach. Does the client check the contents of both cans, or limit himself to just one, demonstrating a restricted, rigid approach? In the sorting of numbers of tiles needed, does the client sort all of the indicated size and color without regard to the correct number needed, possibly indicating loss of the purpose of the selection process to produce a particular design? Or, are time-consuming methods of organization utilized to maintain order and the concept of the whole, such as constant checking and counting of tiles in the sample and in his production? Lack of control and organization is also indicated if the work space becomes cluttered, with different size tiles becoming mixed together, tiles being left out and not returned to the proper cans, and in some cases, tiles being spilled onto the floor. Such responses may also be an expression of hostile feelings towards the examiner or the test situation.

Observation of the placement of the tiles shows the interrelatedness of the conceptual and organizational functions. The ability to perceive the total configuration, or Gestalt, to see the relationship of the parts to the whole, and then to follow an organized sequence in placing the tiles, is demonstrated. Fragmentation occurs when the Gestalt is seen as a number of separate entities, rather than as an integrated, related whole.[16] The tile design consists of two concentric rectangles composed of an outer border of small maroon tiles and an inner border of larger white tiles, with a center column of one diamond-shaped tile placed below one square-shaped tile. The most common sequence followed in placing the tiles is completion of the outer border first, proceeding inward to complete the pattern of concentric rectangles, followed by placement of the center tiles (Fig. 7.3A). Each row is usually completed before the next row is started. Other responses may be seen, with implications regarding the ability to perceive the Gestalt and organize actions. The client may not place the tiles according to the configuration of rectangles, but may attempt to place the tiles horizontally, by rows (Fig. 7.3B), and in so doing, cut across the visual pattern. Or, an approach may be used in which the tiles are placed segmentally, with no clear sequential order, new rows being started before completion of previous rows (Fig. 7.3C). In both responses, tiles may be placed in related segments, but the pattern of the whole is broken up in the sequence of placement followed. Such segmental, or fragmented placement may indicate problems in the ability to perceive or maintain a concept of the whole, and/or difficulties in organization and planning skills. It is important to assess the

Marsha Goodman Evaskus

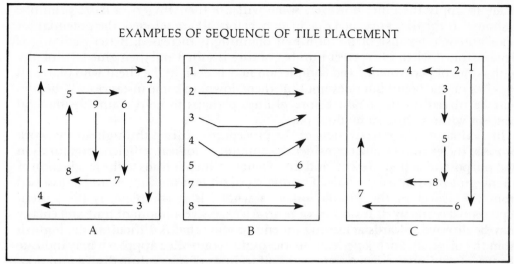

Fig 7.3A: Completion of the outer border first, proceeding inward to complete design. **B:** Placement of tiles horizontally, cutting across the design. **C:** Segmental placement. New rows started before completion of previous rows.

effect of the process utilized on the end-product achieved. A fragmented approach can result in a correct end-product, but at a greater expense of psychic energy and efficiency.

Disturbances in the ability to produce an integrated whole and an inability to respond to the boundaries of the task may be manifested in the stacking of tiles, placement of the tiles overlapping the margins of the wood base, or an incoherent placement of tiles, unrelated to the design configuration. At times, only a few tiles are placed, demonstrating an inability to complete the task. Perseveration, in which the client is unable to make shifts in tile selection to accommodate changes necessitated by the pattern, may be seen in some cases.

Throughout the process of sorting, selecting, placing, and gluing the tiles, problem solving skills must be utilized. The examiner should assess the client's ability to recognize what needs to be done in order to correctly accomplish the task. Is the client able to recognize errors within an appropriate amount of time and to make corrections, or does he feel helpless, unable to act, and give up? Is there externalization of problems encountered? For example, if the spacing is incorrect, does he claim that the wood base is a different size than the model, thereby causing the error? To what degree is the client able to be flexible? Can he formulate alternative plans of action, making necessary changes that lead to the most efficient functioning?

Problem solving and organizational skills are particularly demonstrated in the process of gluing the tiles. The glue is presented in a bowl instead of the regular applicator bottle to further necessitate the use of these skills. Does the client use an appropriate amount of glue and demonstrate an effective method of application? A variety of methods may be seen: 1) glue carefully applied to each tile in a methodical, at times compulsive, manner; 2) glue applied directly to the board, one row at a time, followed by placement of the tiles, a quicker, more efficient approach; or 3) glue applied over the entire board, a more primitive, impulsive approach, usually resulting in a messier end-product. Most clients utilize the available tongue blade to apply the glue; however, some will use their fingers, a more primitive response. If the tiles are glued one by one, before all are selected, the potential for poor outcome because of the minimal planning is increased. Better planning is demonstrated when the correct number of tiles is sorted and then glued. Difficulty with issues of permanency and completion may be seen in the client who places all the tiles on the board but does not glue them down. In some instances, all the tiles will be placed on the board before gluing, perhaps to help maintain the total concept while gluing individual parts.

In evaluating the effectiveness of the procedures utilized throughout the work process, the examiner must consider the amount of logical, efficient organization and purposeful action present, and the extent to which it leads to the production of an integrated, completed whole. The quality of the end-product should be assessed from the aspect of the production as a whole: is it complete, is the pattern represented correctly, is it sloppy, or neat? An excessive amount of time and energy may be directed towards achieving an end-product that is difficult to distinguish from the original. Such a perfectionistic, highly controlled approach may indicate the use of compulsive defenses to ward off feelings of impending disorganization. After completing the mosaic task, the client is asked to think of a use for the tile to assess the ability for abstract thinking. Can the client think flexibly about various uses for the tile? Common responses include coaster, hot plate, or wall decoration.

In addition to assessing cognitive processes, the examiner must assess the affective reactions which influence functioning. What is the feeling tone of the interaction between the client and the task, and between the client and the examiner? What is the level of frustration tolerance and impulse control demonstrated? Is the client able to deal with the limitations inherent in the task, eg, the directions to copy a specific design, the sorting procedure necessary to find the correct tiles, and the gluing process? The ability to delay gratification—to take the time necessary for adequate task completion—should be assessed. Responses to feelings of frustration may range from sighing, grimacing, and groaning, to internally directed declarations of inability or externally directed hostile comments regarding unfair expectations. The degree to which the level of frustration tolerance affects the ability to complete the task should be assessed.

The verbalizations and associations made by the client before, during, and after the work process provide information regarding self-concept and response to authority figures. Is the quality of the interaction with the examiner of a dependent or independent nature, and to what extent? Does the client rely greatly on the examiner, asking many questions, seeking clarification, or requesting help? Are the questions appropriate? Does he wait for directions or begin quickly on his own, conforming to the expectations given in the directions, or creating his own design? The client may seek permission to do the design differently, or there may be a more defiant quality to the response. Are comments regarding the work process and end-product of a self-depreciatory or grandiose nature? Are the client's expectations and perceptions regarding his performance realistic and accurate? In comparing his product to the model tile, is his perception of his capabilities and limitations realistic? Is there over-concern with "getting it right," or externalization of blame for any inabilities?

Therefore, the mosaic tile task allows for assessment of the client's ability to conceptualize a task, plan procedures, and carry the task through to completion. The presence of ego-strengths necessary for functional performance in a structured,

Marsha Goodman Evaskus

task-oriented setting is assessed. The opportunity to evaluate functioning within settings of lessening degrees of structure is present in the drawing and clay tasks of the Goodman Battery.

Discussion of the Spontaneous Drawing Task

In the spontaneous drawing task, the client is presented with a stimulus situation which can be organized and structured in a personally meaningful way. In analyzing the production, the examiner can "gain insight into that individual's private world of meanings, significances, patterns, and feelings."[8] The drawing should be assessed within the framework of the client's ability to conceptualize and organize the task, and the extent to which he is able to produce a comprehensible, related whole. The client's approach to the task, work process, content produced, and verbalizations reveal information regarding level of ego-functioning in response to a task with minimal structure. The verbalizations serve to clarify the meaning and intent of the drawing content, and as such, are an important part of the interpretation process.

The length of time before starting, or latency period, is indicative of the client's ability to organize his performance in a situation with minimal structure and limits. The examiner should note the number and intensity of questions asked during this initial period. Clients commonly ask if they can draw anything or say they cannot draw; however, when given reassurance that it is not a test of drawing ability and with the directions restated, most are able to begin the task. Anastasi and Foley have observed that "abnormals" have a longer latency period than "normals", and show a greater variability in delay.[29] The latency period should be considered in relation to the process utilized and content produced. For example, the client who begins immediately may be impulsive, revealing poor organization and minimal planning skills in the drawing produced, or may quickly and exactly execute a drawing that he has drawn before, thereby imposing a familiar, safe structure to the task. A long latency period could indicate feelings of inadequacy and/or lack of sufficient internal structure and organizational skills to respond to the minimal boundaries present in the task. Is the client asking for more direction and support through questions or non-verbal behavior? The client may appear immobilized by the task, with pencil poised but unable to proceed, or may refuse in an angry, defiant manner, perhaps in compensation for actual or feared inabilities.

The time taken to complete the drawing, and the amount of detail included as related to the energy expended should be considered. A total time of longer than ten or 15 minutes is excessive, and may be seen in cases of compulsive individuals who add excessive detail to the drawing. Minimal time spent and a paucity of details may be seen in clients with low energy levels, or may be indicative of impulsivity if drawn quickly.

The sequence followed in drawing the details is reflective of the client's level of organization and ability to see the relationship between the parts of the drawing and the whole. Is a logical, orderly sequence followed in completing the drawing, or does the client skip from one area or detail of the drawing to another before completing details previously started? Is one idea followed through to completion, or are frequent changes made in the content? The ability to present a related theme as opposed to unrelated objects, and the ability to relate the content and form in a comprehensible manner needs to be assessed. Fragmentation in organization and concept formation is also indicated by parts of the drawing left incomplete and frequent interruptions in the work process.

The use of size and space relationships in the drawing is reflective of feelings of adequacy in relation to the environment.[25,27] The size of the drawing in relation to the size of paper should be noted, eg, if very large, indicating feelings of expansiveness and impulsiveness, or if very small, indicating feelings of restriction or inadequacy. Lack of appropriate proportions within the drawing could be indicative of problems in reality testing or of areas of special significance to the client. Is the total space utilized, or just part? Where is the drawing on the page? Deviations from central placement should be noted. In considering proportions, size and use of space, extremes in presentation, and not minor variances, should be noted.

Areas in the drawing of special significance and/or conflict are indicated when differential treatment is given to that area.[24,25] The client may exhibit unusual concern and emphasis through excessive erasing, especially when the erasing does not produce improved form, by returning to re-work certain details, or by using an excessive amount of time in drawing the detail.[25] Shading and line reinforcement are seen as indicators of anxiety, differentiated from erasures which also show dissatisfaction. Any exaggerations, distortions, and omissions should be noted, indicating conflict related to the area so treated. A deviation from the logical sequence in presentation of details may also be indicative of areas of particular significance. Concerns may be verbalized directly or through refusal to comment on part or all of the drawing.

The graphics, or type of lines utilized in the drawing, have implications regarding the client's self-concept and manner of relating to the environment.[24-27] The pressure of the line, whether sketchy, faint, heavy, etc, and its continuity, whether jagged, flowing, broken, etc, should be noted. The reader is referred to the discussion of graphics on the figure drawing task, for further elaboration. If lines used in one detail of the drawing vary greatly, interpretation should be related to the content so depicted.

The content of the drawing and the method of presentation can reveal information regarding level of functioning, inner drives, and responses. The reader is referred to the work of Anastasi and Foley,[28,29] in which the researchers analyzed and compared the spontaneous drawings of normal and abnormal subjects, finding certain characteristics occurring more frequently in the drawings by abnormal subjects. Is the content realistic or symbolic, comprehensible or idiosyncratic, abstract or concrete, animate or inanimate? Is the content presented in a related, integrated manner? Anastasi and Foley found that fantastic, bizarre compositions and the presence of unrelated objects are indicative of the delusional, idiosyncratic, and disorganized behavior of the subject. Overly schematic or stylized drawings, and the use of stereotypes should be noted. The response of writing in place of drawing, the inclusion of irrelevant words or labelling of parts of the drawing, are also considered abnormal responses. If the client draws objects that are visible from the immediate environment, he may be indicating a need to seek structure from the environment, and/or a "stimulus-bound" response in which the drawing content is influenced by stimuli present in the environment.

The quantity and relevancy of the details presented should be noted. Responses may range from a scarcity of detail, producing a primitive, depersonalized, or empty quality, to over-elaboration and the need to fill in the total space. Problems in thought processes leading to simplistic drawings should be differentiated from problems of an affective nature, as in low energy levels seen in depression. Developmental studies by Goodenough, and Anastasi and Foley have shown that as

Marsha Goodman Evaskus

the individual matures, more accurate and extensive details are utilized in drawings.[25] Omission of essential details and the production of a simplistic, primitive drawing, could indicate interference in this development, or may be indicative of a guarded, evasive attitude.

Through choice of content, the graphics and form used, and verbal associations, the client conveys feelings and attitudes regarding his view of the environment, his role, and the role of others. The feeling tone may be expressive (eg, happy, sad, angry, passive), or the drawing may be non-revealing and guarded. Are the associations appropriate and related to the content and feeling tone of the drawing, or is there looseness of associations? Responses may be very simple and concrete, with the client merely describing the drawing, or he may relate aspects of the drawing to his own life, personalizing the content. Associations may become very elaborate and loosely related to the drawing content, indicating disorganization in thought processes. Or, the client may refuse to comment, in an attempt to keep thoughts and feelings hidden.

In order to correctly interpret the findings from the spontaneous drawing task, aspects of the task must be viewed as a totality: 1) process, including the approach, graphics, and differential treatments, 2) organization and integrity of the entire drawing, 3) content and feeling tone, and 4) verbal and non-verbal behavior. The examiner may then begin to assess the aspects of the inner world of the client revealed through his drawing.

Discussion of the Figure Drawing Task

The figure drawing task is more structured than the spontaneous drawing, in that the directions regarding content are specific, eg, to draw a person. The cognitive processes of organization, concept formation, ability to problem solve, and follow a task through to completion are again needed; however, the affective response to drawing the human body may interfere with the effective functioning of these processes. Excessive time taken before starting the drawing should be viewed as indicative of conflict. Buck reports a latency period of longer than 30 seconds as evidence of conflicting feelings. In some cases, the client may refuse to draw a person, indicating arousal of conscious associations, body image concerns, or difficulties in interpersonal relationships.[25] If the client does not respond to supportive encouragement from the examiner, associations to the task should still be solicited so as to better understand the reasons for refusal.

The ability to organize and to see the relationship of the parts to the whole is demonstrated in the sequence used to draw the parts of the body.[24-26] Is the sequence followed logical or fragmented? Machover emphasizes that illogical sequence can be indicative of disturbances in organization, or a scattering of thought processes.[24] According to Buck, the usual progression is from the head and features, to the neck, trunk, arms (with hands and fingers), legs, and feet (the order of drawing the arms and legs may be reversed).[25] Usually, one set of details is completed before others are started, eg, features of the face are completed at the same time, rather than drawing the eyes, then arms, then returning to add the nose, mouth, etc. Disturbances in organization and conceptualization are also indicated if details are drawn segmentally, without considering the relationship of the details to each other or to the finished whole. Once drawn, the drawing is not usually returned to. The examiner should note if much reworking or reinforcing of lines occurs. The relationship between the sequence followed and the organization of the end-product should be noted. Though the client may be able to present an organized whole, organizational difficulties may still be observed in the process.

The size of the figure, proportions within the whole, and the location of the drawing on the paper, reveal information regarding self-esteem and manner of relating to the environment.[24-27] Extremes in the size of the figure drawn should be noted. For example, is the drawing very large, possibly touching or cut off by the margins of the paper, or is the figure drawn very tiny? The larger figures are often drawn by expansive, aggressive individuals in response to an environment felt to be restrictive. Feelings of grandiosity and an egocentric view of the self in relationship to the environment may also be present. If the legs are cut off by the margins, however, feelings of immobility may exist. A tiny figure could indicate feelings of inadequacy and the tendency to withdraw from the environment, especially when the drawing is located low on the page. Unusual size relationships should be interpreted based on the meaning of the detail so represented. Extreme deviation from central placement and the relationship of the figure to the margins of the page should be noted and interpreted based on the literature.

The graphics, or type of lines used, have implications regarding ego-integrity, self-concept, and relationship to the environment.[24-27] Machover writes that "the pressure of the line, thickness, flow, constancy, direction, and length of strokes, yield judgments regarding: confidence, self-assertiveness, withdrawal, stability, and degree of conflict in a person."[24] The use of heavy outlines can be indicative of the need to contain and delineate ego boundaries, as in cases of depersonalization, where boundaries are weakened and there is confusion of body image with the environment. Unbroken, reinforced outlines may also indicate an attempt to maintain ego-integrity when dealing with external pressures. Buck found that heavy lines used throughout the drawing may be indicative of organicity. In the literature, faint lines are seen to indicate low energy level, feelings of inadequacy, and indecision. Broken, indecisive, or frequently reinforced lines may indicate insecurity and anxiety, while decisive, well-controlled, free-flowing lines are viewed as indicative of good adjustment.[25] The level of impulsivity can be reflected in the length of strokes utilized, eg, short strokes viewed as impulsive, longer strokes more controlled. The presence of jagged lines could indicate hostile feelings.

As discussed in the previous section on the spontaneous drawing task, differential treatments may be given to areas of the drawing representing conflict or concern to the client. Distortions, omissions, or exaggerations, and the presence of excessive erasure, shading, and re-working should be noted and related to the meaning of the details so treated.[25,27] According to Buck, the details included in the figure drawn can be interpreted based on type (relevant, irrelevant, or bizarre), and quantity (excessive or minimal).[25] However, the importance of considering the total configuration when making an interpretation is also emphasized in the literature.[25,27,42] No one sign or detail should be taken by itself, as the meaning of that sign may vary. Specific details need to be understood in relation to the whole. The validity of the interpretation is found to increase as the "number of indications for the same personality feature increases."[42]

The integrity of the whole, the feeling tone and attitudes conveyed, and the capacity for reality testing revealed should be considered. Buck defines concept formation as the "organization and quality of the completed whole."[25] Of primary consideration is the completeness of the figure drawn, especially as related to the presence or absence of relevant details such as the essential body parts. The amount of differentiation present in the figure drawn should be assessed. Is the drawing primitive, a stick figure, or a simple outline with no details, or is it more complex and differentiated, including facial expression, well-integrated body parts, and clothing? Is the sexuality of the drawn figure indicated appropriately or is it exaggerated or hidden? Usually, the figure drawn is the same sex as that of the client. Opposite-sex drawings may be indicative of sexual confusion or identity conflicts. The drawing of clowns, cartoons, or silly-looking figures can be expressive of feelings of contempt and hostility.[27] The figure drawn may represent a projection of the client's self-concept, ideal self-image, or attitudes toward someone else in the environment. Levy concludes that the figure drawn may be a combination of these and other environmental factors.[27]

Most figures drawn are clothed. A complete lack of clothing may indicate feelings of helplessness and exhibitionism if in a self-drawing, or the desire to degrade another person, if in a drawing of another person.[25] The relationship between the age, sex, dress, etc, of the figure drawn to that of the client, as well as verbal comments and associations to the drawing may reveal information regarding the client's needs and aspirations.

The attitude, or feeling tone of the drawn figure is conveyed through the facial expression, stance, degree of movement, and size of the figure. Does the facial expression convey a particular emotion, eg, happiness, sadness, anger, fear, or does it have an unexpressive, empty quality? Does the figure drawn convey a feeling of strength or does it appear weak and ineffectual? The stance of the body, the position of the arms and legs, and the size of the figure combine to project a postural tone. The rigidity or flexibility of the figure, and the content of any actions portrayed should be noted. The perspective presented, whether full-face, profile, or rear view, will convey either an open, guarded, or hidden attitude.

Indications of poor reality testing and thought disorder as discussed in the previous section on the spontaneous drawing task, may also be present in the drawing of a person. As discussed in the literature, [25,42,43] such indications include the loss of perspective, bizarre representations (eg, three eyes, disconnected body parts), transparencies (especially if internal organs are depicted) and labeling. The presence of highly personalized, idiosyncratic symbolism, excessive symmetry, mechanical-looking figures, and empty, depersonalized drawings should also be noted.

The client's ability to communicate effectively and appropriately through verbalizations should be assessed. Are the associations related to the drawing content, or are the associations loose and inappropriate? Are the comments made excessive or minimal, open or guarded? Level of self-esteem may be expressed through comments of a self-depreciatory or grandiose nature, and should be considered together with such indicators as graphics, size, and placement.

Therefore, in the figure drawing task, an assessment is made of the client's level of organization and concept formation, self-concept, view of others, and reality testing ability. Needs, conflicts, and defenses are revealed through the analysis of the work process, content, and verbalizations.

Discussion of the Clay Task

When asked to "Do something with the clay," the client is presented with the task of imposing a structure or form upon a substance that is highly amorphous, plastic, and unstructured.[8] The ability to conceptualize a form and set limits regarding the work, so as to achieve a controllable end-product is needed.[41] Through observation of the approach to the task, work process, and the configuration produced, the ability to organize and cope with the changeability of the clay medium is revealed.

A variety of responses may be seen in the client's approach to the task, ranging from starting immediately without hesitation, to refusal to touch the clay. The amount of hesitation present may reflect the ability to organize and plan procedures in reaction to the minimal limits inherent in the task. The client who touches the clay tenuously, or refuses to touch it, unable to proceed, may be indicating a fear of lack of structure and the potential for loss of control. The client who begins immediately may be reflecting impulsivity in his approach or, in some cases, comfort or familiarity in dealing with the clay medium. Though the ego skills necessary to conceptualize the task may be present, the ability to follow through and complete the task will be affected by the client's level of impulse control, frustration tolerance, and strength of ego-boundaries.

During the process of working with clay, the use of available materials provides information regarding level of organization, needs, and defenses. What amount of the clay provided is utilized in the production? Usually, all the clay is used. The use of only a small portion could indicate low energy level, or a timid, less aggressive approach. The relationship between the amount of clay used and the end-product achieved may also be observed in terms of organization and planning skills. Can the client work within the limits of the amount of clay provided, or does he attempt a project that requires more clay? Is the client able to adjust the size of his product in accordance with the clay available, demonstrating good reality testing skills?

To what extent and purpose does the client utilize the available tools, and to what degree is the use of tools combined with the use of hands?[34] Is the client vigorous or tentative in his approach? Does he use one or two hands? Are aggressive actions such as cutting, stabbing, or pounding present, and to what extent, or is there more smoothing, and patting of the clay? The manner of handling the clay provides information regarding level of impulse control, the presence of aggressive feelings, and dependency needs. The use of tools only may demonstrate the desire to avoid contact with a messy substance, an attempt to control the medium, or the presence of compulsive defenses. The use of hands only may reflect a more primitive, simplistic response; however, the client may enjoy the tactile experience of the clay, and demonstrate the ability to utilize his hands effectively. The combined use of hands and tools to effectively achieve the desired end-product may reflect a higher level of organizational and problem solving skills.

The ability to conceptualize the relationship of the whole and its parts is reflected in the method of working with the clay. The client may work with the total ball of clay, developing details from the whole, or he may take parts of the clay, develop these parts, and then put them together to form a whole. Is the client able to achieve an integrated whole with the method used, or is there fragmentation and the loss of the idea and intent? For example, a breakdown or fragmentation in purpose occurring in working with the total ball of clay would be reflected in the client who appears to lose himself in the clay, unable to proceed, either through immobilization or becoming over-involved in the process. Fragmentation of thought processes may also be demonstrated by the client who takes parts of the total ball of clay, begins to work with them but is unable to form a meaningful whole, instead, leaving the parts undeveloped and unrelated.

The ability to proceed towards a completed whole, to organize and maintain intent, may be interfered with by the arousal of infantile dependency needs as the client works with the clay. There may be an attempt to gratify these needs through excessive handling of the clay. Over-involvement in the process, with much time spent smoothing, wetting, and reworking the clay, without proceeding, could indicate a primitive involvement representative of early anal-dependent needs.

The client's level of impulse control and strength of ego boundaries is reflected in the ability to cope with the clay medium. The plastic properties of the clay permit change, presenting difficulty for either a too rigid or too loose ego structure. The ability to set boundaries and impose limits so as to maintain intent and the production of a meaningful whole may be interfered with in the highly suggestible client who is easily influenced by the changing form of the clay media. Compulsive defenses may be used as a means of imposing structure and control. The ability to be flexible is demonstrated if the changeability of the clay is dealt with comfortably and appropriately. The client's verbalizations further clarify reactions to working with the clay. The number and quality of changes made should be noted. Are the changes of a constructive or destructive nature? A pattern of destroying and rebuilding may reflect dissatisfaction and low self-esteem, hostility, or problems with issues of permanency, especially if all productions are destroyed.

The end-product should be assessed on the basis of complexity of form and the content represented. Is the level of organization simple or complex? What is the level of form representation achieved? Using a developmental frame of reference, implications for assessing the level of functioning of the client can be seen. In the literature,[35,37-40] a progression is described in the development of object representation, from a tactile, process orientation to experimentation with taking apart and putting together, leading to the formation of coils and balls, and the first objects: balls, pancakes, snakes, columns, snowmen, etc. What form does the client achieve? Is it a two-dimensional graphic representation (eg, separate parts laid out on the table as though "drawing" with clay) or is the object three-dimensional? Is the form produced realistic or abstract? What is the nature of any symbolic content present? Are the associations related to the content produced?

In summary, the client's ability to conceptualize and organize unstructured media, his needs and defenses, can be observed. The level of impulse control and strength of ego boundaries become apparent through the attempts to cope with the frustrations inherent in working with so changeable a form as clay.

Case Presentations

The following three cases illustrate a variety of test responses, and the process of analyzing Goodman Battery results. Names have been changed to maintain confidentiality.

Case 1

Joe was a 16 year old male, the second oldest of four children. He was tall, muscular, and older looking than his actual age. His behavior was verbal and arrogant.

Clinical Summary

Reason for Admission. Joe was admitted for a one month diagnostic evaluation, after not responding to one year of outpatient psychotherapy. His symptoms included withdrawal and depression, day-night reversal, increased drug usage, truancy, and acting out behavior.

History. He was described by his parents as having been an outgoing child, with many friends. No problems were reported until the age of 13, when Joe began dating an 11 year old girl. He was possessive and physically abusive of his girlfriend. After having a miscarriage, the girlfriend terminated the two year relationship. Joe became depressed and severely withdrawn, sleeping during the day and listening to music in the dark all night. Behavior also included truancy from school, increased drug use, involvement in group delinquent activities, and an inability to get along with his family. Paranoid ideation and hallucinations were noted under the influence of drugs. Joe did not respond to outpatient treatment.

His parents had been married for 18 years, and were reported to disagree over childrearing practices.

Diagnosis. Joe's diagnosis was borderline schizophrenia, with hallucinogen drug dependency.

Goodman Battery Results

Joe approached the evaluation in a compliant manner. He worked quickly on each task, taking only 40 minutes for the entire battery.

Mosaic tile. The process phase took 12 minutes and the association phase took eight minutes (Fig. 7.4). Joe was able to reproduce the pattern using the correct number of tiles, but with some inaccuracy in spacing and color choice. He pointed out the differences, externalizing the cause by blaming the materials (eg, "a different size wood" base was the cause of the inaccurate spacing). His initial response to the instructions to copy the tile was uncommon and concrete, in that he started to draw the tile design on paper. The task was understood only after the directions were reworded several times. His use of the drawing materials could indicate difficulty in screening out stimuli.

Joe asked questions to clarify the need to use the same color tiles and sought permission to pour the tiles out. He worked quickly, using a trial-and-error method of problem solving, his work process indicating low frustration tolerance and impulsivity. Glue was applied over the entire board to "do it faster". After placing

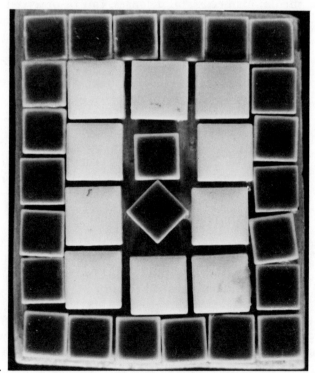

Fig 7.4: Case 1; mosaic tile.

the outer border of small tiles, Joe continued to search the pile of small tiles before finally checking the contents of the other can for the larger tiles. The large size tiles were then poured on top of the small tiles—a disorganized and/or hostile response. Joe was grandiose during the process of returning the tiles to the cans, stating he could resort the tiles because he could remember where he put them; instead, he proceeded to return handfuls of tiles mixed in size. His associations to the task were depreciatory and hostile, eg, "a garbage can can hold it". Though complying with the directions to copy the design, Joe continued to comment that a design using colors of his choice would be nicer. His uses for the tile were to: put it on the wall, use it as a demonstration piece, or show it to little kids "because big kids wouldn't be interested".

Spontaneous drawing. This task had a four minute process, with a six minute association (Fig. 7.5). Seeking clarification and permission, Joe asked if he could draw or write, and proceeded to request a ruler. When told to use the available materials, he used the edge of a clay tool to draw lines, thereby adding structure and greater control to the task. His drawing was personalized and symbolic in content, consisting of a band of closely drawn, heavy, dark lines with a triangular design in

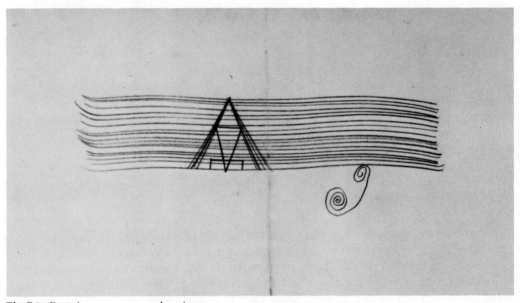

Fig 7.5: Case 1; spontaneous drawing.

the center, and a scroll-like sign below. Associations to the drawing were personalized, loose, and difficult to follow. Joe talked about the lines being "life-lines, roads to travel. . .how things look (all in rows) when you're tripping. . .the peak is when everything pulls together. . .then can come apart in pieces." He talked about finding a "heart in the road"—some caring along the way. His speech was rapid and difficult to interrupt. The association phase finally had to be terminated by the examiner.

Figure drawing. This task had a three minute process, with a four minute association (Fig. 7.6). When directed to draw a person, Joe asked, "Regular, or in my mind?" Initially, he drew the head only, stating that if he drew the body it would

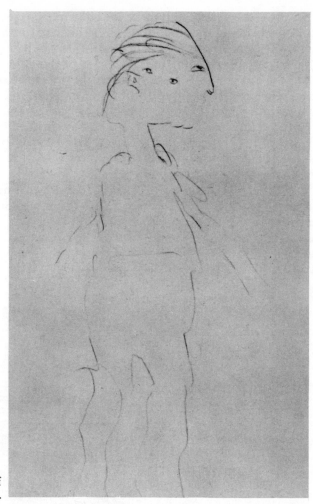

Fig 7.6: Case 1; detail of figure drawing.

"turn out like an animal; a person is an animal." He attempted to complete the figure after being requested to try. Sketchy, broken, faint lines were used to draw the figure, with the head in profile, body in front view. The figure was incomplete and distorted, eg, one arm, no hands or feet, mouth barely visible, and three eyes, with the figure seemingly facing in two directions at one time.

Associations were again rambling. Joe asked, "Ever think someone has eyes in the back of the head—looking at you—can have powers?" and proceeded to talk about an older friend who had powers. He described the person drawn as "paranoid with a messed up physique—you can blame me for that, I created him—long neck, no feet or hands, hair going back." In both the drawing and the associations, there is the representation of an ineffectual, non-communicating individual with weak ego boundaries, distorted and depreciatory self-concept, and paranoid features.

Clay. This task took four minutes (no photograph). In response to the clay task, Joe became increasingly testing toward the examiner, negative, and sarcastic. His comments while working included: "Does it have to be appropriate? Do I have to wet it? I don't want to. There, a ball—done. Not too creative—okay, an ashtray. No? A flower." The productions were primitive; Joe quickly changed and destroyed each, stating. "I can't get invested, make something good, unless I am going to glaze it."

Comparisons. Joe preferred the tile task because "[I] didn't have to get involved— you told me what to do." He liked the clay least: "It didn't seem to fit in right now."

Summary. Joe functioned best within the structure of the tile task; he was able to conceptualize and reproduce the pattern, though initially, he interpreted the directions concretely. His work process was characterized by low frustration tolerance and impulsivity, with the use of a trial-and-error method of problem solving, and a disorganized approach. Though complying with directions, Joe tested limits, and was often hostile in his responses. Weak ego boundaries and a lessening of control were demonstrated in his response to the less structured media, with productions personalized and symbolic, associations loose and rambling. Responses to the clay were primitive and destructive. Joe appeared to have an unrealistic view of his capabilities, with a fluctuating self-esteem, alternatingly grandiose and self-depreciatory.

Case 2

Robert was a 16 year old male, fifth in a sibship of nine; he looked his stated age. His appearance was rigid, with a flat affectless smile.

Clinical Summary

Reason for Admission. Robert displayed acute deterioration, precipitated by a beating received from a gang of youths six weeks prior to his admission. Changes in behavior were noted by his mother: he was bothered by noises at home, he developed rolling motions of the eyes, sleep disturbances and nightmares, and he complained of headaches and seeing things.

History. Robert was described by his mother as kind-hearted and good, and close to her; he was a loner who liked to read, draw, and work puzzles. School difficulties were first noted in third grade, and IQ testing revealed a below average intelligence (IQ 70). Robert's parents had divorced prior to his birth, and his mother remarried when he was four. His mother was reported to be inconsistent and unavailable. Two years prior to admission, Robert's stepfather left home. Robert responded with increased truancy, fist fights, and threatening behavior. He exhibited bizarre behavior, hallucinations, uncontrolled laughter, and wandering off from home. There was a drop in his grades one year before admission. One month prior to admission, his mother disappeared, and all the children were placed in protective custody.

Chief Defenses. These were denial and projection.

Diagnosis. Childhood schizophrenia.

Goodman Battery Results

Initially, Robert refused the evaluation, stating he could not work with clay, then finally agreed to do what he could.

Mosaic tile. The process phase took 20 minutes, and the association phase took 4 minutes (Fig. 7.7). Robert did not complete the task, gluing only one partial row of tiles. Much time was spent sorting the tiles, yawning often, using slow movements, and stilted speech. Rigidity was demonstrated in the selection of tiles: for the first five minutes, Robert used only one hand and one container, leaving the tiles in the can while sorting. He was aware of size differences, but sorted more white tiles than needed. Poor organization and planning ability

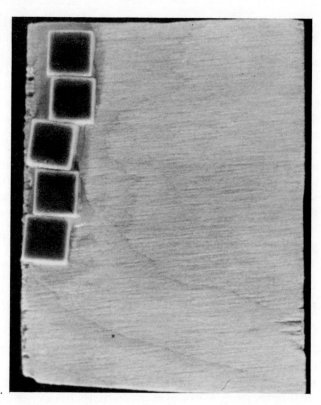

Fig 7.7: Case 2; mosaic tile.

were indicated, as Robert first piled all the selected tiles on top of the wood base. He then poured them off and began to place them. Robert expressed difficulty with the task, stating, "[I] can't do it. . .finding all the tiles is hard." After sorting tiles for 13 minutes, he asked permission to glue, but had difficulty devising a method for applying the glue. Robert externalized his difficulty with the glue process and sought a means for greater control, protesting that a paintbrush had been used to apply glue on the tile model, and that he needed a paintbrush, too. After direct suggestions from the examiner, he proceeded with difficulty and continued negativism. Robert's frustration tolerance and energy level were low, and he was unable to follow through and complete the task. Problems in concept formation and problem solving ability were also present. "See—I'm messing it up—[It's] not turning out right. I tried, but can't do it." Associations were self-depreciatory, regarding his inability and the difficulty of the task. He stated the tile could be used as "a souvenir of decoration. It was made by someone else."

Spontaneous drawing. This task had a nine minute process, and a 30 second association (Fig. 7.8). Robert again yawned a great deal, hesitated, unsure of what to draw, and sought suggestions from the examiner. He proceeded to draw a box with squares, attempting to draw the tile model, but unable to accurately reproduce the design configuration. Robert appeared to be highly suggestible and concrete in his attempt to structure the task by copying the mosaic design. Coordination was poor in both the drawing and erasing, adding to the difficulty in correcting drawing errors. He stopped before completing the drawing, stating, "I did that thing." His suggestibility was demonstrated as he continued to draw again after being asked if he was sure he was finished. Robert stopped again, saying he could not

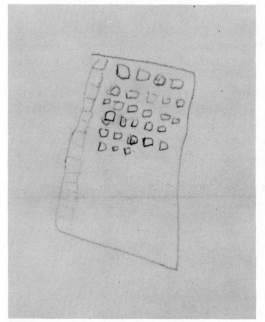

Fig 7.8: Case 2; spontaneous drawing.   **Fig 7.9:** Case 2; figure drawing.

finish; "[I] don't know how to do it—hard to draw squares—[I'm] drawing too many squares." Though he was able to recognize the error, he made no attempt to correct it.

Figure Drawing: This part had a one minute process, and a four minute association (Fig. 7.9). After briefly hesitating and again yawning, Robert drew a primitive, one line outline of, "a man", stating concretely that he was, "thinking of how a man would look on paper." The form representation was poor, incomplete, and had few details; the arms were ineffectual and stump-like, with no hands. The only differentiating details (the simplistic cap and gym shoes indicated by circles at ankle area) were added during the association phase when Robert described the figure as, "a baseball figure...a great baseball player." In describing his favorite baseball player, Robert showed some positive affect and enthusiasm.

Clay. Robert refused the task, stating he "never touched clay before."

Comparisons. Robert liked the tile task best. When asked which he liked least, he responded, "the drawing—I like it. But the tile more."

Summary. Low energy level, poor frustration tolerance, and negativism characterized Robert's approach throughout the evaluation, affecting his level of functioning on all tasks. The productions are all primitive, incomplete, and impoverished, indicating a low level of organization and concept formation. Robert's problem solving ability was poor; his actions were rigid and slow, his speech stilted. Robert's associations and comments were negativistic, focusing on his inability, and the perceived difficulty of the tasks. He functioned at a low level with both the structured and less structured tasks, refusing the clay task completely.

Case 3

Peter was a 15 year old male, petite for his age. He was neatly dressed, soft spoken, with rigid posture and a flat affect.

Clinical Summary

Reason for Admission. Peter was unable to sleep for several days. His symptoms included believing the devil was after him, sleeping on the floor of his mother's room because of fear of his own room, intense anxiety, withdrawal, and preoccupation with evil and death.

History. Peter was described as withdrawn, passive, friendless, anxious, and seldom outdoors. He was interested in activities appropriate for younger children. Peter often complained of headaches and dizziness. He had many phobias, including cats, tornados, and being attacked. His parents divorced when he was four years old, and he has not seen his father since. He was described as having a symbiotic relationship with his mother.

Chief Defenses. These were denial, depression, rationalization, and projection.

Diagnosis. Schizoid personality with obsessive features.

Goodman Battery Results

Peter worked slowly, approaching the evaluation in a willing, though controlled, manner.

Mosaic tile. The process phase was 35 minutes, with five minutes for association (Fig. 7.10). Peter worked in a highly controlled, slow, silent manner, and was able to correctly reproduce the mosaic pattern. However, the process utilized indicated possible difficulty in organization skills and concept formation. He worked

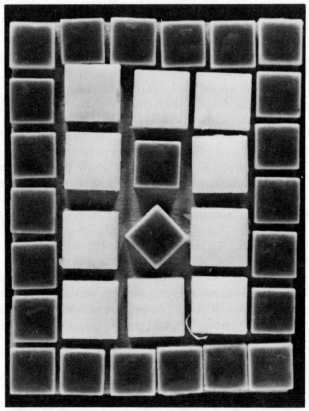

Fig 7.10: Case 3; mosaic tile.

Marsha Goodman Evaskus

without planning ahead, gluing tiles as he found them. He followed a fragmented sequence in placing the tiles, working in several directions at one time, and completing the rows in segments (Fig. 7.3C). The sequence may also represent a compulsive need to establish or set boundaries of the total pattern at the same time in order to maintain the structure. His placement of tiles from right to left was an unusual response.

Though appearing to methodically search for tiles, Peter actually utilized no efficient method for sorting through the pile. He pushed tiles around but did not turn any over to check for color, selecting only from the tiles that were already facing color side up. Except for muttering under his breath when he fumbled and spilled some tiles, and occasionally smiling to himself, Peter maintained a controlled exterior. When many tiles dropped on the floor during clean-up, he smiled and asked if he should pick them up.

During the association phase, Peter said he was thinking about whether his tile product "would be the same or different—exact?" He pointed out the crooked rows on his product, but reflected positive feelings for its use: "hang it up to look pretty, or put it on your shelf."

Spontaneous drawing. This part of the task had a three minute process, and a four minute association (Fig. 7.11). After questioning what he should draw, Peter said, "I'll just draw the face—I don't know how to draw." He then quickly drew a profile using light lines, smiling as he worked. He drew a witch, aggressive in tone, as conveyed through angry-looking eyes and inclusion of teeth and fingernails. Heavy lines emphasized the hair and hat; the nose was long and phallic. The body was cut off by the bottom margin of the paper, leaving no room for the legs. Though hostile in appearance, the figure was immobile, perhaps representing an attempt to control hostile feelings and/or feeling ineffectual in the expression of anger.

Peter smiled and laughed at the drawing, stating that a witch was easiest for him to draw, but the witch "looked stupid 'cause head so big." When asked to make up a story about the drawing, he told an elaborate tale about "children going through the woods to a haunted house—really wasn't haunted so witch wasn't there," again appearing to need to cover or to retract the anger represented.

Figure drawing. This part had a four minute process, and an eight minute association (Fig. 7.12). Peter asked if he should draw "a boy or a girl? The whole self?" He proceeded to use an unusual sequence for drawing the figure. Laughing, he first drew, then erased the head. He then completed the body with detailed clothing before returning to draw the features, adding the top of the head and hair last. He became increasingly secretive, hiding his drawing while completing the face, doing much erasing on the left eye, while making furtive glances at the examiner. Upon completion, Peter laughed, hiding the face of the figure and stating, "It's awful—I messed it up...doesn't even look like a person—like a monster—look at the fingers." His story about the figure he drew: "Once there was a boy who didn't want to get a haircut—didn't listen to his mother. So he let hair grow long. Has twin brother—looked the same, but different interests—this one is dumber, badder, likes fishing, and tennis—other likes football, baseball, smarter, good." When asked if he thought he was like one or the other, he asked, "You mean am I bad? In between."

Peter's verbalizations reflected a poor self-concept and identity conflicts, eg, sexual identity concerns and struggles between a good-bad self. He appeared to feel the wish to be more defiant and autonomous, but at the same time, wanting to please, to control his anger.

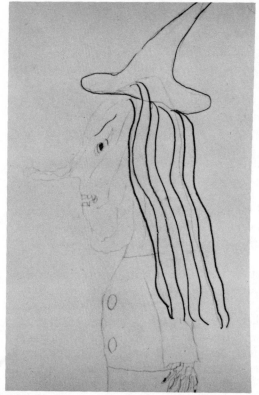

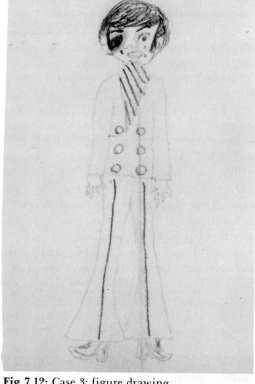

Fig 7.11: Case 3; spontaneous drawing.   **Fig 7.12:** Case 3; figure drawing.

Clay. This part had a ten minute process, and a five minute association (Fig. 8.13). Peter had difficulty controlling the clay, his work process characterized by frequent changes. He first made a small head, then started over, making a witch's face as in his drawing, using cutting actions with the tools. He expressed difficulty in controlling the form: "I never worked with clay, it's falling apart—it won't stay." He continued to change the form, hiding his work more, and finally was told to finish. His associations: "It's a man—it's just what it came. First it was to be a turtle—and then came into this form—clown, turtle, witch, man." The final form was that of a two-dimensional, slab-form of a man's bearded face.

Comparisons. Peter was self-depreciating in his comparisons, stating that his productions were the same, in that all were sloppy. For differences, he concretely stated, "One is clay, one drawing, one tile." He liked the tile best because it was least messy, and the clay least because it was "hardest to form".

Summary. Though the work processes utilized indicated problems in organizational skills and concept formation, Peter was able to achieve integrated, organized end-products. He expended much energy, using time-consuming, inefficient methods. Peter presented a highly controlled, secretive exterior, with indications of underlying hostility, identity struggles, and feelings of inadequacy, as seen in the productions and verbalizations. He appeared to have difficulty expressing his anger—he would smile and laugh instead. He was highly suggestible in response to the lack of structure in the clay task, making many changes in form, and expressing discomfort with the lack of control.

Marsha Goodman Evaskus

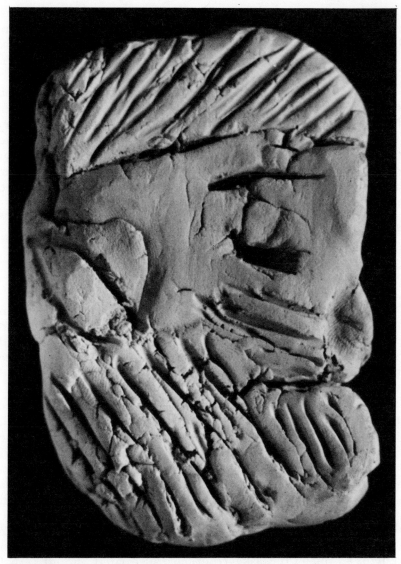

Fig 7.13: Case 3; clay (actual size 2½ x 3¼ x 1 inch).

Suggestions for Research

In the literature on psychological testing, there is agreement regarding the difficulty of scoring projective tests using a quantitative method. Because of the less structured, more ambiguous nature of projective tests, reliability and validity standards are difficult to meet.[44,45] Also, affective aspects of personality are not as precisely measurable as cognitive variables.[44] Anastasi suggests that the value of projective tests emerges when they are regarded as clinical tools, emphasizing interpretation by qualitative, clinical procedures.[45]

According to Buck, qualitative analysis and interpretation are the most productive of valuable diagnostic and prognostic material. However, he also speaks of the need for qualitative standardization studies, "to replace the former system of 'qualitative analysis by inspection' with a more formalized and more objective approach."[25] Schafer has cautioned that scores do not represent the total test responses of the client.[46] Therefore, while there is the need for test standardization, in the attempt to apply standards for objective scoring systems to projective techniques, there may be the danger of losing some of the clinical usefulness of the tool.

The Goodman Battery has a standardized procedure for test administration, and an outline for the analysis of results. However, the additional use of standardized rating scales for the interpretation and scoring of responses to the Goodman Battery would increase clinical reliability in the interpretation of qualitative findings, and enable validity studies to be conducted. To meet these needs, four rating scales have been developed to aid the occupational therapist in organizing and interpreting observed client responses to the tasks presented in the Goodman Battery. Included are the following four scales:

1. Ability to Organize
2. Independence
3. Self-esteem: Performance
4. Self-esteem: Verbal

These can be found in Appendixes H, I, J, and K. From these scales the therapist can also gain information about the client's impulse control, body boundaries, and need for structure. The scales convey the concept of continuums of function, and the extremes in response that may be observed. It is important to emphasize that the present Goodman Battery scales are still in need of further development and refinement to facilitate clinical use.

In the present scales, the responses listed provide a frame of reference for the therapist; behavioral examples are given, but all may not apply to each client tested. The response most nearly describing the behavior observed is checked. The comment section is available for any clarification of the ratings checked.

On all the scales, #4 indicates the most functional response to the task as related to the specific behavior being rated. Responses progressing away from #4 towards either end of the scale show increased levels of dysfunction, as indicated by increased interference with the work process, culminating in the absence of any productive work. As a general guide, in items #1 and #7, the task is not completed. In items #2 and #6, there is difficulty in completing the task, though greater effort is shown than in #1 or #7; in items #3 and #5, the task is completed adequately, though verbal and/or non-verbal cues indicating some difficulty are present.

The scales are designed with a dual progression to accommodate the varying responses of clients having a particular deficit. Items #3 to #1 on each scale indicate an increasingly dysfunctional state that is of an internalized, inner-directed, passive nature. Items #5 to #7 on each scale indicate an increasingly dysfunctional state that is of an externalized, outer-directed, aggressive nature.

In a preliminary study for inter-rater reliability, highest agreement was found with the organization scale, which measures the more cognitive functions, while the scales measuring affective functions showed less agreement. The difficulties that exist in applying the current scales, indicate the need for further development and research studies. A thorough study is needed in which a selected sample is used to identify specific problems in the current scales, and to direct the further refinement of the scales. The need for the development of additional scales should also be assessed. After refinement of the rating scales, recommendations for further

Marsha Goodman Evaskus

research include a study of inter-rater reliability and validity studies comparing Goodman Battery test findings to those of other psychological tests measuring similar functions.

Conclusion

The Goodman Battery evaluates the level of cognitive and affective ego-functioning in clients with psychiatric disturbances. Administered in a progression of decreasing structure, the media in the Goodman Battery combine the highly structured mosaic tile task, with its fixity of form and directions to copy a specific design, facilitating observation of cognitive functioning, with the less structured spontaneous and figure drawing tasks that have the potential for eliciting responses of a more projective nature. The clay task offers a tactile experience with an amorphous media, with the potential for eliciting regressive and/or aggressive responses more graphically than in the other media. The client's responses are assessed within the framework of the ability to function within varying degrees of structure. The Goodman Battery offers the advantages of comparatively brief time for adminstration, and materials that are readily accessible, portable, and inexpensive.

A review of the literature on the use of these media for personality assessment and findings from related psychological tests have been discussed, and related to the interpretation of responses to the Goodman Battery. The standardized procedure for administration of the Battery as well as problems encountered has been presented. The "Outline for Analysis of the Goodman Battery", discussion of each task, and rating scales, provide a framework and guide for the observation and interpretation of responses. Three case examples have been presented. Recommendations for future research emphasize the need for refining the current Goodman Battery Scales, with an assessment of need for additional scales. The use of such standardized rating scales would increase the reliability in the interpretation of responses to the Goodman Battery and enable validity studies to be conducted.

References

1. Azima H, Azima F: Outline of a dynamic theory of occupational therapy. A J Occu Ther XIII (No. 5):215-221, 1959.
2. Azima H: Dynamic occupational therapy. Dis Nerv Syst, Monograph Supplement 22 (No. 4):138-142, 1961.
3. Fidler GS: Diagnostic battery, scoring and summary. In Mazer J (ed): Materials from the 1968 Regional Institutes sponsored by the American Occupational Therapy Association on the Evaluation Process. Final Report R.S.A.-123-T-68. New York, American Occupational Therapy Association, 1968.
4. Androes L, Dreyfus E, Bloesch M: Diagnostic test battery: for occupational therapy. A J Occu Ther XIX (No. 2):53-59, 1965.
5. Cumming J, Cumming E: Ego and Milieu: Theory and Practice of Environmental Therapy. New York, Atherton Press, 1962, pp 13-29, 60-61.
6. Polansky NA: Ego Psychology and Communication—Theory for the Interview. New York, Atherton Press, 1971. pp 48-72.
7. Lazarus RS: Ambiguity and nonambiguity in projective testing. In Murstein BI (ed): Handbook of Projective Techniques. New York, Basic Books, Inc, 1965, p 90.
8. Frank L: Projective methods for the study of personality. J Psychol 8:389-413, 1939.
9. Morris WW: Other projective methods. In Anderson HH, Anderson GL (ed): An Introduction to Projective Techniques. Englewood Cliffs, NJ, Prentice-Hall, Inc, 1951. pp 528-529.
10. Wertham F, Golden L: A differential diagnostic method of interpreting mosaics and color block designs. Am J Psychiat 98:124-131, 1941.

11. Wertham F: The mosaic test. In Abt LE, Bellak L (ed): Projective Psychology. New York, Alfred A Knopf, 1950, pp 238-247.
12. Kerr M: The validity of the mosaic test. Am J Orthopsychiat 9:232-236, 1939.
13. Diamond BL, Schmale HT: The mosaic test. I. An evaluation of its clinical application. Am J Orthopsychiat 14:237-250, 1944.
14. Shoemyen CW: Occupational therapy orientation and evaluation. A J Occu Ther XXIV (No. 4):276-279, 1970.
15. Woltmann AG: The Bender Visual-Motor Gestalt Test. In Abt LE, Bellak L (ed): Projective Psychology. New York, Alfred A Knopf, 1950, pp 322-356.
16. Halpern F: The Bender Visual-Motor Gestalt Test. In Anderson HH, Anderson GL (ed): An Introduction to Projective Techniques. Englewood Cliffs, NJ, Prentice-Hall, Inc, 1951, pp 324-340.
17. Lerner EA: The Projective Use of the Bender Gestalt. Springfield, IL, Charles C Thomas, 1972, p 6.
18. Wechsler D: Manual for the Wechsler Adult Intelligence Scale. New York, The Psychological Corporation, 1955, p 39.
19. Matarazzo JD: Wechsler's Measurement and Appraisal of Adult Intelligence, 5th ed. Baltimore, Williams & Wilkins Co, 1972, pp 488, 206-207, 212-214.
20. Mayman M, Schafer R, Rapaport D: Interpretation of the Wechsler-Bellevue intelligence scale in personality appraisal. In Anderson HH, Anderson GL (ed): An Introduction to Projective Techniques. Englewood Cliffs, NJ, Prentice-Hall, Inc, 1951, pp 550-558.
21. Rapaport D, Gill MM, Schafer R: Diagnostic Psychological Testing, revised edition. Universities Press, 1968, pp 99-101, 137-152.
22. Wechsler D: The Measurement and Appraisal of Adult Intelligence, 4th ed. Baltimore, Williams & Wilkins Co, 1958, pp 79-81.
23. Machover K: Personality Projection in the Drawing of the Human Figure. Springfield, IL Charles C Thomas, 1948.
24. Machover K: Drawing of the human figure: a method of personality investigation. In Anderson HH, Anderson GL (ed): An Introduction to Projective Techniques. Englewood Cliffs, NJ, Prentice-Hall, Inc, 1951, pp 341-369.
25. Buck JN: The House-Tree-Person Technique, Revised Manual. Beverly Hills, CA, Western Psychological Services, 1969, pp 3-13, 80-165.
26. Hammer EF: The Clinical Application of Projective Drawings. Springfield, IL, Charles C Thomas, 1958, pp 59-72.
27. Levy S: Figure drawing as a projective test. In Abt LE, Bellak L (ed): Projective Psychology. New York, Alfred A Knopf, 1950, pp 257-297.
28. Anastasi A, Foley JP: An analysis of spontaneous artistic productions by the abnormal. J Gen Psychol 28:297-313, 1943.
29. Anastasi A, Foley JP: An experimental study of the drawing behavior of adult psychotics in comparison with that of a normal control group. J Exp Psychol XXXIV:169-194, 1944.
30. Swensen CH: Empirical evaluations of human figure drawings. Psychol Bull 54:431-466, 1957.
31. Swensen CH: Empirical evaluations of human figure drawings: 1957-1966. Psychol Bull 70 (No. 1):20-44, 1968.
32. Hammer EF: Critique of Swensen's "Empirical evaluations of human figure drawings". In Murstein BI (ed): Handbook of Projective Techniques. New York, Basic Books, Inc, 1965, pp 655-659.
33. Robbins A, Sibley LB: Creative Art Therapy. New York, Brunner/Mazel 1976, pp 204-205.
34. Fidler G, Fidler J: Occupational Therapy: A Communication Process in Psychiatry. New York, The MacMillan Co, Inc, 1963, pp 76-97.
35. Bender L, Woltmann A: The use of plastic material as a psychiatric approach to emotional problems in children. Am J Orthopsychiat VII (No. 3):283-300, 1937.
36. The Objectives & Functions of Occupational Therapy: compiled by American Occupational Therapy Association, Dubuque, IA, William C Brown Book Co, 1958, p 133.
37. Lowenfeld V, Brittain WL: Creative and Mental Growth, 4th ed. New York, The MacMillan Co, Inc, 1967, pp 106, 115-117, 165-166.
38. Lowenfeld V: Creative and Mental Growth. New York, The MacMillan Co, Inc, 1952, pp 71-73.
39. Hartley RE, Goldenson RM: The Complete Book of Children's Play. New York, Thomas Y Crowell Co, 1963, pp 47-48, 77, 120, 200.
40. Golomb C: Young Children's Sculpture and Drawing. Cambridge, Harvard Univ Press, 1974.
41. Gillette N: Occupational therapy and mental health. In Willard H, Spackman C (ed):

Occupational Therapy. Philadelphia, JB Lippincott Co, 1971, pp 80, 95-96.
42. Hammer EF: Guide for qualitative research with the H-T-P. J Gen Psychol 51:41-60, 1954.
43. McElhaney M: Clinical Psychological Assessment of the Human Figure Drawing. Springfield, IL, Charles C Thomas, 1969, pp 3-5.
44. Aiken L: Psychological Testing and Assessment, 3rd ed. Boston, Allyn & Bacon, Inc, 1979, pp 258, 267.
45. Anastasi A: Psychological Testing, 4th ed. New York, MacMillan Co, Inc, 1976, pp 476, 586.
46. Schafer R: The Clinical Application of Psychological Tests. New York, International Universities Press, Inc, 1958, pp 17-19.

Acknowledgment

I wish to thank my colleague and friend, Elaine S. Novak, O.T.R., for her encouragement and many constructive comments and suggestions offered throughout the writing of this chapter.

Finally, I am grateful to my husband, David, and daughters, Jenny and Leta, whose support and patience made this undertaking possible.

Marsha Goodman Evaskus

8
The BH Battery

Barbara J. Hemphill, M.S., O.T.R.

My interest in evaluating psychiatric clients as an occupational therapist resulted from several years of experience. In fact, it started 12 years ago with the first client who came for treatment. I believed then (and am more firmly committed to it now) that in order to plan treatment, the therapist must first evaluate. However, at that time projective tests such as the Fidler and Azima Batteries were the only evaluations available that assessed the psychological area of human functioning. These evaluations were too time consuming, too subjective, and too difficult to administer. In addition, these evaluations did not provide a set of standards for which projection could be rated. Therefore, after throwing my hands up in despair, I decided to develop my own evaluation, called the BH Battery.

This chapter deals with the development of a projective test that evaluates the psychological area of human functioning. Particular attention is paid to the sequence of development to give the reader a feeling for the process in which an evaluation such as this is constructed.

Historical Development
Rationale

The development of this evaluation began in 1973 during the time I was employed at Ft. Logan Mental Health Center, a state institution located in Denver, Colorado. A team of health professionals, including myself as the occupational therapist, instituted an evaluation process to assess the client's social, psychological, and physical state of health within five days after admission. The purpose of the occupational therapy evaluation was to: 1) assist in diagnosis, 2) evaluate task skills and level of psychological functioning in a short period of time, and 3) assist in treatment plannng.

With this task in mind, I conducted a literature review to find a suitable evaluation. I found that occupational therapists have elaborated on the combination of media proposed earlier by the Azimas in a variety of ways.[1-3] Even though there is agreement among therapists as to what could be evaluated, the establishment of a set of standards through which projections could be rated had not been developed. "Rating scales had been constructed; none were more than lists of things which may be observed."[4]

Paintings have been used by psychoanalytically oriented workers for some time, but their primary interest has been in content rather than in the process. The content, especially when accompanied by free association, or in conjuction with the client's case history, is valuable. The Thematic Apperception test reveals the content of personality.[5] Both approaches are valuable, but neither the Rorschach nor the Thematic Apperception test allows the occupational therapist to observe the client manipulate materials.

Fidler considers that the process by which an individual completes a task is the basis for personality assessment in occupational therapy.[6] Therefore, in the BH Battery, ratings were constructed that would evaluate both content and process, and yield a score for each behavioral observation.

After the decision was made to convert clinical observations into measurable terms by the use of a rating scale, I selected the following behaviors to be evaluated: 1) ability to follow directions; 2) ability to problem solve; 3) degree of frustration tolerance; 4) ability to perceive parts into a whole; 5) ability to abstract; 6) ability to make decisions; 7) ability to follow through in logical sequence; 8) state of internal organization; 9) awareness of body concept; 10) use of structure; 11) ability to handle limits or boundaries; and 12) state of feeling tone.

Since the BH Battery is designed for clinical use in occupatonal therapy, the media chosen had to evaluate the above behaviors and be familiar to the therapist. Therefore, finger painting and mosaic tiling were chosen.

Finger painting offers the advantages of freeing the individual from motor limitations, age,[7] cultural influences, and social pressures.[8] Painting permits the non-verbal, painfully shy, withdrawn individual to express himself. According to expressive behavior theorists, each individual expresses himself in movement patterns which are characteristic, and reveal the unity of his personality. Allport and Venon use the concept of expressive movement and their understanding of the value of finger painting as a diagnostic tool. The authors state:

> Fundamentally our results lend support to the personalistic contentions that there be some degree of unity in personality, that this unity is reflected expression, and that for this reason act and habits of expression show a certain consistency among themselves...It is surely not unreasonable to assume that insofar as personality is organized, expressive movement is harmonious and self-consistent, and insofar as personality is unintegrated, expressive movement is self-contradictory.[9]

This unity and self-contradictory quality of expressive movement if measured and studied, could provide important information in the study of individual personality. The difficulties of capturing, recording, and measuring the transient qualities of overt movements are obvious.[5]

Mosaic tiling was chosen because it measures the person's ability to conceptualize a whole, to form a mental image, to break that image into component parts, and to reproduce it on a mosaic board. Frank states:

> ...the dynamic conception of personality as a process of organizing experience and structuralizing life space in a field...can reveal the way an individual personality organizes experience in order to...gain insight into that individual's private world of meanings, significant patterns, and feeling.[10]

Frank continues by stating that the personality could be approached by inducing the individual to reveal his way of organizing experience by giving the client a field with structure where the subject builds in accordance to materials offered. The subject reveals in the pattern the building or organizing conceptions of his life at that period, as in block-building, or making a mosaic.[11]

Barbara J. Hemphill

Literature Review

In order to obtain the most effective method of measuring the desired behaviors in mosaic tiling and finger painting, psychological and sociological literature was again surveyed. Studies in the projective use of mosaic come from investigations of the Mosaic Test.[12,13] Wertham and Golden describe the following characteristics of mosaics: 1) number of designs; 2) representation of a definite concrete object or abstract design; 3) harmony of the design as a whole; 4) completeness or incompleteness of design; 5) simple or complex design; 6) compactness or looseness of design; 7) position of design within the mosaic in relation to the margin, general distribution, or all-over pattern; 8) number of pieces used; 9) choice of color; 10) simple geometric design; 11) symmetry; 12) repetition; and 13) what comments the subject makes about the design.

In 1950, Wertham introduced a technique for the study of personality through subjects' mosaic projects. The researcher's hypothesis stated that deficits in the achievement of a recognizable gestalt in the mosaic would reflect significant defects in the basic personality structure of the individual. Evidence is presented to support Wertham's contention. The mosaic performance correlates with the presence of various clinical disorders which reveals the severest disturbance in the mosaic gestalt.

Waehner presented the first attempt at critical analysis of expressive behavior in the literature. The criteria used to match student paintings with Rorschach interpretations was: size of paper, format, symmetry, balance, rhythm, motion, preference for lines or spots, use of color, distribution of form, organization of form, and shading. In 87% of the cases, a student's painting could be matched correctly with the Rorschach interpretations.[14]

Napoli reported in three consecutive articles a five-point rating scale based on expressive behavior in finger painting.[15-17] Napoli divided the rating scale into three major categories: 1) performance observation, which includes all visible, emotional, behavioral, and physical manifestations of the subject in action during the process; 2) the painting analytics—this category is broken down into eight subdivisions: handedness, color, motion, rhythm, texture, composition, order, and symbolism; and 3) verbalizations, which is the story the individual attaches or uses to explain his finger painting. When clients' case histories are compared with their expressive behavior in finger painting, syndrome characteristics of schizophrenic and paranoid personalities can be observed. However, Napoli's studies give no statistical analysis.

Kadis presented a rating scale based on the researcher's review of the literature. The researcher suggested diagnostic considerations in painting and summarized them under the terms *distance* and *involvement*.[7] Distance refers to the behavior the subject shows when he desires to separate himself from the task. Behavior such as keeping one hand behind the back, using fingers with arms outstretched, and using fingers as a pencil, are indicative of distance. Involvement is behavior that indicates participation, such as using entire body movements. Kadis divides the characteristics into the following categories: 1) time—noting pauses, hesitations, and total time; 2) space utilization and location—noting the individual who paints beyond the edges of the paper, uses a small section of the paper, or works from the middle out or vice versa; 3) color—noting whether the individual mixes and combines colors—to do so is considered higher intellectual functioning; 4) shading—noting patting or stroking; 5) strokes—the width, pressure, and multiplicity of strokes, shapes, and texture; 6) content—the organization; 7) movements and motions—noting if the direction is away or toward the individual; and 8) rhythm—noting recurrent use of pattern or themes in a sequence. Kadis' conclusions have been supported by comparing client's responses to finger painting with the client's case history.

Dorken attempted to establish the reliability and validity of a rating scale based on the behavioral aspects of finger painting. The researcher's rating scale, which includes the categories and their values, are illustrated in Table 8.1. The rating scale is arranged so that a score of 8 represents the optimal ratings. In a series of not fewer than four paintings, test-retest reliability coefficients are significant in all categories for chronic schizophrenic (.804—.924), chronic depression (.654—.934) and manic-depressive psychotics (.517-.917).[18] In order to test the hypothesis that all four categories relate to the painter's overt behavior, a comparative statistical analysis shows that psychotic clients are distinguished from normal individuals in all categories. An intratest correlation among the finger painting categories suggests that the internal organization of the personality in the psychotic is

TABLE 8.1

DORKEN'S RATING SCALE FOR FINGER PAINTING

Category	Rating	Category	Rating
I. *Energy ouput*		III. *Content*	
daubing	1	no content	1
dotting	2	indefinable	2
use of thin lines	3	bizarre	3
1/4 use of space	4	unreal	4
coordinated strokes	5	repetition	5
continuous strokes	6	lettering	6
1/2 use of space	7	symbolism	7
variety of design	8	building/ship	8
strong pressure	9	people	9
3/4 use of space	10	creature/plant	10
overlapping	11	object	11
scratching	12		
tearing	13		
		IV. *Clarity*	
II. *Color*		smearing	1
		confusion	2
A. Spontaneous	3	carelessness	3
red or yellow		hazy	4
		poor	5
B. Controlled	2	fairly distant	6
blue or green		distant	7
		accurate	8
C. Somber	1	meticulous	9
black or brown			
D. Combination			
orange	3		
lime	2		
purple	1		

Barbara J. Hemphill

different from that of the personality of normal individuals. Dorken's investigation substantiates this finding. The categories for subjects of the non-psychotic or normal group are independent in both the first and the final paintings. The results indicate that each category measures a separate and distinct aspect of personality.

Interpretation of Behaviors Assessed

After the media was selected, a rationale formulated, and existing rating scales surveyed, another literature review was conducted. This aspect of the literature review consisted of ascertaining the meanings of overt behaviors included in the BH Battery. This review was important, because it gave me an idea of what behaviors had been researched and how they had been measured in the past. It also gave clues to the outcome of subsequent research studies.

For organizational sake, the interpretation of behaviors assessed are presented according to seven major categories in the BH Battery rating scale* (see Appendixes L and M): 1) color; 2) approach to the media—including such items as posture, attitude, format, placement of the first daub of paint, and parts of the hand used; 3) use of space—including surface coverage, motion, texture, order, and overlapping; 4) form and pattern—including such items as detail, shape, size, and distribution of objects, and symmetry; 5) verbalizations; 6) characteristics—including direction, width of lines, and pressure in finger painting, and number of designs, use of space, and position of design in mosaic tiling; and 7) time. The items in each category are interpreted, beginning with research findings in finger painting and followed by mosaic tiling. For definition of terms, there is a training manual for the BH Battery which can be obtained from the publisher.[19]

Research Findings With Regard to Color

The affective tone is known to vary among colors.[18] This is well illustrated by reviews of Precker[5] and Napoli.[17,20] There is general agreement that the use of red and yellow is a more spontaneous form of expression[21] than the blues or greens, which are more representative of controlled behavior.[7] Choungourian has demonstrated that neurotics significantly prefer more red than extroverts, while extroverts prefer significantly more yellow-green than neurotics.[22] Black and brown are common to states of repression[15] and regression.[7] A combined analysis of the first, second, and third most preferred colors yields significant differences in frequency of blue, chosen more often among normals. These findings are supported by other researchers.[24,25] Ulman and Levy report that normals use more color, and colors are mixed and blended.[26] Kadis has stated that mixing and combining colors is associated with higher intellectual functioning.[7]

Maria Brick presented the meaning of various behavioral aspects in art productions of 200 children based upon comparisons and case history material. Unfortunately, no quantitative material was presented. However, the researcher reported that the choice of dark and muddy colors is observed in children in states of anxiety and depression.[27] Weahner examined 760 pictures made by 12 normal and 26 abnormal children which supported Brick's observations. Overlapping—the blotting over or repeatedly going over one layer of the art product with another[24]— is another characteristic that distinguishes the abnormals from the normals.

The studies regarding color in mosaic tile came from investigations of the Mosaic Test. A study by Wertham and Golden which analyzed 1,000 mosaics of adults,

---

*Taken from the thesis, A Research Study in Mosaic Tiling and Finger Painting. Ft. Collins, CO, Colorado State University, 1976.

children, normals, and psychotics showed that psychotics demonstrate no organization of color, and use red more often than any other group.[12] Clients with severe depression use black interchangeably with blue. Designs which contain only black and white are characteristic of schizoid personalities. A characteristic of schizophrenics is the relative lack of color. A large percentage of white is used with yellow, blue, green, or black, but seldom red. Frequently, schizophrenics make a whole design of solid color.[13] Wideman's study is in agreement with these findings.[28]

Research Findings With Regard to Approach to the Media

Posture. The balance an individual experiences in his body movements can be represented in the composition of the finger painting. If the individual's posture is not good but the picture is balanced, then there have been certain compensations.[17] The individual who leans on one hand while painting with the other is self-conscious and fears criticism. Others who shift from one foot to another or wrap one leg around the other are usually shy, timid, and withdrawn.[20]

Attitude. In a series of paintings made by a group of normals and a group of clients, the most prevalent characteristic that differentiated the client group was the refusal to paint.[24] Some subjects plunged into the task immediately; others halted or hesitated. Long reaction time reflected anticipatory anxiety associated with reactions to wetness or dryness of the media.[7]

Part of the hand used. Normal individuals use the whole hand—palm and fingers—while throwing weight on the extremity. Napoli, after comparing case histories, reported that women who dislike washing dishes, and pass the responsibilities of child rearing to others, approach painting with disgust and use their fingertips in a hesitant manner. Others use the palm with their fingers turned up. Individuals possessing vocational and/or social inferiority cup their hands and use the lateral side of the hand to paint.[20]

Research Findings With Regard to the Use of Space

Surface coverage. Nursery school children who paint off the paper tend to show either an immature pattern of dependence or uncontrolled asocial behavior.[29] Rejected and deprived children never use the entire paper, but cram their work close to the bottom.[27] Children who work in small areas tend to show withdrawn, emotionally dependent behavior. From Rorschach interpretations, subjects who show a consistent tendency to stay away from the margin are highly self-controlled. Neglect of margin indicates lack of control. When form elements are kept at a great distance from the margin, anxiety and over-control is usually present.[14] Those individuals who use a small percentage of available space show psycho-motor retardation accompanied by severe depression. When severe psycho-motor retardation is associated with suicidal ideas, the individual uses less than a quarter of the available space.[30]

The principle of space in mosaic tile is the relation of the pieces to the tray. All-over patterns are made by adults,[13] but in abnormal conditions, they frequently represent a primitive factor.[12] Advanced and deteriorated schizophrenics make scattered isolated mosaics.[28] Clinging to the edge of the board and avoidance of the open area of the central space is found in conditions in which anxiety is present. Designs which cling to the margin and take the form of frames occur in neurosis.[12]

Space in mosaic tile is also expressed in terms of compactness or looseness. Compact designs, where all the pieces touch one another are made by matter-of-fact

Barbara J. Hemphill

people. The agglutination of a few pieces that show no discernable organization is characteristic of severe undifferentiated functional psychosis. A compact design is never seen in healthy persons. Loose designs, where space is left between the pieces, are likely to be made by normal people who are impressionistic and imaginative.[12,28]

Motion. This represents a clear and overt expression of an immediate feeling. Motions that reflect aggressive impulses are pulling, slapping, scratching, scrubbing, or tearing. The motions associated with sensuous feelings are patting and smearing. To group motions into *sensuous* and *aggressive* is inadequate according to Kadis, because each motion represents a specific feeling.[7]

The longer an individual smears in a continuous but undirected manner, the more immature and insecure the client is, regardless of his chronological age. Although there is a short scrubbing period in the normal client, prolonged scrubbing is indicative of disturbed personality.[20] A destructive type of scrubbing is illustrated by the individual who is antagonistic to the painting situation and who tenses the body because of inner drives.[17] Likewise, by comparing motion with case histories, Napoli has suggested that scribbling shows defiance, disappointment, and lack of ability in competition.[20]

There are two types of pushing out. One type describes the articulate, extroverted individual and the second type of pushing out conveys the getting-rid-of.[17] The latter individual is defiant, refuses responsibility, refuses to be imposed upon, and is continuously disagreeable. The individual who paints with emphasis on pulling in motion is introverted, selfish, gluttonous, orally dependent, self-centered, and self-conscious. Withdrawn individuals pull their lines down to the very bottom of the paper, and often frame their pictures with this movement.[20] Patting is a motion that depicts something desired or something that is being accepted.[17] This is done by people who show affection and gratitude, and respond to love.[20] Therefore, a slap is a pat with violence attached to it, and is motivated by anger, defiance, antagonism, and inadequacy.[17] A movement made up of single violent slaps is referred to as a slap of violence to kill. Scratching is significant of defiance, rejection, and a wish to destroy something.[20] Picking is considered a teasing or tantalizing form of movement accompanied by guilt.

Texture. The ideal texture for paint is smooth and the amount of water added is indicative of the obedient, cooperative person who wishes to excel in his desire to paint.[17] Any deviation from the smooth and wet texture is considered inadequate.[20] Individuals who use too much paint and not enough water make the material non-obedient, because their attitude is that of non-cooperation in the situation. People who use too much water are responding to the situation in a defiant manner. These individuals need supervision and constant attention.

Order. Order is expressed in form, movement, and content. An individual who does not approach his painting in a sequential manner has a partial disorientation to reality. Lack of order has its base in transient emotional disorganization.[20]

Research Findings with Regard to Form

Details. Waehner reported that students who make minute details are described as over-neat, and are often depressed. Unrelated details and scribbling are indicative of disturbance. In Waehner's study, only three students who had narcissistic disturbance showed this form.[14] Very few details, or no details, occurs more frequently in the unadjusted group and in the groups with academic failure. Few but essential details occur only in the adjusted group.

Shape of objects. Waehner reported that students who consistently make sharp and clear objects have high intelligence ratings, but too great a sharpness is an indication of lack of adjustment. Students who use vague objects have low intelligence ratings. The use of rigid contours is found in those individuals who are occupied with repression of hostile ideas, and occurs among compulsive neurotics.[14]

Size of objects. Objects that are small in relation to the whole format suggest anxiety and over-control. Normal individuals show a mixture of large, medium, and small objects.[14]

Centering and symmetry. Distribution of objects is represented by emphasis on the center, or symmetry in relation to the horizontal, vertical, and middle axes. Normal children show well-balanced distribution of objects in their paintings. Depressive neurotics show rigid symmetry, while psychotics show a lack of symmetry.[14]

There is always a central figure integrated with the rest of the picture in paranoid personalities. This central theme is well balanced, with other objects on either side for the purpose of protecting the central object with which the individual usually identifies.[15]

In mosaics, the distribution of objects is expressed in the presence or absence of symmetry. In schizophrenics, there is an exaggerated and rigid symmetry in both design and color. Wertham defined a marked contrast between a very pronounced symmetry and meagerness or emptiness of design as *super-symmetry.*[13] Super-symmetry is a diagnostic sign of schizophrenia.[12] The diagnostic significance becomes greater as the design becomes more inadequate and emptier. Wertham states that it is merely one expression of the over-emphasis or organization of schizophrenia.

Research Findings With Regard to Strokes

Direction. In finger painting, strokes are considered to constitute the direct expression of the subject's inner psycho-dynamics, for they are a direct continuation of total bodily movements with no intervening tool to retard the momentum of expression.[7] Vertical lines are identified by Alschuler and Hattwick as representing assertive drives, and horizontals to denote self-protection, fear, and overtly cooperative characteristics.[29] Some paintings of children and disorganized clients fail to show a definite direction tendency but produce a jumbled effect. With progressive emotional growth, a more coherent structure emerges from the disorganized jumble.[7]

Width, pressure and multiplicity of strokes. Alschuler and Hattwick describe lines and objects as the best representation of energy expended. Lack of restraint, not only in the motion of the stroke,[29] but in the size of the painting is considered as evidence of aggressiveness or motor release.[21] Pressure is another indication of energy level.[5,7]

Strokes vary from fine and narrow made by finger nails, to wide and heavy lines produced by the palm or elbow. Some subjects exert degrees of pressure by displacing all paint and leaving the lines as a white surface on the painting sheet. Finally, strokes are produced as single strokes with one finger, or double strokes by employing the corresponding number of fingers.[7] Light strokes represent timidity and fear. Fearful neurotics, chronic schizophrenics, and catatonics show little pressure.[24] Heavy pressure represents forcefulness and tension.[7]

Shape and length. Kadis suggests that angular strokes represent an aggressive

Barbara J. Hemphill

pattern, while an angular zigzag direction reflects the subject's indecision toward his aggressive behavior. Long strokes represent controlled behavior, and short strokes are characteristic of impulsive behavior. Strokes less than six inches long are identified with insecurity and anxiety. Closed strokes represent withdrawal, while the degree of openess symbolizes the degree of willingness to communicate with the world.[7]

Research Findings Regarding Verbalization

Kadis stated that the correlation between the content and the client's story about the painting is an index of the degree of ego development. The symbolic content gives clues to dynamic mechanisms, such as identification, projections, rationalization, and sublimation. They also give clues to emotional states such as conflict, wish fulfillment, fear, repression, and anxiety.[15] Napoli suggests that verbalizations take on the form of one type or a combination of many types of stories—fantasy, fiction, fact, culture, and mythology, and these stories are symbolic in their meaning insofar as they involve the projection of mental mechanisms that reflect actual conditions.[17] At the same time, they reveal the subject's adjustive attempts to cope with or justify his existing condition. Verbalization could happen any time during or after the process. Non-verbal individuals who lack security, are overcome by guilt, or are conditioned to questions and answers, remain silent throughout the process. People who ramble reveal their inadequacies, insecurities, and disorganization. Displeasure is shown when the client later denies having painted the picture, because it reveals too much of his guilt. Satisfaction towards the painting is shown by the client whose verbalizations denote asking for approval.[15]

Research Findings with Regard to Content

The literature dealing with spontaneous art productions of psychotic subjects indicate longstanding interest in the unusual contents portrayed in pathological thought processes. Various researchers show that there are significant differences in the content between normal and abnormal paintings.[24,26,31] Productions of the psychotic are apt to be abstract, fantastic, containing unrelated objects, symbolic, and of human content. The productions of manic-depressive psychotics are often themes of prisons, cages, tombs, and coffins. These themes appear during both mania and depression. Similar to the enclosed shapes associated with cages, coffins, and tombs is a configuration of concentrically organized forms. This figure occurs more in obsessive-compulsive clients who produce geometric designs; hysterical personalities do abstract designs; and handprints appear most frequently in the finger paintings of schizophrenic adult clients.[30] Ulman and Levy demonstrate that normal paintings are landscapes and objects that portray reality.[26] The finger paintings of normal individuals are scenes, buildings, plants and trees, and symmetrical abstract designs.[17]

Research Findings with Regard to Use of Time

The degree to which the subject allows himself to be involved in the painting is reflected by the total amount of time. When the time span is short, it is significant of wastefulness and disorganization,[20] or of the desire of the individual to separate himself from the situation as quickly as possible, because it causes anxiety.[7] Those subjects who participate for an unusually long time find relief from anxiety, and are unable to separate themselves from the media. Individuals who take a long time to complete a painting also reflect their overprotectiveness and their striving for perfection. Normals take longer than the abnormals because they show their adaptability in exploration and acceptance of a new situation.[20]

In summary, the entire review of occupational therapy literature involved a survey of evaluations, existing rating scales in finger paintings and mosaic tiling, and interpretations of behaviors assessed. To my mind, the evaluations in occupational therapy were inadequate, and led me to develop the BH Battery. Four rating scales in finger painting, and studies involving the Mosaic Test were reviewed. Many of the studies were either non-experimental or lacking in research methodology. Much of the interpretation of the material is out of date. Therefore, modern research methods and statistical procedures need to be employed to ascertain the meaning of the behaviors assessed in the BH Battery. However, the information does yield assistance to me regarding the method for measuring the behaviors. The last literature review relative to the relationship between the behaviors assessed in finger painting of the abnormal client when compared to the normal individual is as follows: the abnormal client uses dark colors or no color, demonstrates poor posture, refuses or shows reluctance to complete the activity, and uses fewer parts of the hand. In the category regarding the use of space, the psychiatric client uses one half or less surface coverage, uses more paint than needed, demonstrates poor balance with no composition, and works away from self when compared with a normal group. The psychiatric client differs from the normal individual in the lack of openness in strokes, the use of minute detail to unrelated scribbling, the use of small, vague objects, lack of symmetry, no verbalization or too much verbalization, no content, and use of repetitions, abstractions, geometric designs, and lettering in content.

Behavioral aspects of mosaic tiling in the psychiatric individual are associated with the lack of color, incomplete design, lack of symmetry, two or more designs, and very loose or compact designs. Tile placed beyond the edges, edges left vacant, and designs that are plain, or completed in a random fashion separate the psychiatric individual from the normal individual.

Administration

The procedure for administering the BH Battery is written in detail in the training manual.[19] Equipment, materials, and environmental factors essential for giving this assessment tool are explained. The manual describes the following: the size of masonite board, and the color and size of mosaic tile. It also discusses the type, size, and colors of finger paints used; rating scales containing dicotomous and ordinal data; ordinal data arranged so that normal behavior is scored one and abnormal behavior is scored five (see Appendixes L and M). This battery is constructed to provide a method to measure the behaviors cited earlier in this chapter. Two different tasks are used which require no previous experience other than what is provided in the training manual. Each task serves as a subtest, and must be administered in one setting.

The rating scales contain 143 different observations. Therefore, they are constructed to make it easier for the administrator to record all behaviors in less than five minutes. The observations for each subtest are divided into two phases—those that can be recorded during the tasks, and those that can be recorded after the tasks are completed.

It is my suggestion that the assessment be given within 24 hours after the client is admitted. It should be administered to clients who appear to be incapable of being assessed. By giving the testing procedure at this time, it helps to assure that the

Barbara J. Hemphill

results are not affected by drugs, thereby giving a more accurate measure of progress later in the client's treatment.

Research

During the preparation for developing this battery, it became obvious that the first consideration in the process towards standardization is reliability. In order for other occupational therapists to obtain reliable results, it is essential that each item in the battery be examined for ambiguity and stability. Therefore, stability and inter-rater reliability studies were conducted. Inter-rater reliability was achieved both for mosaic tiling (75%) and finger painting (73%). Stability was .73858 at the .05 level of confidence. The research methodology employed is described in the training manual.[19]

Suggested Research

Since reliability of the BH Battery is well established, the next question to address is its validity. The battery appears to have face validity. When clients are asked to participate in the testing procedure, they become aware that it is a projective test to assess their psychological wellbeing; therefore, it is accepted by the virtue of its being a projective test.

By using a correlational research design, criterion validity should be examined. An established assessment tool, such as the Minnesota Multiphasic Personality Inventory could be used to examine its power to distinguish between diagnostic categories. Other assessment tools could determine its ability to measure the behaviors it purports to judge.

Conclusion

In developing an assessment tool, the steps involved are: 1) develop a rationale; 2) do a complete and thorough literature review; 3) develop a method for recording the behaviors; and 4) begin the appropriate research procedures.

Developing the rationale for an assessment tool should begin with a need to evaluate behaviors for a particular population. This should be followed by a survey of the literature to find assessments that are appropriate, relative to the need. Finding none available or finding inadequate tools should then lead the investigator to related literature that contains appropriate material. This phase of the literature review should involve retrieving the early theoretical and statistical information and getting clues to the method of recording the desired behaviors. When developing a means to measure behavior, a scoring system should be constructed. This scoring system should be used to record the behaviors. After a method for recording is established, preliminary research procedures should begin. Reliability studies should be conducted, and particular attention should be paid to ambiguous terminology. Validity studies should involve ascertaining the meaning of the scores obtained.

In the case of the BH Battery, all the steps have been completed except for the last. At this time, no validity studies have been conducted. Therefore, the meaning of the scores have not been determined.

References

1. Llorens L, Young E: Finger painting for the hostile child. A J Occu Ther 14(6), 1960.
2. Androes L, Dreyfus E, and Bloesch M: Diagnostic test battery for occupational therapy. A J Occu Ther 13(5), 1959.
3. Shoemyen C: Occupational therapy orientation and evaluation. A J Occu Ther 24(4), 1970.

4. Gillette N: Occupational therapy and mental health. In the Willard H, Spackman C (ed): Occupational Therapy. Philadelphia, JB Lippincott Co, 1971.
5. Precker J: Summaries: Painting and drawing in personality assessment. J Personality Assessment, 14, 1950.
6. Fidler G, Fidler F: A diagnosis and evaluation process. Occupational Therapy: A Communicative Process in Psychiatry New York, The MacMillan Co, 1963.
7. Kadis G: Projective Psychology. New York, Abt and Bellak, 1950.
8. Hammer E (ed): Areas of Special Advantage for Projective Drawings: The Clinical Application of Projective Drawings. Springfield, IL, Charles C Thomas, 1971.
9. Allport G, Vernon P: Studies in Expressive Movement. New York, The MacMillan Co, 1933, pp 171-182.
10. Frank L: Projective methods for the study of personality. J Psychol. 8:403, 1939.
11. Zubin J, Eron L, Schumer F: An Experimental Approach to Projective Techniques. New York, John Wiley & Sons, Inc, 1965.
12. Wertham F, Golden L: A differential method of interpreting mosaics and color block designs. A J Psychiat 98, 1941.
13. Wertham F: The mosaic test. In Knopf A (ed): Projective Psychology. New York, Abt and Bellak, 1950.
14. Waehner T: Interpretation of spontaneous drawings and paintings. Genetic Psychology Monographs, 33, 1946.
15. Napoli J: Finger painting and personality diagnosis. Genetic Psychological Monograph, 34, 1946.
16. Napoli, J: A finger painting record form. J Psychol, 26, 1948.
17. Napoli J: Finger painting. In Anderson H and Anderson G (ed): Introduction to Projective Techniques. New York, Prentice-Hall, Inc, 1956.
18. Dorken H: The reliability and validity of spontaneous finger paintings. J Projective Techniques, 18, 1954.
19. Hemphill B: The Training Manual for the BH Battery, New Jersey, Charles B Slack, Inc, 1982.
20. Napoli J: Interpretive aspects of finger painting. J Psychol, 23, 1947.
21. Zimmerman J, Garfinkle L: Preliminary study of the art productions of the adult psychotic. Psychiatric Quarterly 16, 1942.
22. Choungourian A: Extroversion, Neuroticism, and Color Preferences. Perceptual and Motor Skills, 34, 1972.
23. Pianetti C, Palacios M, Elliott L: The significance of color. A J Occu Ther 18(4), 1964.
24. Anastasi A, Foley J: A survey of the literature on artistic behavior in the abnormal. J Gen Psychol. 52, 1941.
25. Jacobsen A, Adamson J: Relationship of picture content and patient's age and diagnosis to color choice. A J Occu Ther 27(1), 1973.
26. Ulman E, Levy B: The judgment of psychopathology from paintings, Bull Art Therapy 8(1), 1968.
27. Brick M: Mental hygiene value of children's art work. A J Orthopsychiat, 14, 1944.
28. Wideman H: Development and initial validation of an objective scoring method for the Lowenfeld mosaic test. J Projective Techniques, 19, 1955.
29. Alschuler R, Hattwick L: Easel painting as an index of personality in preschool children. A J Orthopsychiat, 13, 1943.
30. Clower G, Metzler K: Finger painting as an adjunct to psychiatric diagnosis, Bull Art Therapy 5(3), 1966.
31. Langevin R, Hutchin S: An experimental investigation of judges ratings of schizophrenic and non-schizophrenics. J Personality Assessment, 37(6), 1973.
32. Wadeson H, Bunny W: Manic-depressive art: A systematic study of differences in a 48 hour cyclic patient. J Nervous and Mental Disease 150(3), 1970.

Barbara J. Hemphill

9
The Magazine Picture Collage

Carole Lerner, O.T.R.

Collage is a French word meaning gluing. More commonly, the word is used to describe the art of making designs and pictures by gluing bits of cut or torn paper, or other materials to a background.[1]

In this chapter the magazine picture collage—a composite of cuttings from magazines glued to a sheet of construction paper—will be discussed in terms of its clinical and research applications. In addition to its role as an occupational therapy assessment device for evaluating psychiatric clients, I will also review three research studies involving the collage. Two of these studies represent an attempt to assess the construct validity and potential usefulness of a system devised for scoring the collage.

Historical Development

For over 12 years I have used the magazine picture collage as the psychiatric clients' initial activity in occupational therapy. This began at Sinai Hospital in Detroit, Michigan, and has continued for the past six years at Mount Sinai Hospital in Toronto, Ontario. Both of these hospitals are large, teaching, general hospitals with psychiatric inpatient units (about 30 beds). In both hospitals occupational therapy is required for all clients as part of their overall treatment program. A psychoanalytic approach to treatment is the philosophy of both psychiatric departments.

Rationale

The collage has been used as the initial activity for several reasons. The newly admitted psychiatric client is typically quite anxious.[2] By the time the client is seen by the occupational therapist he has already been subjected to a host of verbal and physical examinations which, in and of themselves, are also anxiety arousing. In addition, the occupational therapy setting in which the emphasis is on *doing* as well as on verbal interaction also arouses tension, especially for those clients whose performance skills have faltered because of symptomatology. Thus, amid this context of heightened discomfort and anxiety, a task such as constructing a collage adds minimally to the distress. Further, because the client can see other collages on display, he quickly realizes that it is a routine procedure.

From the occupational therapist's perspective, the collage involves materials that are universally familiar and readily available. The cost is minimal, and it could even be considered that the magazines are being recycled. A sense of attachment is fostered by displaying each client's collage during their hospitalization. Further, this easy first task is a stepping stone to more complex activities in occupational therapy.

Literature Review

Despite its increased clinical usage, studies regarding the collage have appeared infrequently in occupational therapy literature. Holmes and Bauer[3] briefly discuss the collage as a means of assessing selected aspects of an individual's mode of thinking. An extensive discussion of the value of the collage as an assessment technique is provided by Buck and Provancher.[4] These researchers comprehensively evaluated the collages made by 500 adult psychiatric clients. From the collages, the investigators drew inferences to major facets of personality, including self-image, level of psychic energy, level of mental organization, quality of defenses and controls, and nature of symptomatology. The inferences derived from the collages corresponded to the client's diagnosis and related significantly to clinical information appearing in the client's hospital chart.

The use of the collage at Mount Sinai Hospital in Toronto is consistent with the major conclusions of Buck and Provancher.[4] That is, the magazine picture collage is a valid and useful indicator of core aspects of personality organization. Because of the scant material in the literature which consists basically of clinical reports about the use of the collage, I initiated a series of studies to substantiate and to contribute to the theoretical and applied bases of this procedure.[5,6] In the remainder of this chapter I will report these studies and then discuss the respective findings with regard to their clinical, research, and theoretical implications.

Administration and Scoring

The administration of the collage is simple and straightforward. After being supplied with glue, scissors, a selection of colored construction paper (29 x 45 cm; 12 x 18 inches), and a stack of magazines, the client is told, "Select a sheet of construction paper; look through the magazines and cut out whatever appeals to you and then glue it down. There is no right or wrong way to make your collage."

While the client is making the collage, the administrator remains in the background, thus prompting the client to rely on his own resources. Further, this lessened contact permits greater projections on the part of the client. The therapist should observe the following: how the client handles tools and materials, his approach to the task, general organizational skills, memory for directions, capacity to tolerate frustration, and degree of dependency as evidenced by requests for further instructions or reassurances.

After the collage is completed, the client is asked to put his name, the date, and a title for the collage on the back. The collage is then discussed with the client in terms of its personal meaning, why various cuttings were selected, feelings toward the content of the cuttings, and more general feelings about having made the collage. At this point the client's permission to share the collage with other members of the treatment team is obtained.

The collage is presented to the client's planning conference as part of the initial occupational therapy assessment. It represents the only tangible, actual, expression of something from the client. At the conference, it is used as a diagnostic instrument providing information with respect to various aspects of personality (ie, sense of self, quality of relating) including specific ego functions (ie, capacity to integrate and synthesize, organizational skills, level of judgment).

The collage is the only project made by the client that is not kept. The client's collage is filed after discharge for the purpose of comparing collages, should re-hospitalization be necessary, and for teaching and research purposes.

The collage may be likened to the client making his own Rorschach blot or Thematic Apperception Test card, because in all three situations the individual is presented with raw material and asked to fashion a product which reflects conscious and unconscious aspects of himself. All three tasks are further alike in that they are relatively unstructured. Because of this, each allows and even invites an expression of the structuring and organizing principles of the individual's personality.[2]

Scoring system

For research purposes, I developed a system for objectively scoring the collage. It is important to note that the system is in a rudimentary stage and at this point simply represents an attempt to objectify, quantify, and validate specific items which, in my experience, I have found clinically useful. For example, clients are often observed to exhibit unusual behavior while making their collage, such as gluing one picture on top of another, randomly placing pictures in an upside down position, and tearing rather than cutting out pictures. Pictures with little relationship to each other and fragmented arrangements are often observed in the collages of acutely psychotic clients, whereas depressed clients tend to use fewer cuttings and make collages that are bleak and sterile in their overall effect. When pictures of people are included in the collage, they frequently offer clues as to the client's sense of self, prevailing mood, and attitude toward others. While two of the studies reported here involved determining the construct and predictive validity of specific items, future research will be aimed at determining how item scores can be weighed and combined. so that composite scores can be obtained and used.

The scoring system, which is in Appendix N, is based upon the theoretical formulation of Azima and Azima,[7] an organizing framework suggested by Schlesinger,[8] the clinical data of Buck and Provancher,[4] and as noted above, my personal clinical experience. Azima and Azima drew an important conceptual relationship between projective tests as used by psychologists, and projective material (such as the collage) produced in occupational therapy, noting that the theoretical and applied aspects of the former are applicable to the latter. In an attempt to provide a conceptual framework for psychological testing, Schlesinger outlines three sources of information the psychologist has at his disposal: the client's behavior in the testing situation, the content of the client's test responses, and the formal aspects of the tests, including quantitative scores. In line with these distinctions, the scoring system is divided into three sections: formal variables, content variables, and the client-therapist interactional variables.

Because one part of the scoring system involves the assessment of client-therapist interactional variables, when using the system it is suggested that the collage be administered as previously outlined. Further, if research groups are to be compared, then all subjects should be given *identical packets* of magazines and construction paper.

Reliability

Consistent with its stage of development, reliability studies called for the determining of inter-rater agreement in scoring collages with the system. Such reliability findings are available. In one study (Study B) the collages of 10 clients were selected and scored using the system. Five of the collages were used for practice and discussion of scoring problems between two raters. The remaining five collages were scored independently. From the five collages scored, the raters achieved 92%

agreement on the formal variables and 94% agreement on the content variables. A second reliability study, in which the collages for the final sample were used, yielded highly consistent results.

Research

In this section three studies will be reviewed, each of which was designed to contribute to the theoretical and applied basis of the magazine picture collage. The first study involves an investigation of the collage as a means for clinical-impressionistic inferences, whereas the other two studies directly relate to the scoring system.

Study A

This study was designed to assess the level, types, and accuracy of clinical inferences trained professionals can draw from the collage. The study was initiated from the responses and predictions that were often discussed by the treatment team when the collage was presented at the client's initial conference. Although this process had become somewhat of a tradition, no one had stopped to question the efficacy of this procedure or whether the collage should be used in this way.

In this study, 12 psychiatric workers, representing six disciplines, were asked to distinguish the collages of 12 hospitalized clients from those of 12 paired controls. They were instructed to record descriptive and dynamic features about the client that could be inferred from the collage, and to document those specific aspects of the collage that were used in drawing the inferences.

With respect to distinguishing client collages from control collages, the judges tended to be relatively unsuccessful. On the 12 judges, the selections of only three of the raters were significant using a .06 level of probability. When the ratings of the judges by discipline were compared, the only one found to be significant (p < .05) involved the comparison of the ratings of the clinical psychologists with the ratings of the group as a whole.

To determine the number of times each individual collage was selected as a client collage, a frequency matrix was developed. In reviewing this matrix, it was found that when a collage was selected by nine or more judges it was a client collage; however, all collages selected by two or fewer judges were always control collages. Four of the 12 clients were selected by at least 10 of the judges. A review of the individual cases indicated that of the client group, these four clients were the most severely disturbed, suffering from either acute psychotic episodes or severe bouts of depression. Thus, it was concluded that the judges, on the basis of the collage, were sensitive to more severe forms of psychopathology.

To identify and organize the multitude of inferences the judges drew from the collages and the accuracy of the inferences, a framework used for the organization of diverse psychological data was adopted.[9] This framework consists of the following broad topics, all of which are clinically relevant and are rooted in psychoanalytic theory: thought organization, affect organization, defensive structure, sense of self, quality of object relations, and instinctual conflicts.

The 12 judges drew a total of 88 inferences. While each of the specific categories (ie, thought organization, affect organization) was used, more than one third of the total inferences related to aspects of thought organization. Fewest inferences related to the categories of sense of self and instinctual conflicts.

To determine the accuracy of the derived inferences, two raters, neither of whom had participated in other aspects of the study, were independently furnished 12

Carole Lerner

scoring sheets. On each sheet was included the client's name, a list of the inferences drawn about him, and a set of instructions. The rater was instructed to carefully review each client's psychiatric chart and then to rate the accuracy of the inferences. Each inference was rated on a 3 point scale ranging from supported, through neither supported or contradicted, to contradicted. The results, based upon a pooling of the two raters, were quite dramatic. Of the 88 inferences generated, using material in the client's chart as a criteria, 60 were supported, 22 neither supported or contradicted, and only 6 contradicted.

The final purpose of this study was to identify what it was about the collage that served as a basis for the inference. A classification system based on whether the inference came from formal properties of the collage (ie, number of cuttings, placement of cuttings, overall neatness), the content of the specific cuttings (ie, tone of feeling conveyed by the picture, expression, or activity of the people) or a combination of both, was employed. A review of these findings indicates that, in general, the judges based their inferences on a combination of both formal and content aspects of the collage. Further, if only one of these two aspects is employed, it tends to be the formal aspect.

The major findings in this study may be summarized as follows: "1) in general, experienced psychiatric staff are not able to distinguish hospitalized psychiatric clients from controls solely on the basis of a global impression of the individual's collage; 2) experienced psychiatric staff are highly accurate in deriving varied descriptive and dynamic inferences about a person's collage; 3) the majority of inferences made by the group of judges pertain to the nature and quality of the subject's thinking; and 4) in drawing inferences these judges relied on a combination of both formal and content aspects of the collage."[5]

Study B

In this study an attempt was made to investigate the construct validity of scale items by identifying individual indexes that differentiated collages made by psychiatric inpatients from those made by a control group, and to relate the scores to certain dimensions of personality.

The sample included 24 subjects divided into two groups, each consisting of six males and six females. One group included 12 clients who had recently been admitted to a psychiatric unit. The diagnosis of these clients varied, ranging from severe anxiety and depressive reaction to and including borderline states. The control group included 12 individuals who were each individually paired with the psychiatric clients on the variables of age, sex, educational level, socio-economic status, and marital status.

Using chi square analysis, it was found that the two groups differed significantly on the following scores: number of cuttings, number of people, number of animals, overall balance, framing, central theme, and search for direction and reassurance. "Specifically, the client group used fewer cuttings, chose more cuttings with animals and fewer with people, were less able to achieve an overall balance, and produced collages that lacked a central theme."[6] Further, the client group seeks directions more frequently and requires more expression of reassurance that the task is being completed correctly. Although no statistically significant differences on the other variables were found, certain trends are evident. "For example, colors appearing in the client collages tend to be more subdued and when pictures of humans are included the humans were often in a state of relative inactivity. Controls tended to use shaping (cutting in a contour fashion or in detail around the subject) more often than the clients. In general the control collages were neater. Tearing out a picture, using excessive glue, and cutting in a haphazard fashion were observed in several client collages but rarely appeared in a control collage. Finally, whereas only controls took less than 30 minutes to complete their collage, only clients required more than an hour."[6]

Study C

Study C[10] also involved an investigation of the construct validity of the scoring system. In this study I attempted to determine if specific scores were sensitive to change in psychiatric clients concomitànt with hospitalization.

The sample consisted of 18 clients admitted to the same psychiatric facility described in the previous studies. Included in the sample were eight males and 10 females. Clients ranged in age from 18 to 59 years with a mean of 27.9 years. While various diagnoses were represented, the majority of clients were diagnosed schizophrenic. Length of hospitalization was relatively short, ranging from 20 days to 9 months with a mean of 5.1 months.

In this study each client made two collages, one soon after admission and another shortly prior to discharge. On both occasions, the client was presented identical and intact issues of 4 magazines (*McCall's, Playboy, Better Homes and Gardens*, and *People*) and eight different colored sheets of 29×45 cm (12×18 inches) construction paper of which the subject was to choose one. Immediately after the client completed the collage, the occupational therapist recorded the following: 1) time taken to complete the collage; 2) repeated directions requested; and 3) reassurances requested by the client. In addition, upon discharge the psychiatrist most familiar with the client was requested to indicate on a four point rating scale the degree of improvement (no, slight, good, significant).

Changes in the various individual scores were subjected to the chi square analysis. The results are presented for the format, content, and client-examiner variable in Tables 9.1, 9.2, and 9.3 respectively. Although several of these findings are significant, other important but non-significant findings are obscured and not reflected in the statistics. For example, *fragmentation* in Table 9.1 shows that nine clients on their first collages manifested signs indicative of this score. A review of the second collages indicates that eight of these clients no longer show such signs. This finding is most important, yet is not reflected in the statistics. Therefore, to better address the question of the sensitivity of the collage to changes in psychiatric clients after hospitalization and to shed light on the psychological processes underlying various items in the scoring system, discussion will be focused on an analysis of individual items.

With respect to the *number of cuttings,* a review of Table 9.1 reveals that a significant number of clients changed. Upon closer examination eight used more cuttings on their second collages, whereas five used fewer cuttings. Buck and Provancher found a relative paucity of cuttings in their client sample and interpreted the finding in terms of concept of psychic energy.[4] That is, they argued, "If it is assumed that any individual has but a limited quantity of psychic energy available, then when energy is expended to ward off alien impulses and painful feelings, little is left for investment in the outer world."[4] In a previous study, I also found that clients, as opposed to controls, made collages with fewer cuttings. From a slightly different theoretical vantage point, however, this may indicate a sign of remission marked by a reinstating of previously faltering controls and defenses. To reconcile these somewhat different interpretations, each client's

Carole Lerner

TABLE 9.1

CHI SQUARE VALUES BETWEEN COLLAGES FOR FORMAL VARIABLES*

	# of clients who changed†	X^2	P
Background Color	17	6.3	<.01
Number of Cuttings	13	1.4	<.10
Color of Most Cuttings	6	.7	NS
Overall Color Effect	6	.7	NS
Manner Cuttings are Cut Out	7	.3	NS
Degree of Neatness	10	.1	NS
Pictures Upside-down or Sideways	2		NS
Overlapping of Cuttings	8	.1	NS
Pictures Glued Completely Over Others	5	1.4	NS
Overall Balance	3		NS
Fragmentation	9		NS
Dimensionalizing	1		NS
Cutting Out & Use of Words	7	.3	NS
Framing	3		NS

*Being assessed here are the number of clients whose scores changed from the first to the second collage.
†Out of a total of 18.

TABLE 9.2

CHI SQUARE VALUES BETWEEN COLLAGES FOR CONTENT VARIABLES*

	# of clients who changed	X^2	P
Number of People	13	1.4	<.10
Age & Sex of People	3		NS
Feelings People Expressed	2		NS
Activity State of People	5	1.4	NS
Emphasis on Body Parts	2		NS
People Clothed in Costumes, etc.	—		NS
Achievement of Central Theme	7	.3	NS
Number of Animals	7	.3	NS
Emphasis on Objects	8	.1	NS
Type of Objects	11	.3	NS
Use of Appropriate Title	7	.3	NS

*Being assessed here are the number of clients whose scores changed from the first to the second collage.

TABLE 9.3

CHI SQUARE VALUES BETWEEN COLLAGES
FOR PATIENT—EXAMINER VARIABLES*

	# of clients who changed	X^2	P
Seeking Repetition of Directions	7	.3	NS
Seeking Reassurance	6	.7	NS
Time Taken to Complete	8	.1	NS

Being assessed here are the number of clients whose scores changed from the first to the second collage.

individual hospital chart was reviewed. Each of the five clients whose second collage had fewer cuttings had been hospitalized in the midst of an acute psychotic episode, and as the hospitalization progressed, there was a remission of the psychosis. Thus, for these clients, the drop in cuttings accompanied a movement toward greater control. By contrast, many of the clients whose second collage revealed an increase in cuttings were hospitalized with a variety of symptoms including depression, and, as their hospitalization progressed, a lifting of the depression was noted. Thus, in these cases the number of cuttings seemed more related to the client's affective state rather than the issue of control. An increase in cuttings from the first to the second collage is illustrated in Figures 9.1 and 9.2.

The findings regarding *degree of neatness, pictures glued on upside down or sideways,* and *pictures glued completely over another* are not statistically significant. Nevertheless, changes found on these items are noteworthy. Of the 10 clients whose neatness was judged differently on the second collage, nine were rated as having neater collages. Two clients on their first collage glued pictures in an upside down or sideways fashion. On the second collage, such placements were absent. Again, both clients were hospitalized in acute psychotic states and the observed collage changes coincided with their remissions. To *glue one picture completely over another* is unusual and peculiar, a process which has come to be associated with a psychotic level of functioning. Of the five clients whose score on this item changed, four displayed completely overlapping placements on their first collage but not on their second. The fifth client changed in the opposite direction; however, there was little information·in the client's hospital chart to help explain this shift.

Five of the 18 clients were unable to achieve an overall *balance* on their first collages. Of these five, three were able to achieve balance with their second collages. In previous work, Lerner and Ross found that this score clearly distinguished client collages from the collages of controls.[6] In the discussion of the finding, we felt that such ego functions as planning ahead, thinking before acting, and tolerating frustration were reflected in the score. A review of the clients' charts in this study supports the original speculation, in that the consistent behavioral changes were noted among the clients whose scores changed.

Fragmentation and *dimensionalization* were included in the scoring system as further indicators of quality of thinking. In the earlier study, these items did not distinguish the client and control group.[6] In neither group were these processes

Carole Lerner

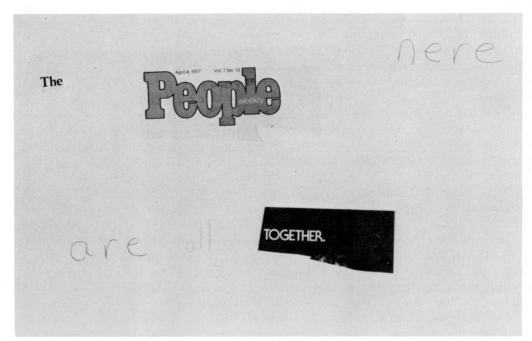

Fig 9.1: Paucity of cuttings.

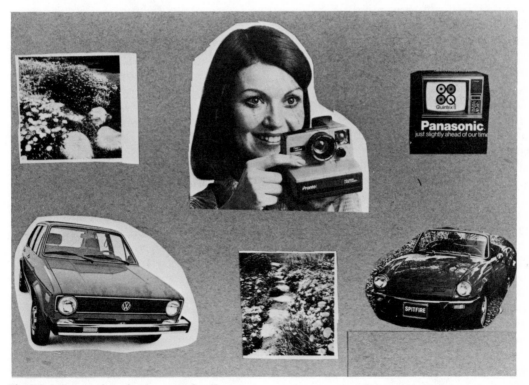

Fig 9.2: More cuttings in the second collage.

The Magazine Picture Collage

evident, probably owing to the consideration that the client group consisted of basically neurotic and character disorders. In this present sample, which by contrast included 13 clients diagnosed as schizophrenic, fragmentation was found in the initial collages of nine clients. Of these nine clients, the second collages of eight changed in that fragmentation was no longer evident. Fragmentation is evident in the first collage, Figure 9.3. It is absent in the second collage, Figure 9.4. One client's first collage was scored for *dimensionalization;* this was not scored on the second collage.

The final item among the formal variables is *framing.* Changes with regard to this item were found in the collages of three clients. In each case, framing was observed in the first collage but not in the second. From a psychodynamic perspective, framing may be viewed as an attempt to impose external boundaries or controls on the basis of one sensing that internal controls cannot be relied upon. Typically, the need to monitor, regulate, and control the outer world is found in individuals who experience their inner controls as tenuous and shaky, chaotic, turbulent, and in a state of disarray. If this conceptualization is accurate, then one would expect that clients who no longer find it necessary to impose outside limits will also feel less chaotic and more able to regulate their own thoughts, affects, urges, and behaviors. A review of the hospital records of the three clients whose framing score changed lent strong support to this proposition.

The first item among the content variables involves the *number of people* appearing in the cuttings. In the earlier study the collages made by clients contained significantly fewer people than the collages made by the controls.[6] A review of Table 9.2 indicates that 13 of the 18 clients changed on this item. Whereas the second collages of 8 clients had more people, the second collages of five clients had fewer. This finding is puzzling, especially in light of the results of the previous study. However, when comparing changes in the number of people with changes in the total number of cuttings, those clients who had fewer people in their second collages also had fewer cuttings in their second collages. This relationship between number of people and total number of cuttings is not as clear among those clients whose second collages included more people.

With respect to *achievement of a central theme,* five clients on their initial collages were able to construct their collages around a central theme, while 13 were not able to do so. Of these 13, six achieved a central theme with their second collages. This finding is believed to be reflective of psychological changes concomitant with hospitalization. In the earlier study, the collages of the control subjects included a central theme significantly more often than did the collages of the clients.[6] On the basis of both studies, the achievement of a central theme requires that the individual be able to organize and integrate a variety of detail into a meaningful whole that can be shared with another. No central theme is evident in the first collage, Figure 9.3. Central theme is evident in the second collage, Figure 9.4.

In Table 9.2, the content variable which relates to the *number of animals* included in the cuttings, the score of seven clients changed, with five having fewer animals on their second collages, and two having more. The direction of the change (toward fewer animals) is consistent with earlier research.[6] In the earlier study, the controls included significantly less animals than did the clients. The original finding was interpreted as indicating a preference for relationships that involved less commitment, less demand, and greater security. The clients in the current study moved in the direction of including more people and less animals in their second

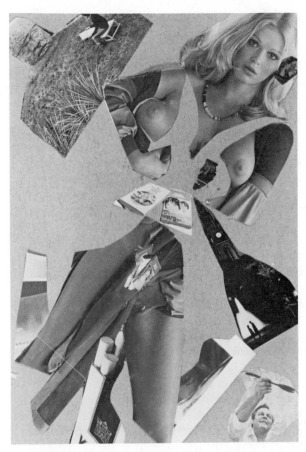

Fig 9.3: Fragmentation and no central theme.

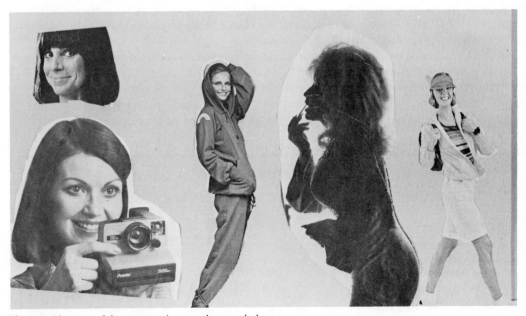

Fig 9.4: Absence of fragmentation, and central theme present.

The Magazine Picture Collage

collages. This could indicate a greater readiness to trust, to relate to, and to humanize their world.

With respect to *use of appropriate title,* 12 clients either did not title or inappropriately titled their first collages. Six of these 12 clients were able to appropriately title their second collages. To appropriately title a collection of pictures and words, necessitates organizational and integrative capacities. An inspection of the hospital records of those clients who changed on this variable supported this inference.

Three items comprise the *client-therapist section.* The first two items are designed to assess a certain aspect of the interaction, specifically asking for repeated directions and seeking reassurance. This may be considered reflective of a tendency to seek dependent relationships. With respect to the first item, the scores of seven clients changed from an asking on the first collage to not asking for more directions on the second. A similar shift occurred with item 2. That is, of the six clients in which the change was noted, five moved in the direction of not seeking reassurance. Compared, these two items suggest that several clients within the larger sample, over their period of hospitalization, moved toward greater independence and more autonomous functioning.

In the final part of this study, an attempt was made to relate changes in scale items with the degree of clinical improvement. On the basis of ratings made at the time of discharge, one client was judged as not improved, eight as slightly improved, seven as having shown good improvement, and two as significantly improved.

These sub-groups were compared with each other in terms of the overall number of items in which change was found. The mean number of items in which change was observed, by sub-group, is presented in Table 9.4.

Although the number of cases per sub-group is unfortunately low, a review of Table 9.4 indicates a marked difference in the mean number of scale items (5 vs. 13.5) between the one client who is rated as not improved and the two clients who are judged as having improved significantly. Of note here is that this finding pertains only to the sheer number of items that changed and does not involve a consideration of the direction of the change.

To determine if specific items were directly related to level of improvement, a frequency matrix was developed in which each variable was examined in terms of scale changes for each client per improvement category. A review of the frequency matrix reveals no discernable patterns. That is, when looked at strictly quantitatively, not one item change is related to degree of improvement.

TABLE 9.4

MEAN NUMBER OF ITEMS CHANGED PER IMPROVEMENT CATEGORY

Category	# of clients	x̄ n of changes
Significantly Improved	2	13.5
Good Improvement	7	9.1
Slight Improvement	8	11.9
No Improvement	1	5.0

In contrast with the quantitative analysis, when each item is examined qualitatively in terms of the direction of the change, several indentifiable and interesting patterns emerge. For example, with respect to *number of cuttings*, a linear relationship is found between an increase in cuttings (as opposed to a decrease in cuttings) and level of improvement. Specifically, 100% of the clients judged as significantly improved showed an increase of cuttings; 80% (four of five) of the clients who revealed good improvement showed an increase of cuttings on the second collage, and 50% (three of six) clients judged as slightly improved changed in the direction of an increase of cuttings. With respect to the items, *degree of neatness* and *number of people*, similar linear relationships were found between changes in the direction of greater neatness, increase in cuttings with people, and level of judged clinical improvement.

Clinical Implications

Study A[5] represents an attempt to study the validity and usefulness of the collage when it is approached in an impressionistic way, as is the case in most clinical situations. That is, an attempt was made to ascertain the level of clinical assessment at which the collage can be most accurately and helpfully used.

In keeping with this purpose, Weiner made an important distinction between the assessment of personality variables or processes as contrasted with the prediction of behavior.[11] I have noted that personality variables, such as ego structures and core intra-psychic dynamics, are directly measurable by means of conventional and current psychological diagnostic methods. The prediction of behavior is more complex, and depends on more than an evaluation of the person. An evaluation of the relative impact of significant interacting situational variables is also needed. Holt, in an illuminating discussion of the controversey over clinical versus statistical prediction, made a similar point.[12]

Therefore, it is not surprising that the judges, despite being experienced psychiatric workers, had difficulty distinguishing hospitalized psychiatric clients from non-client controls strictly on the basis of the collage. The need and decision to hospitalize is based upon more than personality factors. Situational variables such as availability of family and community supports, skill of outside therapists, and stability in employment are typically considered.

By contrast, in this study, the level of accuracy the judges attained with regard to their descriptive and dynamic inferences is striking. It might be recalled that of the 88 inferences generated, 60 were clearly supported by information in the client's chart, six were contraindicated, and 22 could not be supported or refuted. In carefully scrutinizing the latter 22 inferences, it was found that most were so subtle that their verification required a more intimate understanding of the client than was available from existing hospital chart material.

In summary, findings from this study indicate that the collage, when used in a clinical-impressionistic way by skilled and experienced psychiatric workers, does yield valid inferences, and that the collage is best used as a method of assessing psychological processes (ie, quality of thinking, nature of object relatedness, experience of self) in contrast with attempting to assign a diagnosis or predict behavior.

Research and Theoretical Implications

Studies B[6] and C[10] were designed with the intent of assessing the construct validity and research usefulness of a system for objectively scoring the collage. In developing the scale, an attempt to organize and quantify formal and substantative dimensions of the collage was found to have clinical value. Findings from both studies have contributed to an understanding of the psychological processes underlying many of the specific items, refinements in the scale as a whole, and a greater appreciation of the potential uses of the scale.

Behaviors Assessed

The following items were included in the scoring system to assess the individual's level and style of *cognitive-perceptual functioning:* manner in which most cuttings were cut out, degree of neatness, pictures glued on upside down or sideways, overlapping of cuttings, pictures glued completely over others, achievement of an overall balance, fragmentation, dimensionalizing, achievement of a central theme, and use of appropriate title. Cognitive and perceptual functioning refers to the quality of an individual's thinking and his distinctive way of perceiving the external environment. It involves various facets of mental functioning, including attention, memory, language development, concept formation, and integrative capacities. The interest is in the individual's unique thought style. For example, the way in which tasks are approached, the degree of emphasis accorded neatness and accuracy, the client's reaction to frustration, and the effects of various conditions (structure vs. non-structure) upon thinking and perceiving. Also included under this heading would be indications of disturbed thinking and distorted perceptions.

Several items were intended and found to measure what might be termed *nature and quality of defenses*. This heading refers to the individual's openess to new experiences, as well as his characteristic way of managing feelings and impulses. Items assessing this psychological process include number of pictures or cuttings, cutting out and use of words, and framing.

Closely related to the quality of defenses is the third major psychological dimension, *affect organization*. This refers to feelings, and includes the way in which the feeling is experienced and expressed. The concern is with predominant affects, and with the individual's range of feelings. The following items relate to this topic: *color of most cuttings, overall color effect, feelings people expressed,* and *activity state of people.*

Two final factors involved in the choice of scale items were *sense of self* and *quality of object relations.* Sense of self refers to those conscious and unconscious identities and roles that comprise the individual's experience of the self and that help direct his actions. It involves the person's self-image, including wishes and fears, and the extent to which he accepts it or externalizes it onto others. Closely related to sense of self is how the person experiences others. This refers to both the content and the structure of relational tendencies. For example, the therapist is interested in the types of relationships formed (ie, cooperative, competitive, dependent) and in the individual's ability to see relationships as stable and long-lasting as contrasted with fleeting and transitory. Items designed to assess these factors include *number of people, age and sex of people, people clothed in costumes, uniforms or unusual attire, number of animals, emphasis on objects, seeking repetition of directions* and *seeking reassurances* of doing task correctly.

Revisions in the Scale

Data from Studies B[6] and C[10] have led to several revisions in the scoring system. For example, Item 1, formal variables, pertains to the *color of construction paper* selected. In Study B, this item did not distinguish the client from the control group, and in Study C significant changes were noted; however, the changes appeared totally random. Because of these observations the item was deleted.

The item, *emphasis on body part,* was included with the intent of determining whether the individual was preoccupied with a certain part of the body and whether this would be manifest on the collage. For example, it has been found that clients with paranoid pathology frequently attune to eyes. In both studies this item proved ineffective. Recent advances in psychoanalytic object relation theory[13] have pointed to a major distinction between individuals who relate to others as total human beings and those who relate to others as part objects (less than totally human). Based on this consideration this item was revised as an emphasis on body parts (without specifying the part) or full human figures.

The item, *type of objects,* was included with the intent of assessing dominant themes in an individual's personality make-up. For example, an individual who constructs a collage laden with cuttings of food would be expected to manifest many oral-infantile features. Although consideration of the non-peopled aspects of a collage is important, for research purposes this item was found to contribute little. Thus, it was decided to exclude it.

Future Research

The scale so far has been used in two types of studies. One involved a comparison of client collages with those of controls, while the other involved an attempt to assess changes in psychiatric clients concomitant with hospitalization. Future research is to apply the scoring system to the collages of clients in various diagnostic groups (ie, schizophrenics, borderlines, depressive reactions) with the intent of determining if specific patterns are associated with particular diagnoses. If specific patterns can be identified, then clearly, the scoring system would have much to contribute to differential diagnosis.

Conclusion

Increasingly, the magazine picture collage is being used in psychiatric occupational therapy settings as an important assessment technique. The only research regarding this technique consists basically of clinical reports. As a result of this, a series of studies designed to contribute to the theoretical and applied bases of the collage was carried out. One study involved an investigation of the collage as a source of clinical-impressionistic inferences. The other studies investigated the construct validity of a system devised for objectively scoring the collage. Based on the results of these three studies and my clinical experience, this chapter has attempted to outline the clinical and research uses for the magazine picture collage.

References

1. Hall D: Collage: The Art of Painting with Paper & Paste. Tustin, Walter Foster Art Service, 1960.
2. Rapaport D: The theoretical implications of diagnostic testing. Congr Int Psychiatric 2:241-271, 1950.
3. Holmes C, Bauer W: Establishing an occupational therapy department in a community hospital. A J Occu Ther 24:219-221, 1970.
4. Buck RE, Provancher MA: Magazine picture collage as an evaluation technique. A J Occu Ther 26:36-39, 1972.
5. Lerner CJ: The magazine picture collage: Its clinical use and validity as an assessment device. A J Occu Ther 33:500-504, 1979.
6. Lerner C, Ross G: The magazine picture collage: Development of an objective scoring system. A J Occu Ther 31:156-161, 1977.

7. Azima H, Azima FJ: Outline of a dynamic theory of occupational therapy. A J Occu Ther 13:215-221, 1959.
8. Schlesinger H: Interaction of dynamic and reality factors in the diagnostic testing interview. Bull Men Cl 37:459-517, 1973.
9. Applebaum S: A method of reporting psychological test findings. Bull Men Cl 36:535-545, 1972.
10. Lerner C, Waltman G: Changes in collages during hospitalization. (In preparation for publication).
11. Weiner I: Approaches to Rorschach validation. In Rickers-Ovsiankina M (ed): Rorschach Psychology, ed 2. New York, Robert E Krieger, 1977.
12. Holt R: Yet another look at clinical and statistical prediction; or is clinical psychology worthwhile? Am Psychol 25:337-349, 1970.
13. Kernberg O: Borderline Conditions and Pathological Narcissism. New York, Jason Aronson, 1976.

Carole Lerner

10
Comprehensive Assessment Process: A Group Evalution

Frances Ehrenberg, O.T.R.

Historical Development
Rationale

This chapter is a description of an assessment process used by occupational therapists in a short-term, acute care psychiatric facility. Prior to the initiation of the evaluation program in 1975, occupational therapy consisted of daily client "activities" programs. Progress notes were recorded in each client's medical chart. Treatment planning was not done systematically; nor was it based on any formal, structured client evaluation.

This occupational therapy assessment program has been designed to evaluate overall client behaviors as efficiently and effectively as possible; the resulting information provides the basis for individualized treatment plans. An examination of previously published techniques for evaluating specific client skills reveals that no single evaluation encompasses all the critical areas of individual client behaviors observed in the occupational therapy setting.[1-8] Activities of daily living[4] or work skills[1-3,6,8] are usually emphasized.

Behaviors Assessed

Using some existing procedures for reference, I decided to evaluate each client in terms of seven general characteristics:[9]

1. *Quality of one-to-one interactions:* Ability to be self-disclosing, cooperative, and responsive during interviews; eye contact.
2. *Insight:* Recognition of dysfunctional symptoms.
3. *Self-esteem:* Being on good terms with the super ego.[10]
4. *Use of leisure time:* Productive use of free time; ie, when not working or in school.
5. *Basic living skills:* Independent functioning in the areas of personal hygiene, child care, food and money management, cleaning, laundering, sewing, transportation, minor home repairs, etc.[11]
6. *Work skills:* Demonstration of skills needed for productive performance at work and/or school.
7. *Interpersonal skills:* Productive and constructive functioning in group situations.

Administration

All clients admitted to any of the three adult psychiatric inpatient units (68 total beds) are referred to occupational therapy. The most common presenting diagnoses among the clients are: paranoid psychosis; schizo-affective psychosis; bipolar affective disorder; psychotic depression; reactive depression; adolescent adjustment reaction; and personality disorder. During a two-week assessment period, each client is interviewed twice and observed in group activities. The Initial Evaluation Interview (Appendix O) includes general information on educational background, work history, and use of leisure time at home. This interview is also used to evaluate the client's one-to-one interaction skills, level of insight, and self-esteem.[11]

The second interview covers activities of daily living skills (Appendix P). The responses indicate whether a client is independent in a specific area or dependent upon others; the client's desire to attend a specialized activity of daily living group to learn or improve specific skills is also determined. Questions focus on personal hygiene, child care, food and money management, homemaking tasks, sewing, minor home repairs, and transportation.[11]

Clients are interviewed individually in a reasonably distraction-free private area. The client's primary occupational therapist (registered occupational theraptist, certified occupational therapy assistant, or occupational therapy technician) explains the general purpose of the interviews, reads the questions aloud, and records the client's responses. If necessary, the Activities of Daily Living Questionnaire can be completed by a relatively intact, self-motivated client; in such cases the therapist and client jointly review the form to clarify any ambiguous or incomplete responses and allow the client to ask questions (see Appendix Q, Standardized Assessment Procedure, for complete outline of the intitial interview procedure).

These inteviews help the therapist to establish rapport with the client, appraise the client's psychological status, reinforce and encourage the client's participation in treatment planning, and gather specific information.[9,12,13]

In addition to the interviews, clients are assigned to evaluation groups. The client is told that the occupational therapy staff wants to observe his work and interactions skills to determine whether any of the department's other treatment groups might be beneficial. Except for severely anxious or resistant cases, this evaluation is conducted within two weeks of hospital admission. During a one week period, a closed group (ie, no new members are added for the duration of that group) of five to 10 clients meets for 3 one-hour sessions. The three sessions involve a carefully structured series of tasks which make increasing demands on each client's ability or willingness to interact with other group members. Two therapists observe and take notes on each client in the evaluation group (two registered occupational therapists or one registered occupational therapist and one certified occupational therapy assistant). The registered occupational therapist is in charge of the group. Two therapists are used to enhance the reliability of the observations.[11] At the end of each day of assessment, the two therapists discuss each client's behavior; after dividing the client group between them, each therapist independently enters these observations in the occupational therapy charts.

Session 1. The goals of the evaluation group are reviewed with the clients. In order to ensure regular attendance, clients are requested to reschedule any leaves of absence or other appointments. Before the group task is begun, the therapists introduce themselves and ask each member to do likewise.

The first assignment is to construct a mosaic tile hot plate—a simple, structured, individual task. Written instructions are provided (Appendix R); a 50 minute time limit is announced. The clients are seated around a large table furnished with the following supplies: enough six-inch square masonite boards and bottles of white

Frances Ehrenberg

glue for each client; four containers of ⅜ inch square ceramic tiles separated according to color: black, white, blue, and maroon (the choice of four colors allows some creativity). These containers, masking tape, and three pens are shared by the group. The group leader will initially refer a client back to written instructions if there are questions. If the client appears unable to follow the written directions, a staff member will give oral instructions. If oral directions are not understood, a staff member will demonstrate the procedure. The remaining time is announced after 25 minutes have elapsed, and when only five minutes remain. Clients' questions about the remaining time will be answered at any point during the session. Those who do not complete the task within the allotted time are allowed to finish later that same day.

The mosaic tile hot plate task was chosen because it could be completed by clients with widely varying levels of function. According to Wertham and Golden,[14] it is a "useful diagnostic aid, can be quickly done, [and] is independent of language. . . ." Almost all clients are able to complete the tile hot plate—though quality varies markedly.

Session 2, Part 1: The therapist intiates name introductions after clients assemble. Clients use the first half hour of the session to complete the grouting on their tile hot plates, while the therapists continue to assess work skills and casual interactions. The group members are told to cover the work table with newspaper and collect their hot plates. They are again handed written instuctions (Appendix R) and given a 30 minute time limit. The remaining time is announced after 15 minutes have elapsed, and on request. Clients are provided with a container of white grout and six grout colors. There are also enough paper cups and tongue depressors (for stirring the grout) for each client; the room contains a sink. Again, a client asking for assistance is first referred back to the directions; the staff's oral input and/or demonstrations are provided only when necessary. After 30 minutes have passed, the group is asked to put their hot plates away to dry. Incompleted tasks may be finished at another time during activities therapy.

Session 2, Part 2: The clients now begin the second assignment of the evaluation group process. The group is asked to choose one of the following three activities (Appendix Q): 1) An individually completed magazine collage with the theme of how each client would like to be viewed by others. Clients select one or more pictures from magazines provided by occupational therapy and glue them onto a piece of construction paper. At the end of the session, clients are asked to discuss the meaning of the pictures. 2) A group mural of a Utopian Place—ie, a place of ideal perfection. The clients are given a large sheet of paper and magic markers for drawing. At the end of the session, each client discusses his individual contribution. 3) Hypothetical Problem—the clients are told they will be given a problem which has nothing to do with their personal or emotional problems and is not mathematical. The group must solve the problem. After repeating the titles of the activities, the leader gives the group the remaining time (about 20 minutes) to decide on the third day's tasks (the staff is not involved in their decision). Clients usually have to be reminded about not involving staff members.

The completion of each activity requires varying degrees of group interaction—ie, the individual magazine collage requires minimal interaction, the group mural—minimal to moderate, and the hypothetical problem—moderate to extensive. Therefore, both the chosen task and the client's expression of the choice—ie, whether the client spontaneously expresses a choice, waits to be called upon by another group member, professes indifference, acquiesces easily, debates—

are significant. While not used specifically as projective techniques, the collage and mural may be used to make inferences regarding the client's psychodynamics.[5,15,16]

On the very rare occasions when a group is unable to reach a decision, the evaluation group leader selects the magazine collage, because it is the most structured and potentially least threatening task (in terms of self disclosure and interaction)

Session 3. The group's selected activity is completed on the third and final day of the evaluation program. The methods of implementation are:

1. *Individual Magazine Collage:* The therapist places a variety of magazines (*National Geographic, Life, Ebony, Sports Illustrated, Family Circle,* and others), a 12 x 18 inch sheet of white construction paper, a pair of scissors for each client, and four bottles of rubber cement on the table. After the name introductions, the clients are instructed to select pictures from the magazines that best illustrate how they would like to be seen by others. The group members are told they have 40 minutes to find the pictures and glue them onto the construction paper. The clients are told when only 10 minutes are left. After 40 minutes have elapsed, each client is asked to explain the significance of their chosen pictures with other group members.[5]

2. *Group Mural—Utopian Place:* Before the group assembles on the final day, the evaluation group leader places a large sheet of white paper (about 3 x 5 feet, depending on the number of clients in the group) and magic markers in a variety of colors and tip widths on the table. After name introductions, the clients are told they have 40 minutes to complete the mural. The group must decide whether the actual drawing will be an individual or group effort. The chairs are removed from around the table to allow for easier access to the paper and markers. The remaining time is announced at the midway point. After 40 minutes have elapsed, the clients are instructed to: a) affix the mural to a wall; b) discuss the significance of their individual contributions to the mural; c) decide what should be done with the mural—eg, display it on one of the wards or in the occupational therapy department. The clients are also asked to evaluate their functioning as a group. The staff can then determine how clients perceive the group process; eg, which clients may be either overtly or covertly angry because other client(s) are too controlling.

3. *Hypothetical Problem:* After the reintroductions are completed, the evaluation group leader hands each client a pencil and an individual exercise sheet (Appendix S).* A volunteer from the group is asked to read the instructions. Participants are told they have 10 minutes to individually rank the items listed. After 10 minutes have passed, the group is given 30 minutes to arrive at a consensus on the rank order of the items. Time reminders are given after 15 minutes have elapsed and when only five minutes are left. When the task is completed, the participants are asked to evaluate their performance as a group. Prior to terminating the session, the "correct" NASA list of items is read aloud (Appendix T). Before the clients return to their wards, they are told that their primary occupational therapist will meet with each of them individually to discuss the results of the evaluation and subsequent treatment goals.

In addition to the previously described procedures, clients usually participate in an activities therapy program while they are hospitalized. These sessions facilitate the informal assessment of work and interaction skills; these observations are added

---

An alternate hypothetical problem can be found in Jones JE, Pfeiffer JW (eds): The 1975 Annual Handbook for Group Facilitators. La Jolla, CA, Univ Assoc, 1975.

Frances Ehrenberg

to those noted during the formal assessment process. The activities groups meet five days per week for one-hour sessions. An occupational therapist who is familiar with the client's diagnosis and ward behaviors encourages the client to choose an activity. Activities may include crafts, reading, helping the staff organize supplies, etc.

Aside from being therapeutic, the activities group presents an opportunity to supplement the evaluation group observations. The activities group provides a much less demanding, more relaxed milieu than that of the evaluation group, thus enhancing the potential variety of behaviors that may be used to assess "the patient's level of mental and physical functioning in occupational therapy."[7]

The Evaluation Report

Evaluation observations are recorded at the end of the assessment period, and a checklist (Appendix U) is included in the client's medical chart. Specific behaviors are grouped under four major categories: General Appearance; Interaction Skills; Work Skills; and Activities of Daily Living. The first three categories include 26 specific behaviors which are rated as "good" or "needs improvement":

1. *Grooming:* The quality of personal hygiene and appropriateness of dress.
2. *Level of awareness:* Is the client responsive to stimuli in his immediate surroundings (conversations, questions, noxious stimuli)?
3. *Orientation:* In relation to person, place, date.
4. *Affect:* The character and range of the client's emotional expression.
5. *Motor level:* The level of activity displayed by the client; eg, slowed, hypomanic.
6. *Self-esteem:* The client's ability to acknowledge and appreciate his personal strengths.
7. *Attendance:* Regular, prompt.
8. *Self-direction (motivation):* The ability of the client to stimulate himself to complete the task.
9. *Task investment:* The client's expressed or inferred interest in a task.
10. *Independence:* The ability to work on a task without requesting staff or peer assistance.
11. *Concentration:* The ability to focus and maintain attention on the task for a prescribed time limit.
12. *Following instructions:* Competence in following written, oral, and/or demonstrated instructions.
13. *Problem solving:* The capacity to find solutions to difficulties that interfere with the efficient and effective completion of a task.
14. *Decision-making:* The ability to make choices or judgments in selecting a task or subtask; eg, choosing materials to complete a task.
15. *Frustration tolerance:* The ability to cope with delayed gratification.
16. *Work tolerance:* The ability to work on a task during an entire treatment session.
17. *Planning/Organizing:* The ability to develop a planned, systematic method or approach to a task.
18. *Workmanship:* The quality of a client's work.

19. *Relationship to authority:* The quality of a client's interaction with staff members in their role as authority figures.
20. *Eye contact:* The ability to make and maintain eye contact during interactions.
21. *Effective use of verbal and nonverbal expression:* The presence or absence of correspondence between the client's verbal and nonverbal expressions of emotion.
22. *Casual interaction:* The character of nonspecific, chance spoken interchanges between a client and the staff or other client(s).
23. *Meaningful interactions:* The character of significant, purposeful spoken interchanges between a client and the staff or other client(s).
24. *Self-assertion:* The client's capacity for forceful or bold self-expression.
25. *Group membership:* The character and extent of the client's spoken interactions in the specific context of their role as a group member.
26. *Leadership:* The ability of a client to manage and/or guide others.

Treatment Program

At the end of the assessment period (interviews and groups), individual treatment plans are written and discussed with each client. The client is then assigned to the appropriate treatment groups, which range from relatively intense group experiences; eg, communication-task group; work group, to more traditional treatments such as activities therapy. The following five groups are offered:

Activities of Daily Living. This consists of a series of one-hour sessions in the following areas: application of make-up; nutrition; hand and machine sewing; cleaning and laundering; using a bank; budgeting; smart shopping; minor home repairs; getting a driver's license; public transportation (see Appendix O). A three-hour cooking group which focuses on meal planning and preparation is also available. When appropriate, an occupational therapist will take a client into the community to go grocery shopping or use the public transportation system.

Activities Therapy. This provides daily one-hour treatment groups tailored to a client's specific need(s). Goals might include: increasing self-esteem; developing vocational interests; improving the quality of casual interaction; improving general work skills.[17]

Communication-Task Group. This is designed to increase insight, self-awareness, assertiveness, self-esteem, self-expression, etc, through structured exercises.[18-20] (Three one-hour sessions per week.)

Relaxation Groups. These are used to teach clients to become consciously aware of their body tensions and to learn techniques for their relief.[21] (Two one-hour per week.)

Work Groups. These are organized to help the client learn the kinds of behaviors that are expected in work situations and to begin developing good work habits through 1) basic work experience; eg, horticulture; clerical work; and assembly line projects; and 2) discussion groups; eg, teaching tapes; filling out applications; and role playing.[9] (Three one-hour sessions per week.)

Case Study

The following case study will illustrate the use of the total assessment in developing a comprehensive treatment program.

C.H., a 35 year old, married, white female employed as a librarian, was hospitalized in August, 1979. Although it was the client's first admission to this institution, she had had two previous psychiatric hospitalizations at other institutions. One day after admission, the client's private psychiatrist referred her to occupational therapy with a diagnosis of depression. The occupational therapy department was requested to "assess and treat" the client.

On the second day after her voluntary hospitalization, the client's primary occupational therapist conducted the Initial Evaluation Interview (Table 10.1) in an area apart from the client group. The client also completed the Activities of Daily

TABLE 10.1

INITIAL EVALUATION INTERVIEW

Division _____ HP_____

Name _____C.H._____ Age _____35_____ Marital Status _____M_____

Number of children _____none_____ Ages _____

With whom were you living prior to hospitalization? _____husband_____

What type of residence: Home _____X_____ Apartment _____ Other _____ (Specify) _____

Why are you seeking treatment? _____depression/frustration_____

What would you like to change about yourself? _____increase self-image (self-confidence)_____

EDUCATION

High School grade completed _____graduated_____ College years completed _____under-graduate and graduate completed_____ Major and Degree _____BA, MSLS_____

Vocational Training/Other Education

Do you have future educational plans? If so, what? _____none definite_____

WORK HISTORY

What type of work do you do?/Full or Part Time _____librarian (full-time)_____

How many jobs have you held in the past 10 years? _____one_____

How long has it been since your last employment? _____2 weeks prior to admission_____

If you could work at any type of job, what would it be? _____librarian_____

RECREATIONAL

Approximately how much free time do you have per day? _____most of the day_____

What do you do in your free time for entertainment and/or relaxation?
(Hobbies, sports, community involvement) _____reading, sleeping_____

What do you consider your outstanding abilities, talents, or strong points?
What do you think you do well? _____communication with others_____

What do you think you will be doing 6 months from now? _____back to work/feeling good_____
_____ One year from now? _____back to work/feeling good_____

Therapist _____LS OTR/L_____ Date _____8/27/79_____

Comprehensive Assessment Process

Choose a typical weekday in your life, for example, Monday. Fill in the following schedule which deals with how you spend the day.

This is a typical day prior to the summer (recently, increased sleeping, no activity).

Time Period	Schedule
6 am — 8 am	get up at 7:00
8 am — 10 am	8:15 arrive at work 9:00 begin teaching
10 am — 12 pm	teaching 11:35 lunch
12 pm — 2 pm	lunch 1:00 teaching beings
2 pm — 4 pm	teach until 3:30 work with kids informally to 4:00 - 4:15
4 pm — 6 pm	go to after school meetings or home
6 pm — 8 pm	eat dinner read and do school work
8 pm — 10 pm	read and do school work talk on phone sometimes
10 pm — 12 am	retire any time between 10:00 p.m. and 1:00 a.m.

Living Questionnaire at that time (Table 10.2). The therapist and client reviewed the questionnaire together to clarify the client's activities of daily living requests; ie, to improve her knowledge of nutrition, food preparation, cleaning and laundering, sewing, minor home repairs, budgeting, and smart shopping. The client was also told that she would be participating in the evaluation group during the following week; the therapist briefly explained the group's purpose and goals. The client participated in the formal assessment group at the scheduled time.

During this initial evaluation period it was noted that the client's eye contact, one-to-one interaction, and insight were good. She demonstrated poor self-esteem and poor use of her leisure time at home (increased sleeping time). The client indicated independence in all areas included on the Activities of Daily Living Questionnaire except money management, for which she depended upon her husband.

During the evaluation group, C.H. demonstrated good work skills; ie, she was not easily frustrated, worked during the entire treatment session, planned and organized her tasks, followed written directions independently, and was able to focus and maintain attention. Although she did not socialize with peers or staff members, she was an active group member. She provided logical and spontaneous input during the hypothetical problem—which was her first choice, as well as the group's, during the second part of Session 2.

Frances Ehrenberg

TABLE 10.2

ACTIVITIES OF DAILY LIVING QUESTIONNAIRE

Name _____CH_____ Age ___35___ Date ___8/27/79___ Division ___HP___

Interviewer ___LS___

I. *Personal Hygiene*
   1. Do you take care of your personal hygiene independently? (bathing, care of hair, teeth, nails, shaving) ___yes___

II. *Child Care*
   1. Are there any children living at home with you? ___no___
   2. Which member/members of the family takes care of the child's:
      a. Hygiene _____
      b. Food requirements _____
      c. School requirements _____

III. *Food Management*
   1. How many meals a day do you eat? ___2-3___
   2. Where do you eat most of your meals? (home or out) ___home___
   3. Who does the grocery shopping? ___me___
   4. Do you know how to cook? ___not very well___
   5. How often do you cook? ___4-6 times per week___
   6. What is the number of people you are accustomed to cooking for? ___2___
   7. Who does the majority of the cooking at your residence? ___me___
   8. Would you be interested in attending a group discussion on nutrition in O.T.? ___yes___
   9. Would you be interested in planning and cooking a meal in O.T. with a small group of patients? ___yes___

IV. *Homemaking Tasks*
   1. *Cleaning*
      a. Who does the housekeeping at your residence? ___me___
      b. Do you see a future need for learning or improving cleaning techniques? ___yes___

   2. *Laundering*
      a. Who does the laundry at your residence? ___mostly me___
      b. Do you do your own ironing? ___yes - minimal___
      c. Do you see a future need for learning or improving ironing and laundering techniques? ___yes___

V. *Sewing*
   1. Who does the basic sewing repairs? (hems, buttons, seams) ___me___
   2. Can you use a sewing machine? ___yes___
   3. Are there any sewing techniques you would like to learn? ___machine button holes___

   4. If you answered yes, check which ones you would be interested in learning:
      a. How to sew buttons, hems, seams _____
      b. How to read a pattern _____
      c. How to lay out and cut a pattern _____
      d. How to sew a pattern _____

VI. *Home Repairs*
   1. Who does the basic home repairs in your house or apartment (ie, repairing leaking faucets, lamp cords, lamp switches, broken window panes)? ___husband___
   2. Would you like to attend a minor home repair group? ___yes___

Comprehensive Assessment Process

VII. *Money Management*
    1. *Banking*
       a. Do you have your own savings account?   X
                         checking account?   X
       b. Can you balance your checkbook with the monthly statement?   --
       c. Would you like to learn how to get a checking or savings account? _____
    2. *Budgeting*
       a. Who handles your or your family's money?   husband
       b. At the end of the month do you usually have more bills than money? only sometimes
       c. Would you like to increase your skills in budgeting?   yes!
    3. *Smart shopping*
       Would you like to learn hints for smart shopping?   ie, food, household articles, energy conservation   yes!

VIII. *Transportation*
    1. Do you have a driver's license?   yes
    2. Would you like to learn how to get a driver's license? _____
    3. Are you familiar with how to use public transportation? (rapid, buses) _____
    4. If not, would you like to learn? _____

As a result of the overall evaluation sessions, the following goals and methods of treatment were established by the two evaluation group observers, and discussed by the client and her primary occupational therapist.

1. The client was to participate in appropriate activities of daily living groups to increase her skills in food planning and preparation, nutrition, minor home repairs, and smart shopping.

2. The client's self-esteem was to be increased through mastery experiences in activities therapy and positive feedback in the communication-task group.

3. Exposure to various leisure time tasks in activities therapy was designed to increase the client's interest in avocational activities; ie, to increase her productive use of leisure time at home.

4. By participating in the communication-task group and being encouraged to interact with staff and/or clients in activities therapy, the client would increase both her casual and meaningful self-expression.

During the remainder of her hospitalization, C.H. attended activities of daily living groups dealing with food planning and preparation, nutrition, minor home repairs, and smart shopping. She refused to attend a group on sewing. Though intitially hesitant to share her thoughts, she became an active group member. She seemed eager to learn and assist in various activities. C.H. sat with her group members while working on several projects in activities therapy. She initiated meaningful peer and staff interactions more frequently than during her initial sessions. Offering assistance to another client was considered indicative of enhanced self-esteem. When first seen in the communication-task group, the client was preoccupied, withdrawn, and did not openly discuss her feelings. At the time of her discharge, C.H. appeared increasingly spontaneous and self-disclosing. She seemed alert to the group experiences and less hesitant about sharing her own thoughts and feelings.

                                                   Frances Ehrenberg

Her behavioral changes during occupational therapy indicated that most of the established goals had been achieved. The client herself reported that the communication-task group had been one of her most helpful experiences during hospitalization. It is difficult, however, to assess the specific effects of the occupational therapy program in relation to that of other treatments; ie, group, individual, and chemo-therapies. There is also no follow-up information on whether the behavioral changes were maintained after discharge.

Suggested Research

The assessment process described in this chapter enables the occupational therapist to analyze a client's level of functioning in terms of a broad range of behaviors. Further research should be directed toward the evaluation of the procedure itself, as well as of the occupational therapy treatment program. Clearly, both the reliability and the validity of the assessment process must be determined.

An evaluation of the reliability of the assessment instruments would ascertain whether behaviors were being measured in a consistent fashion. Specific aspects of reliability include:

1. *Inter-rater reliability:* Are clients rated consistently by different therapists? In cases where target behaviors are precisely defined, independent observers should arrive at approximately the same ratings. Inter-observer reliability studies should be useful in determining which behaviors can be consistently measured.

2. *Inter-item reliability:* What is the correlation between observed behaviors? Behaviors with a very high degree of consistent correlation should not be rated separately. The relative independence of the rated behaviors increases the predictive value of the evaluation process; eg, response to treatment.

3. *Stability of ratings over time:* How stable are these ratings over various periods of time? Obviously, some behaviors represent relatively enduring characteristics which are not usually influenced by various environmental or internal changes; others reflect more transient adjustment characteristics. Those behaviors which appear completely unstable during a relatively static period; eg, from the beginning to the end of the assessment group, should be eliminated from the protocol.

After determining reliability, the validity of the assessment process must be verified. Does the process measure both behaviors that are significantly related to independent criteria (eg, psychiatric diagnosis; various outcome criteria, such as duration of hospitalization or frequency of rehospitalization) and more specific factors (eg, client's ability to function in various occupational therapy programs; client's subjective responses to hospital therapy programs)?

If the behaviors being evaluated represent a set of relatively independent factors, the pattern of ratings can be used to compile a behavior profile of each client. These profiles could then be used to classify clients according to various types of problems. The extent to which clients with similar rating patterns function effectively in specific occupational therapy treatment groups is an important measure of successful utilization of the procedure to develop individualized treatment programs. This will enable an assessment of the treatment outcomes, since not all groups are equally valuable for all clients. The evaluation research would serve the dual purpose of determining the validity of the assessment process and demonstrating the utility of the entire occupational therapy treatment program itself.

Obviously, there is much work to be done before the assessment process can be considered a reliable research instrument for use with a diverse group of clients. Yet it is incumbent upon a profession dedicated to the treatment of psychologically disturbed individuals to develop a relatively objective means of specifying target problems and evaluating treatment effectiveness. It is hoped that the present program will be considered an initial step in that direction.

Conclusion

Several problems were encountered in establishing this assessment program. Nonoccupational therapy staff members seemed especially resistant to the new occupational therapy program, possibly due to a general fear of anything new or different. In particular, concern was expressed about the omission of the traditional occupational therapy activities. In fact, activities therapy was relatively de-emphasized when it became part of a broader program. Misgivings were also expressed concerning the "nontraditional" roles proposed for occupational therapists. Although this apprehension probably extended to all new groups, it focused on the communication-task group, a program similar to traditional group therapy programs conducted by other services.

Schedule conflicts were a major problem in the expansion of occupational therapy programs. Clients undergo a variety of diagnostic procedures when they are first hospitalized—eg, physical and laboratory examinations; interviews; and psychological testing. Clients may be unavailable during their scheduled occupational therapy sessions or actually removed from a group. This is especially disruptive if it occurs during the evaluation group, as it interrupts the continuity of group process.

There have been various specific difficulties with the assessment processes. The number of referrals occasionally subjects the therapists to considerable time pressure. This pressure is particularly evident in individualized client interactions; eg, administering the Initial Evaluation Interview and/or Activities of Daily Living Questionnaire; or discussing the individual treatment program with the client. The occupational therapy staff has also questioned the validity of the clients' responses to questions on the Activities of Daily Living Questionnaire. Often, however, these responses have been corroborated through ward observations by nursing staff and/or information aquired from the client's family. Another problem is the tendency of the occupational therapy staff to vary the standardized assessment procedure. Though each staff member is provided with guidelines for administering the various evaluations and observing client behaviors, therapists sometimes depart from those procedures; they must be frequently reminded of the correct assessment method. Lastly, there have been no evaluations of the validity of the therapists' observations during the assessment period. The effectiveness of the individualized treatment programs based on the assessment procedures has also not been confirmed. Nevertheless, I feel confident that the program can potentially evolve into a comprehensive, quantified occupational therapy assessment process.

References

1. Brayman SJ, Kirby TF, Misenheimer AM, et al: Comprehensive Occupational Therapy Evaluation Scale. A J Occu Ther 30:94-100, 1976.
2. Androes L, Dreyfus E, Bloesch M: Diagnostic Test Battery for Occupational Therapy. A J Occu Ther XIX:53-39, 1965.

Frances Ehrenberg

3. Shoemyen CW: A Study of Procedure and Media Occupational Therapy Orientation and Evaluation. A J Occu Ther XXIV:276-279, 1970.
4. Casanova JS, Ferber J: Comprehensive Evaluation of Basic Living Skills. A J Occu Ther 30:101-105, 1976.
5. Buck RE, Provancher MA: Magazine Picture Collage as an Evaluation Technique. A J Occu Ther 26:36-39, 1972.
6. Wolff RJ: A Behavior Rating Scale. A J Occu Ther XV:13-16, 1961.
7. Allard I: Our Professional Judgment Sound or Haphazard? A J Occu Ther XVIII:104-107, 1964,
8. Ethridge DA: Pre-Vocational Assessment of Rehabilitation Potential of Psychiatric Patients. A J Occu Ther XXII:161-167, 1968.
9. Mosey AC: Activities Therapy. New York, Raven Press, 1973.
10. Hinsie LE, Campbell RJ: Psychiatric Dictionary (Fourth ed). New York, Oxford Univ Press, 1967.
11. Hopkins HL, Smith HD (Eds): Willard and Spackman's Occupational Therapy (Fifth Edition). Philadelphia, JB Lippincott Co, 1978, pp 304-313.
12. Gill M, Newman R, Redlich F: The Initial Interview in Psychiatric Practice. New York, International Univ Press, Inc, 1954.
13. Fenlason AF: Essentials in Interviewing (Revised Edition). New York, Harper and Row Publishers, 1962.
14. Wertham F, Golden L: A Differential-Diagnostic Method of Interpreting Mosaics and Colored Block Design. A J Psychiat 98:124, 1941.
15. Lerner C, Ross G: The Magazine Picture Collage: Development of an Objective Scoring System. A J Occu Ther 31:156-161, 1977.
16. Lerner C: The Magazine Picture Collage: Its Clinical Use and Validity as an Assessment Device. A J Occu Ther 33:500-504, 1979.
17. Corry S, Sebastian V, Mosey AC: Acute Short-term Treatment in Psychiatry. A J Occu Ther 28:401-406, 1974.
18. Simon SB, Howe LW, Kirschenbaum H: Values Clarification. New York, Hart Publishing Co, Inc, 1972.
19. Pfeiffer JW, Jones JE (Eds): A Handbook of Structured Experiences for Human Relations Training, Volume I, II, III, IV, V. California, Univ Associates Publishers and Consultants, 1974, 1975.
20. Malamud DI, Machover S: Toward Self-Understanding (Fourth Printing). Springfield, IL, Charles C Thomas, 1975.
21. Jacobsen E: You Must Relax. New York, Whittlesey House, 1948.

Acknowledgment

I wish to express deep appreciation to the following staff members of the University Hospitals of Cleveland who assisted with the preparation of this chapter: Jeanne Wohl, O.T.R./L. and the late Elizabeth Dineen, O.T.R. for their assistance in the development of the evaluation process; James L. Mack, Ph.D. of the Department of Psychology, Maxine Landers, O.T.R./L. of the Occupational Therapy Department, and Barbara Juknialis, M.A., of the Department of Psychiatry for their editorial assistance, and Laraine Croson and Marcy Geraci for their expert typing.

Frances Ehrenberg, O.T.R/L.

11
The Person Symbol As An Assessment Tool

Lorna Jean King, O.T.R., F.A.O.T.A.

Specifically, what is meant by the "person symbol"? The person symbol is an individual's representation of the human body. While it may be a three dimensional figure, a sculpture, or construction, in general, reference is to a two-dimensional figure drawn with a pencil on paper.

Literature Review: General Characteristics of the Person Symbol

Anthropological Factors

Certain characteristics of the person symbol make it a useful means of assessing various aspects of human function. In the first place, it is a universal symbol, transcending time, cultures, and races. Ancient person drawings have been found as pictographs on rock, and painted or incised on pottery. In fact, wherever primitive

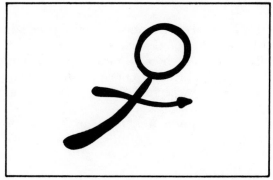

Fig 11.1.

men used materials which have endured, the person symbol has been found. It was stylized into the archaic Chinese written character for "child" (Figure 11.1).

Primitive Chinese writing came into widespread use in China over 4,000 years ago. It is of interest that the capsule of the Pioneer 10 spacecraft—the first craft to leave the solar system—carries a plaque on which are inscribed (in addition to some mathematical formulae) the figures of a man and woman.

Humanity is but one species, ie, capable of interbreeding, and the variations in the human form such as hair characteristics, eye folds, skin color, etc, are insignificant compared to the universality of body parts, proportions, and movement characteristics. It is not surprising that an attempt to have raters differentiate black from white subjects on the basis of person drawings failed,[1] since the minute details that differentiate race are seldom an important part of the individual's mental "map" of his body.

Two-dimensional representation through drawing is also a widespread human activity familiar to people growing up in almost any culture. Whether the drawing is done with a stick in sand or mud, with charcoal or on a piece of bark, incised in a soft rock, or drawn with a pencil on paper, the process is easily generalized, and is widely familiar. Thus the individual who is asked to "Draw a person," is confronted with a familiar activity and a familiar subject and the results, therefore, have a sound basis for comparison.

Consistency Across Individual Time

In addition to its anthropological characteristics, the person symbol is significant in other ways which are vital to its use as an assessment tool. First is its consistency across time in the normal person. The fact that the adult with a stable personality configuration (normal or otherwise) will produce remarkably similar person symbols across lengthy periods of time, makes changes in the person symbol significant indicators of change in personality, mental status, or body concept. Cohn, who studied over 8,000 drawings as part of neurological examinations wrote:[2]

> It was most instructive to observe that when the symbol of a person was achieved by the adult, there was little change in the symbol during the ensuing years, distortions only became manifest as the result of disturbance of brain function...This fixity of the normal adult picture or restricted repertoire of graphic expression is central to the idea that a picture production is the individual's unique symbol of "a person". Even in subjects where distortions of the symbol are the result of structural lesions and metabolic disturbances of the brain, the pre-morbid and the recovery patterns show remarkably similar characteristics.*

Machover comments, "Occasionally drawings of clients obtained over a period of years are so remarkably alike as to constitute a personal signature."[3] Figures 11.2 and 11.3 illustrate this point. The two drawings in each example are separated by a three year interval. Figures 11.2a and 11.2b are produced by a normal adult. Figures 11.3a and 11.3b are the work of a psychiatric client who had not shown significant change in psychiatric status in the interval.

Since consistency is one of the criteria of a good test, one can have added confidence in the person symbol in measurement because of this constancy across time.

Sensitivity to Changes in Central Nervous System Function

The second characteristic of the person symbol important to its use in patient evaluation is that it is sensitive to dysfunction in the central nervous system, whether induced by trauma, or by endogenous or exogenous chemical changes. The task of drawing a person is cognitive, ie, it depends on knowing and remembering, as will be discussed more fully later. It involves the ability to abstract and to use symbols, but also involved are visual-motor feedback loops, spatial organization, and sequencing. Thus functions of both hemispheres, cortex, brain stem, and

---

*From Cohn, R: The Person Symbol in Clinical Medicine, 1960, courtesy of Charles C. Thomas, Publisher, Springfield, IL.

Lorna Jean King

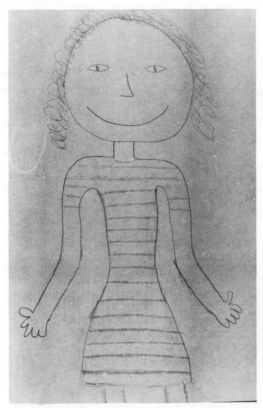

Fig 11.2a.

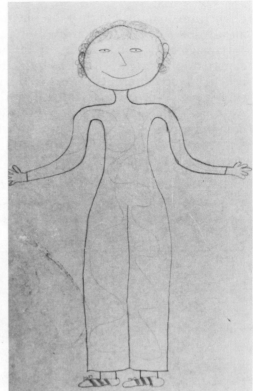

Fig 11.2b.

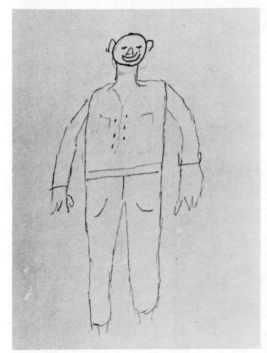

Fig 11.3a.

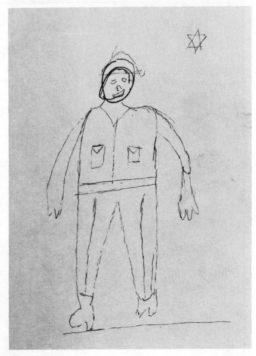

Fig 11.3b.

The Person Symbol

cerebellum, to name but the most obvious structures, are all involved in producing an integrated whole—the symbol of a person.

Damage or dysfunction in any of these areas, or connecting pathways, can be expected to interfere with the production. It follows from this that changes in a beneficial direction in CNS function will also be reflected in improvements in the expression of the person symbol. Figure 11.4 is a series produced by a young man who had suffered a concussion and was unconscious for several days. The first drawing was done within 24 hours after he regained consciousness. The others were done at intervals of one week until time of discharge. He was able to return to his previous employment.

Use of the Person Symbol

Occupational therapists are relative newcomers to the use of the person symbol as an evaluative measure. It has been used for decades by psychologists, but for entirely

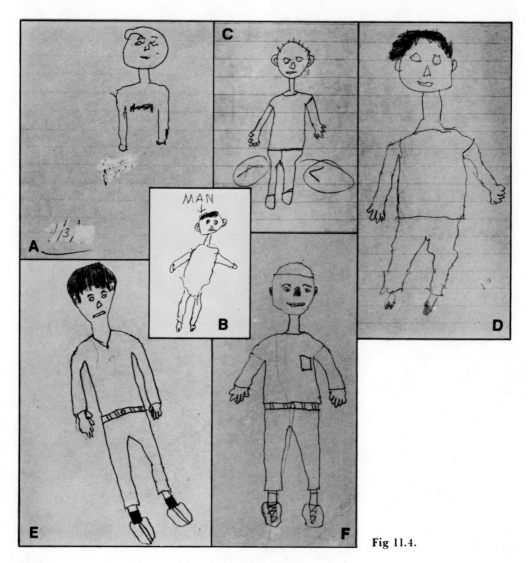

Fig 11.4.

Lorna Jean King

different reasons than those suggested here for the occupational therapist.

Measure of Mental Maturity. In the early 1920s, Florence Goodenough became interested in the correlations between children's drawings and chronological age, school grade, and other evidences of mental capacity, such as the Stanford Binet Intelligence Test, which had been standardized and put into wide use at that time. It seemed clear from Goodenough's investigations that the spatial relationships, size, proportions, and the amount of detail that children put into their human figure drawings did, in fact, have some correspondence to whatever mental capacities were measured by various tests.[4] In the 1960s, Dale B. Harris, a student and associate of Goodenough's, conducted painstaking research based on Goodenough's original work. He acquired new data from thousands of children, distributed among each age group and widely representative of various geographic and economic samples. His book, *Children's Drawings as a Measure of Mental Maturity,*[5] gives a detailed account of his research, as well as thorough review of the literature. Harris constructed standard scores, and these and the scoring guides and criteria can be found in the above mentioned book, as well as in test booklets and manuals.

Unfortunately, some users of the Goodenough-Harris test have assumed that Harris' term, *mental maturity*, was equivalent to *intelligence*. Rather, it seems that conceptualization of the body is one component of cognitive function, but only one. The true nature of intelligence still eludes precise definition. The finding that in normal children there is a general correspondence between maturity of body concept and other measures of cognition should not obscure the fact that the child with inadequate body concept may still function at an average or above average level on other cognitive measures.

The use of the Goodenough-Harris scale in assessing adult drawings will be discussed in a later section of this chapter.

Projective Test. It was also in the 1920s that the work of Sigmund Freud and his theories of psychoanalysis emphasized the conflict between the *id* (instinctual drives) and the *super-ego* (the socially and culturally determined conscience). The super-ego was conceptualized as repressing instinctual material so that the conscious mind (ego) was not aware of it. The id was thought to be continually striving to express its needs in disguised form so as to escape censoring by the super-ego. Dreams and creative productions of all kinds were thought to provide vehicles for the unconscious expression of id-related feelings and fantasies. It was quite natural, therefore, that psychologists should begin to look at the person symbol— an expressive individual creation—as a likely vehicle for the expression of otherwise repressed emotions.

The book, *Personality Projection in the Drawing of the Human Figure,*[3] describes a detailed and subsequently widely used method of interpreting person drawings according to a psychoanalytic framework. It is an atomistic approach, in that it looks at small parts of the drawing in making inferences. For example, a figure with teeth showing is said to indicate "oral aggression". Hammer,[6] in an extensive review of the literature points out that numerous investigators have failed to replicate Machover's findings, and that the interpretation of drawings according to Machover's criteria is of questionable validity and reliability.

Another way of looking at person drawings is according to holistic or stylistic elements. An example of this approach is Johnson's study, which showed a positive correlation ($p < .01$) between placement of the entire figure in the upper left quadrant of the paper and high scores on an anxiety scale.[7]

In addition to figure placement on the page, other stylistic elements on which evaluation has been attempted are such things as realism, symmetry, rhythm, firmness of line, etc. Stewart used these elements in looking at the "personality style" of adolescents.[8] It should be noted that these elements would require clear and concrete definitions if inter-rater reliability were to be attained. Placement on paper, on the other hand, is easily defined. In Johnson's study, the criterion was that in order to consider the figure in the upper left quandrant, it should not touch either the horizontal or vertical middle line of the paper.

The House-Tree-Person (H-T-P) Test looks at commonalities and differences in the three drawings.[9] Interpretation tends to be subjective and intuitive; however Margolf and Kirchner report that the H-T-P drawings of normal adults, like the person drawing alone, show consistency across periods which ranged from four to six weeks.[10] Analysis showed agreement in the sets of scores ranging from 65.8% to 95.9%. This was true of drawings done by both men and women.

Egal and Lindgren demonstrated that H-T-P scores correlated positively and significantly with vocabulary test scores for university women and grade school girls, but not for university men and grade school boys.[11] This suggests a higher correlation between graphic and verbal abilities in women than in men.

It remains for someone to devise a precise scoring system for the H-T-P Test, and it, like Machover's signs, has yet to demonstrate validity in assessment of signs of psychopathology or emotional status. The test is widely used by psychologists, and is undoubtedly useful to the trained evaluator.

In spite of the lack of statistical data confirming the usefulness of the person drawing in assessing emotions and personality characteristics, Sundberg reports that the person drawing is second only to the Rorschach in popularity with psychologists, as a projective test.[12] Wade and Baker confirm its popularity with psychologists who believe that psychological training should include interpretation of person drawings.[13] While it is obvious that psychologists find the projective aspects of the person drawing useful, it is equally clear that the validity of this use of the drawings depends in great measure on the training, experience, and sensitivity of the interpreter. Occupational therapists, as a rule, are not trained in the use of drawings as projective measures, and therefore should not use person drawings for that purpose.

Diagnostic Tool. Neuropsychiatrists have long utilized the person drawing in the diagnosis and evaluation of neurologically impaired clients. In 1950, Schilder discussed aberrations in body concept as shown in drawings.[14] In 1956 Reznikoff, Marvin, and Tomblem discussed the differentiation of organic pathology from schizophrenic or neurotic syndromes with the use of person drawings.[15]

Probably the most exhaustive exploration of the subject is Cohn's book, *The Person Symbol in Clinical Medicine.*[2] Cohn used the person drawing as part of a neurological examination in over 8,000 cases. His book is chiefly useful to the therapist in emphasizing some of the more frequent and reliable indications of organicity.

Use of the Person Symbol by Occupational Therapists

The use of the person symbol as an assessment tool by occupational therapists must be considered as part of a total framework of evaluation and treatment. Like any other one test, it is of little value when taken alone. However, when considered along with clinical observations and other evaluative measures, it can provide considerable useful information. The exposition of the person symbol test in this chapter needs to be considered in the framework of my view of psychiatric occupational therapy, which is summarized as follows:

The functional ability of psychiatric clients, like that of other individuals, is built into a hierarchical development structure in which higher levels of function rest on a foundation of more primitive, less differentiated abilities. The successive mastery of developmental levels leads to maturation and adult function. The developmental hierarchy is characteristic of motor, cognitive, and emotional realms, which are not separate, but interlocking elements of total personality.

While dysfunction or malfunction may occur at any level, the neurochemical abnormalities which are now widely accepted as being characteristic of the major psychoses, seem often to impair lower level or foundation abilities as well as more mature functional abilities. In the case of process schizophrenia, it is not so much a case of impairment of developed function, as of an early failure to develop. Restoration of, or development of, function, as the case may be, needs to begin with foundation abilities rather than with higher level, more discrete functions. Therefore, a neurodevelopmental or sensory integrative approach which focuses on foundation level abilities, is frequently an appropriate level for beginning treatment. Intervention will then proceed to higher levels, and more mature and discrete skills as the client develops. Thus the therapist is not in the position of having to choose between a sensory integrative approach and other approaches, but can apply sensory integrative programs where they are appropriate, and proceed to other aspects of treatment as the client is ready.

Administration

Person Symbol Assessment Procedure

Materials and Equipment. A table and two chairs are needed. White, unlined paper, 8½ x 11 inches, of typing paper grade (not onion skin), and two or three pencils, #2½, fairly long, with usable erasers, completes the equipment.

Directions. Seat the subject comfortably at the table. Place the paper directly in front of the subject and lay the pencils above the top of the paper, erasers toward the subject so that he can easily pick a pencil up with either hand.

Say, "I'd like you to try a pencil and paper task. Take a pencil please, and make a person, a whole person." If the subject responds that he can't draw, say, "It doesn't really matter how well you can draw. We are just interested in how you handle pencil and paper tasks."

Any further questions should be answered casually and non-commitally. For example, if the subject asks, "Male or female?" reply, "Whichever you want." If the subject asks, "With or without clothes?" respond, "It doesn't matter," etc.

The therapist should sit in the other chair and look busy, so as not to appear to be watching the subject too closely. Nevertheless, observe such things as great pressure, (breaking the lead), signs of discomfort with the task, such as frequent erasures, fidgeting, overflow, tongue thrust, or lip biting. Exaggerated speed and carelessness, flushing, perspiration, or other signs of stress should be noted. Note also such things as turning the paper so that the subject is drawing sideways, frequent turning of the paper, covering or closing one eye while drawing, etc. When the subject is finished, return overt attention to him and say, "Good," "That's fine," or, "Thank you." Put the paper away without further comment and go on to other assessment tasks, or else chat casually with the subject for a few moments. It is important not to ask questions about the figure as that is, in effect, "teaching" the subject what you are looking for in a drawing, and to a degree would invalidate the subsequent use of the task as a post-treatment evaluation measure.

As soon as possible after the subject leaves, record *on the back* of the drawing the date, name, sex, age, and hand used for drawing. All this information is absolutely vital for research purposes, and failure to record it will likely render the drawing useless for scientific purposes. Diagnosis and length of hospitalization should also be included if known. Other information which might be recorded is educational level, any physical handicaps such as visual problems, glasses, tremors, history of seizures, etc. A separate sheet should be used for clinical observations, and it should be attached to the drawing.

If the subject indicates that he is finished but has only drawn a head, say, "That's fine." Lay down another sheet of paper and say, "Now make a *whole* person, please." Whether or not the second attempt produces a complete figure, it should be accepted without further comment and the subject thanked pleasantly.

Scoring. If a quantifiable score is desired, it is suggested that the Goodenough-Harris rating scale be used. It is important to establish the sex of the person symbol drawn, since the scoring is different for male and female figures. If there is doubt as to which sex is intended, assume that the drawing is the same sex as the subject. The most reliable use of the numerical score is to compare the subject with himself. Before and after drawings can reveal substantial changes in score.

Behaviors Assessed

Body Concept

The person symbol provides a means of evaluating one basic or foundation ability, namely the ability to conceptualize the body accurately which, in turn, is the basis for praxis or motor planning.[16,17] Impairment of body concept could be expected to disrupt motor planning, especially for non-automatic and complex motor skills. Impairment of praxis can lead to the need to compensate by cortical motor planning, which is slow and cumbersome, and results in psychomotor retardation and greatly increased fatigue. The ability to conceptualize a "map" of the body and understand its movement capacities is, then, a foundation or prerequisite for all the higher functions which are implied in object relationships, occupational role behavior, and even interpersonal relationships. Since manipulation of the self and of objects is the core of the activity or occupation, and occupation is, in turn, the core of occupational therapy, the therapist clearly has a vital interest in the client's body concept as it forms the basis for praxis.

Occupational therapists are deeply indebted to Ayres not only for elucidating the theoretical relationships between sensory input, body concept, and praxis, but also for demonstrating the practicality of developing body concept, and hence, remediating motor planning deficits through appropriate sensory and motor experiences.

In 1961, Ayres discussed the person drawing as a reflection of body concept and cited an interesting case study of a nine year old girl who showed substantial improvement in body concept after 21 days of activities designed to promote development of body scheme through proprioceptive and tactile input.[18] The improvement in body concept was accompanied by marked improvement in motor planning. This child's person drawings progressed in 21 days from a lop-sided oval with three scribbles which might have been features, to a figure with head, eyes, nose, mouth, a body, arms, and an attempt at fingers. This case illustrates the importance of intensive daily treatment in achieving rapid improvement.

In 1969, Mosey discussed the role of occupational therapy in treating distortions of the body image as seen in psychiatric clients.[19] Her suggestions for treatment included sensory-motor experiences, body awareness exercises, and cognitive exploration of personal and cultural attitudes toward the body. Her discussion of means of evaluating body image distortion centered on observable cues such as clothing, dark glasses, hair, clumsiness, rigidity, self-mutilation, and accident proneness. She did not mention the person drawing in the assessment of body image.

The Cognitive Nature of Body Concept

Frequently, *cognition* is used as if it were synonymous with *thinking*—the partly conscious scanning of memory traces and juxtaposing of different bits of information which is the core of the problem solving process. However, cognition means, "the act of knowing,"[20] and much knowing is unconsciously acquired and also used without conscious awareness. This is particularly true of knowing about the body. The feedback from movement, pressure, and touch starts even before birth to build blocks of knowledge about the physical self; what feels pleasant or unpleasant, what moves, and how it moves. As the infant lifts its head, turns, crawls, and walks, these blocks of knowledge expand and integrate into the knowing what is body concept.

Only occasionally it is possible to glimpse the *gaps* in body knowledge of the young human. A normal six year old who was told that her arm was broken after a fall, became very frightened, and revealed that "broken" to her meant falling apart like a broken dish, and she expected her arm to fall off. She was somewhat reassured by being told that her arm would not fall off, but only when she saw it emerge from the cast six weeks later, did she really know that her arm was still intact, and that broken body parts do not fall off.

Children become conscious of body concept and motor planning when introduced to an unfamiliar trick, like trying to pat the head while rubbing the stomach. There is generally an expression of surprise as the child experiences difficulty in controlling the body, which has responded automatically. Body concept is also brought into awareness when an individual is asked to draw a person.

The person drawing task has several components. First there must be the cognitive component just discussed—the mental picture, map, or concept which accompanies the word *person*. With young children, the therapist may need to say, "Draw a man or woman or a boy or girl," since *person* may be an unfamiliar word. Next, there must be an ability to organize the concept spatially. Decisions must be made about where on the page to start, what part of the body to draw first, how large, etc. This ability is not strictly cognitive, since the person may be able to recognize spatial errors in other's drawings but not be able to correctly manipulate space himself.

Then follows the ability to guide the pencil (fine motor planning and/or control). There is at this point the visual-motor feedback which guides and corrects the hand movements. And finally, there is the judgment or critical facility which leads the individual to be satisfied or dissatisfied with what he has produced. Judgment or self-criticism may be considered a component of cognition.

The ability to produce a person symbol may be interfered with at any of these points—cognitive, spatial, or motor. Thus, the very young child (approximately age three) often draws a circle for a head, two circles on the page for eyes, and two lines completely unrelated spatially which could be called arms. The child has no overall map of the body, no cognitive gestalt, but he is aware of various parts. As Luquet pointed out, the child draws what he knows, not what he sees.[21] He knows about the parts, so that is what he draws, not the relationships.

An individual may be unable to get the complete drawing on the page due to starting much too large, or too close to the edge of the paper. In this case it is at the point of spatial organization where the impairment occurs. In an individual with athetoid movements, it is the lack of motor control which disrupts the task. Lack of critical faculty is seen in small children and in adults with some types of neurological dysfunction.

Therefore in evaluating body concept, the therapist must first make a judgment about motor control, visual-motor feedback, and the ability to handle spatial relationships before deciding whether or not adequacy of body concept can reasonably be inferred from a drawing.

The Person Symbol as a Reflection of Physical Status

The body concept just discussed is chiefly important as a basis for praxis. It is an abstraction which could reflect knowledge of any human body, not just that of the person who drew. An individual's person symbol is also, however, a very personal reflection of his own body, and as such can be used as a starting point for investigating aspects of physical status which may be important in treatment planning and/or prevocational evaluation. Machover states:

> The body, or the self, is the most intimate point of reference in any activity. We have in the course of growth, come to associate various sensations, perceptions, and emotions with certain body organs. This investment in body organs or the perception of the body image as it has developed out of personal experience, must somehow guide the individual who is drawing in the specific structure and content which constitutes his offering a "person". Consequently, the drawing of a person in involving a projection of the body image, provides a natural vehicle for the expression of one's body needs and conflicts.[3]*

Berman and Laffal reported a correlation significant between the .05 and .01 levels, between body type of individuals and body type of the figure drawn. "The parallelism may indicate that individuals when given free rein to draw a figure, draw one they are most familiar with—their own. The findings also tend to support the hypothesis that the figure drawing represents, at least in part, a projection of the body image."[22]

In looking at the drawings of obese children at three different age levels (7, 10, and 13) as compared with matched controls, Nathan found that the data strongly supported the hypothesis that the obese children would draw figures considerably more global and less differentiated than the non-obese controls.[23]

In my experience, there is a strong tendency for individuals to mirror, often unconsciously, their own body characteristics in their drawings. A young man drew a figure with one normal appearing eye, the other a mere line (Figure 11.5). Subsequent questioning revealed that the man was blind in that eye. He was unaware that he had drawn the two eyes differently. Figure 11.6 was produced by a

---

*From Machover, Karen: Personality Projection in the Drawing of the Human Figure, 1949, courtesy of Charles C. Thomas, Publisher, Springfield, IL.

Lorna Jean King

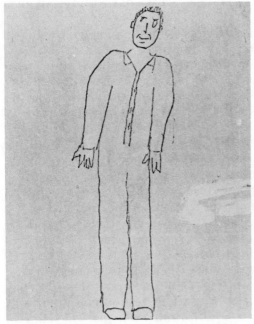

Fig 11.5.

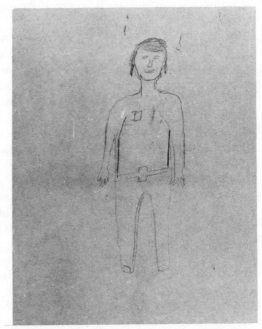

Fig 11.6.

man with chronic pleurisy. One can note the heavy emphasis on the chest wall.

At this point it should be noted that the observer is viewing the drawing as one would observe a person—the hand on the right side of the paper is the figure's left hand and vice-versa. Schilder says, "For this purpose we create a mental point of observation opposite ourselves and outside ourselves and observe ourselves as if we were observing another person."[14] Cohn corroborates the right-left orientation outlined above.[2] This orientation should be kept in mind in using the person symbol as a point for possible inquiry about physical conditions.

Two other examples should suffice to emphasize that individuals put their own physical characteristics into their drawings, albeit often unawares. A right-handed boy of 16 was drawing a person. His left hand was broken and was in a cast. He drew with little difficulty until he came to the figure's left hand. He erased and redrew the hand several times until, with an exclamation of disgust, he drew a hook instead of a left hand and added a pirate's hat to the figure! Only later did he think about the parallelism to his own temporary disability.

A 25 year old depressed man drew a figure that was unremarkable except that part of the lines indicating the right thigh were missing. They had not been erased; there was simply a gap in the lines. A search of the chart disclosed nothing in the physical exam or history which would explain this. When questioned about his right leg, the client revealed that he had recently been released from a hospital after lengthy treatment of a complicated fracture of the right femur. It had failed to heal properly and finally a metal plate had been fastened to the two sections of the bone to secure it. The client was unaware that he had left a gap in the lines in his drawing.

As can be inferred from the foregoing examples, the person symbol can serve as a basis for asking questions, not making assumptions. The infinite variety of human responses suggests that one person may leave out an ailing or defective part, while another may emphasize it with heavy lines. While the therapist can usually surmise

The Person Symbol

that something is amiss, it is not possible to know exactly what without asking questions.

Among other clues to physical status which might be explored are those regarding hearing: are the ears missing, very large, emphasized with dark lines, misplaced on the head? It should be remembered that poor auditory discrimination and auditory defensiveness as well as acuity may be problems to be explored.

Another kind of clue which can be observed is illustrated by a right-handed 18 year old client who drew a figure in which the left side was smaller and less formed than the right. Subsequent muscle evaluation revealed that there was, in fact, a very mild left spastic hemiplegia which had never been diagnosed.

Sensory-integrative Dysfunction. In addition to frank physical problems, the person symbol often provides clues to more subtle problems involving the organization of sensory input and motor responses in the central nervous system. As was suggested with regard to physical problems, the therapist should never assume on the basis of a drawing that a problem exists, but should use the clues it provides as a basis for further assessment, either through additional testing or clinical observation of response to various treatment activities.

Equilibrium Responses. Because of the importance of the vestibular system in the processing of input,[16] the therapist is concerned with the adequacy of vestibular responses. The person symbol does not substitute for specific vestibular testing, but may act as a screening device to provide clues to equilibrium problems. The slanted figure which is not aligned with the borders of the paper may indicate balance problems (Fig. 11.7). Jordan[24] believes that the projective drawings such as person, and H-T-P may be more sensitive to cerebellar disorders than the Rorschach or the Bender. All three cases cited in his study "listed heavily to the right". Another indicator of equilibrium problems is the tripod symbol, in which the line of the trunk is extended downward to form a "third leg" (Fig. 11.8). While most frequently seen in the stick figure, it is occasionally seen also in two-dimensional drawings such as Figure 11.9, which combines the tripod with a figure whose exceedingly wide stance also raises the question of balance control.

Balance my also be in question in the symbol with extremely small or pointed feet

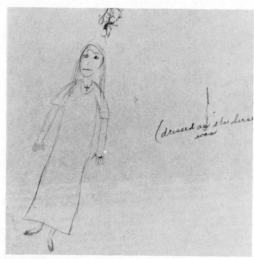

Fig 11.7

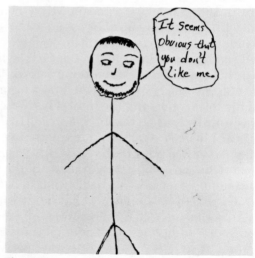

Fig 11.8.

Lorna Jean King

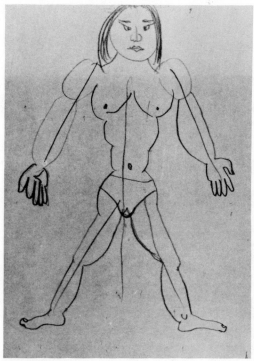

Fig 11.9.

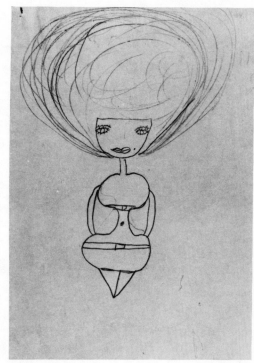

Fig 11.10.

which are very close together, giving the impression that the figure is about to topple over. This type of drawing (Fig. 11.10), also raises the question of adequacy of proprioceptive input; is the individual well-based? Is he aware that the ground is there and is supporting him? Is he aware of feet and legs, or is his awareness centered almost exclusively in the head and upper extremities? Similar questions arise about the figure with no feet, and the figure which "floats" above a line seemingly intended for the ground. The therapist might ask about the person who produces these kinds of drawings, if a few weeks of activities such as jumping rope, marching, dancing, or trampoline work would result in a different kind of drawing, and more importantly, in improved function?

Shoulder Girdle Stability. Figure 11.11 suggests confusion about how the arms are attached to the body and would lead to exploration of shoulder girdle stability and co-contraction as a prerequisite for fine motor control of the upper extremities. In Figure 11.12, the very ineffectual appearing arms as contrasted to the legs might suggest the desirability of proprioceptive input and co-contraction activities such as pushing, pulling, clapping hands, wedging clay, kneading clay, or bread dough, etc.

Midline Problems. Another basic element in central nervous system functioning is the coordination of the two hemispheres of the brain and the two sides of the body. In my experience, problems in crossing the midline of the body are frequently found in a schizophrenic population. Even more frequent is the inability to cross the midline visually with any degree of smoothness. Midline problems can interfere with the normal sequence of motor planning, and therefore sharply cut down motor efficiency. A personal symbol which emphasizes the midline with a heavy row of buttons or other lines should be a clue to look for midline crossing problems

The Person Symbol

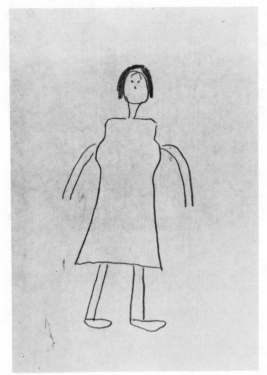

Fig 11.11.

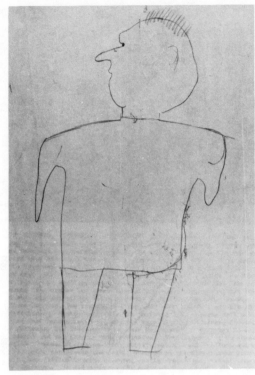

Fig 11.12.

(Figure 11.13). A body midline which is off-center with the midline of the face may also be suggestive of coordination problems.

Coordination of top half and bottom half of the body is frequently overlooked, but is an important factor in functional ability. The observant therapist should be aware of mismatches in body build in individuals and in their drawings. In the person symbol a therapist may see undue emphasis on the top half or bottom half, or one may see a very definitive division such as heavy emphasis on a belt (Fig. 11.14 and 11.15).

Tactile Responsiveness. Because skin responsiveness is not a stable factor, but is in a constant state of flux, there are relatively few clear-cut indications of tactile problems in the person symbol. In most humans, skin responsiveness varies with temperature and humidity, with electro-static conditions in the environment, with the individual's state of alertness or sleepiness, and so forth. The figure without body boundaries, which literally seems to be flying apart (Fig. 11.16), calls for boundaries to be reintroduced through pressure touch (wrapping, sleeping in a sleeping bag, etc). These activities can help to put the skin back on these individuals, and exert a calming, soothing effect. Figure 11.16 was drawn by a manic client who responded very well to pressure touch on a short-term basis. Effects were not lasting, but might have had a cumulative effect if they could have been repeated frequently. In my experience, this type of drawing is typical of those produced by manic clients.

Figure 11.17, with its double skin or border, also would indicate the need for exploration of tactile system responses. Beyond such obvious clues, it can also be pointed out that in my experience there is such a consistent relationship between

Lorna Jean King

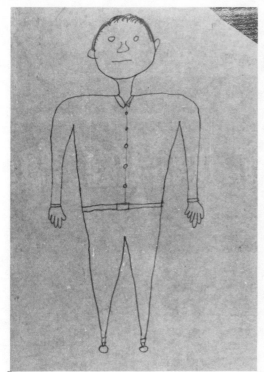

Fig 11.13.

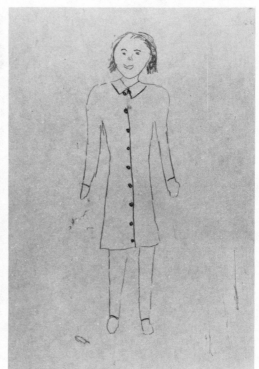

Fig 11.14.

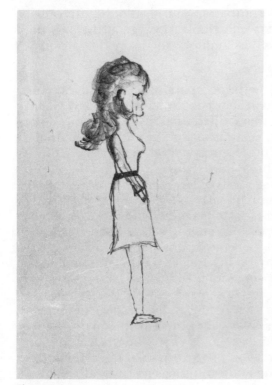

Fig 11.15.

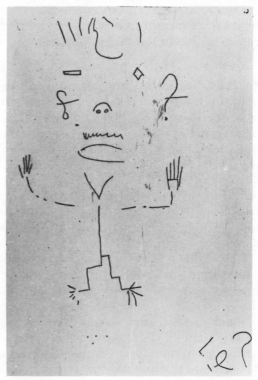

Fig 11.16.

The Person Symbol

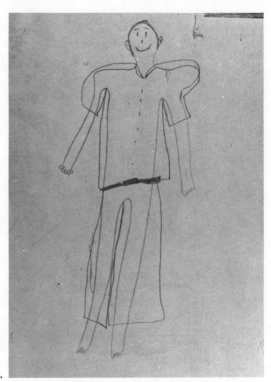

Fig 11.17.

auditory defensiveness/poor auditory discrimination and tactile defensiveness/ poor tactile discrimination, that it might be well to look at exaggerated or missing ears as a clue to test tactile functions as well as auditory adequacy.

Organicity

While diagnosis is not the responsibility of the occupational therapist, there are many occasions when information gathered in an occupational therapy assessment may prove useful to the physician in making a differential diagnosis. One of the most common types of cases where this may occur is that of the middle aged (in the 50s) individual who acts confused, disoriented, agitated, and/or depressed. Since the person is usually considered "too young" to have had a stroke, and there is no visible motor involvement, the tentative diagnosis is often "involutional psychosis" or "adjustment reaction of adult life". Not infrequently, however, a person drawing will show definite signs of organic problems. McDonald dealt with this with regard to the body concept deficiencies of adults with cerebral vascular accidents.[25] She developed a standardized test to assess body scheme in this population.

I have often used the Winterhaven Copy Forms and Visual Retention Test to corroborate the findings on the person drawing. Some of the typical signs in such cases are extremely bizarre or fragmented body concepts (Figure 11.18). A child-like drawing in a person whose history suggests a reasonably high level of achievement, or many perseverative, scribbly types of lines is also indicative of organicity (Figure 11.19). Some of the same characteristics can be seen on the Winterhaven, plus an inability to remember the simple forms and complete the partial figures. Figures 11.20a and 11.20b shows the person drawing and Winterhaven of an individual of this type.

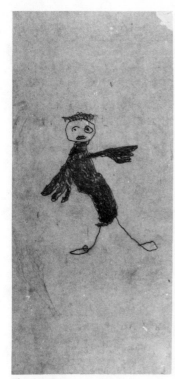

Fig 11.18.

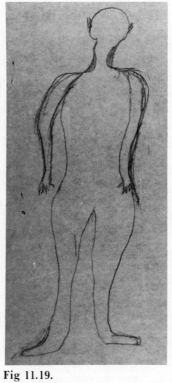

Fig 11.19.

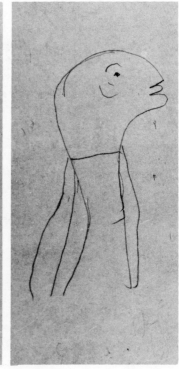

Fig 11.20a.

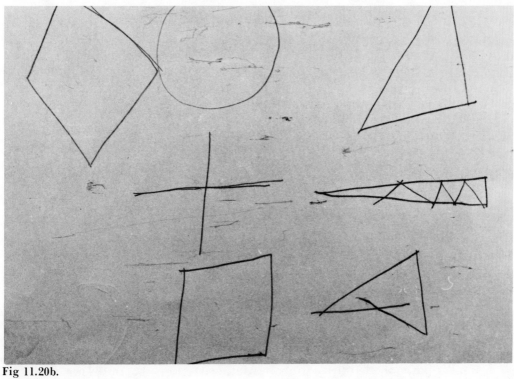

Fig 11.20b.

The Person Symbol

185

A 58 year old woman was admitted to the state hospital because her daughter complained that she had refused to talk for several weeks, was agitated and tearful, and appeared to be confused. The diagnosis was involutional psychosis. On being assessed by the occupational therapist, the woman did not speak, but shook her head and nodded. When asked if she would fill out an interest inventory sheet, she nodded and took the pencil. Her writing was legible, but consisted of "word salad" types of responses. Her person drawing was bizarre and perseverative, and the Winterhaven showed similar findings. These results were taken to a staffing the following day, but in the meantime the patient had collapsed and had been taken to the county hospital where she died. The autopsy showed a tumor which had invaded the left temporal lobe.

Sometimes a client's history includes an automobile accident or other trauma resulting in unconsciousness. Since there may also be family problems and various emotional factors, the possible significance of the head injury may be discounted or overlooked, especially if there were no noticeable motor sequelae. Again, the person drawing and the Winterhaven may indicate the likelihood that the individual has neurological damage which needs to be considered, and if confirmed, taken into account in treatment planning.

A 35 year old woman was admitted to the hospital because of incidents of child abuse. These incidents had taken place following her recovery from a sub-arachnoid hemorrhage. She had no motor sequelae and in ordinary conversation showed no apparent abnormalities in speech or thought content. The question was: is there a primary psychiatric problem or is there some damage resulting from the hemorrhage? The person drawing (Fig. 11.21) shows very definite abnormalities in the person concept. The misspelling of "leg" by a woman who is a college graduate, as well as the labeling of parts per se, are further indications of probable neurologic impairment as a result of the cerebral accident.

It is important to be aware that neurological disorders do not always result in pathological person drawings. Cohn reports that the majority of seizure patients do not show abnormal person drawings and that correlation of abnormal EEG readings with abnormal person drawings is lower for seizure disorders than for any other clinical category.

One might speculate that this is true because the left temporal lobe is the most common site for focal lesions resulting in seizures, while space-form-graphic abilities center chiefly in the right hemisphere.

The therapist must exercise discretion in using person drawings as an aid to diagnosis, and the first element is to gain a background of experience. It is best to suggest possibilities or ask questions rather than making flat statements. Drawings, at best, are indications, not evidence. A drawing can be added to the results of a neurological examination and laboratory results, but by itself it is only suggestive, not conclusive.

The Person Symbol and Sexual Identity

What significance can be attached to the fact that the person symbol is of the same sex or the opposite sex as the person who is drawing? Several authors have considered this question. Levy states that of 5,000 adult subjects, 87% drew their own sex first when asked to "draw a person", and subsequently to "draw a person of the other sex".[26] There is no information however, about the composition of the sample as to males and females.

A smaller but more definitive study by Mainord reports that of 164 male subjects,

Lorna Jean King

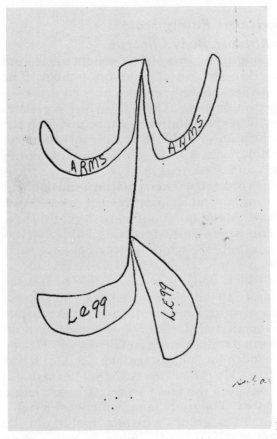

Fig 11.21.

82.3% drew the self-sex first. Of 105 females, 60.9% drew the self-sex first.[27] These differences between male and female responses lend credence to the idea that cultural factors related to male and female status in a society influence the choice of the first figure drawn. A cross-cultural investigation by Fawzi also supports this theory.[28] He found that a relatively larger number of females than males drew the opposite sex first, and that this effect was more pronounced in cultures where male dominance reached exaggerated proportions.

To the degree that a society is male dominated, it is "normal" or expected for a substantial number of females to draw male figures. In most societies it would be expected that fewer males would draw female figures first. It should be noted that in Mainords's study a substantial number of normal subjects drew the opposite sex first (39.1% females and 17.7% males). It is, therefore, risky to draw conclusions about the sexual orientation of the subject on the basis of the sex of the figure drawn.

Hassell and Smith, in a study of female homosexuals noted that as a group they tended to sexualize and embellish drawings of the female figure.[29] They emphasize that this *cannot* be used as a clinical predictor of homosexuality, but only as a possible source of speculation.

The Goodenough-Harris rating scales are different for male and female figures and it is important to make a determination at the outset as to which sex is represented. If the sex is unclear, the rater should assume that the person has drawn the self-sex.

The Person Symbol   187

The Goodenough-Harris Rating Scale
as a Means of Quantifying Body Concept

As has been discussed earlier, Goodenough, and later Harris, sought to measure the mental maturity of children as expressed in the person symbol. The Goodenough-Harris rating scale represents the end product of their work—a quantification of the elements in the person drawing. The scale, which correlates very satisfactorily with other measures of mental ability, is concerned with the elements of body concept. It measures the number of details that are incorporated, the appropriateness of proportions, and the expression of movement possibilities through the accurate depiction of joints and of movement.

Quantifiable tests are always desirable in order that statements can be made about how much development has taken place, or how much improvement or regression has occurred in a given amount of time. Many questions must be considered, however, in using any scoring system. This is even truer when using a scale that was developed for one population with a group for which it was not originally intended.

What, then, are the considerations which make it seem feasible to use the Goodenough-Harris rating scale with adults? In the first place, it has a wide enough spread of points to accommodate even a superior adult production. The possible points are 71 for women, 73 for men. In a small study I recently completed, the mean score for thirty-eight 20 to 39 year old normal right-handed females was 44.47. The range of points was from 13 to 67. The mean for females age 20 to 29 (n =18) was 44.33. The mean for females age 30 to 39 (n = 11), the mean was 37.18. The small size of the two older groups may well account for the lower scores. A much larger normative sample will eventually be tested. The study sample included 8 right-handed males and 3 left-handed females. These groups were too small to provide meaningful average scores. Further studies are currently underway with a more representative and much larger group. It is possible that the means may prove to be somewhat different, but it seems that there is little likelihood of adults topping out at or above the top of the scale.

Another advantage of the Goodenough-Harris scale is that it is independent of artistic ability. While the artistic drawing may earn a relatively high score, a meticulous, detailed, but unartistic drawing may score high. Figures 11.22a and 11.22b are a case in point. Figure 11.22a scored 58 while Figure 11.22b scored 56. Harris mentions research demonstrating that art training has little or no effect on person drawing scores in children.[5]

The Goodenough-Harris scale has the additional advantage of demonstrating inter-rater reliability. Harris reports that various tests of inter-rater reliability ranged from the low .80s to as high as .96. Values commonly exceeded .90.

Research

I conducted a study comparing inter-rater reliability of inexperienced raters who had only one hour of training, with the inter-rater reliability of experienced raters. Using Spearman's rank correlation the inexperienced raters had reliability of .883 while the experienced raters scored .849. Both correlations are quite satisfactory. It seems probable that the inexperienced raters were paying closer attention to scoring criteria because of their lack of experience.

The Goodenough-Harris scale is useful because drawings can be scored quickly with its use. Directions are clear and demand only that the rater follow directions literally.

Lorna Jean King

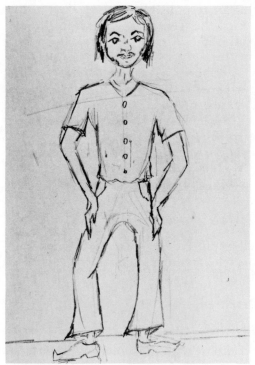

Fig 11.22a.

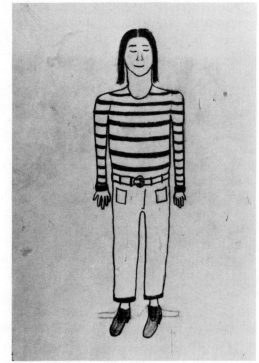

Fig 11.22b.

Usefulness With Schizophrenic Population

The instruction, "Make a person, a whole person," is interpreted literally and concretely by children. This tends to be true of a schizophrenic population—especially those classified as non-paranoid. These clients usually do not indulge in philosophizing or psychologizing about the task, but make a straight-forward concept as the individual knows it. It appears that the more chronic the client, the more likely he is to be concrete and literal about the task of drawing a person.

Concreteness is not necessarily typical of the normal adult, the neurotic, or the marginally ill person, where frequently the self-critical or judgmental aspects of cognitive function lead to the, "I can't draw" response. The individual may then resort to a stick figure which does not invite judgment of artistic ability. Or the person may resort (infrequently) to an abstraction and report that it represents "soul", or essence.

Plateauing of Scores

Harris points out that Goodenough-Harris scores appear to plateau between the ages of 12 and 14. By adding detail points to Goodenough's original rating scale, Harris was able to extend the normative scores to 14 years 6 months.

The data from the normative sample of adult females ages 20 to 39, previously referred to, was in agreement with Harris' finding that scores do not increase beyond the age of 14. The mean for the group of females, 44.4, is very close to Harris' mean for female subjects age 14 years 6 months. (45 for female subjects drawing males, 48 for female subjects drawing females.)

Harris seems to feel that two major factors are responsible for the lack of further progress in scoring after the early teens. First, he feels that expression through speech and language is so much more versatile and satisfying by early adolescence that there is little drive to self expression through art or other creative media. Secondly, he mentions the development of self-critical or judgmental faculties which leads most individuals to be dissatisfied with the drawings they produce.

In a recent work, Edwards states that drawing attempts are shut off at an even earlier age by self-criticism.[30] The researcher cites hemisphere specialization studies as indicating that the "naming" left hemisphere loses interest and therefore does not observe objects as soon as it can classify and name them. The right hemisphere which is concerned with space and form is chiefly involved with drawing. It is interesting to speculate that the tendency of brain-injured clients to name or even label body parts as they draw may result from the need for the left hemisphere to assist with the task which was formerly principally the province of the right hemisphere.

Whatever the reasons, the person drawing test scoring with the Goodenough-Harris scale is most useful with individuals who are literal and concrete about the task, and who are not unduly inhibited by self-criticism.

Future Research

Scores of Psychiatric Clients

How do the scores of psychiatric clients compare with those of normal adults? At present there is relatively little data available to answer this question. The person drawing as scored by the Goodenough-Harris scale was used as a pre- and post-test with 25 chronic non-paranoid schizophrenics in Illinois in 1977.[31] The pre-test means for the experimental and control groups were 21.5 and 21.2 respectively. If this group was typical of a chronic group, it can be inferred that chronic schizophrenics will score less than half the points earned by normal adults. Further studies are proceeding with clinical material.

Use of the Goodenough-Harris Scale to Measure Change

Until trustworthy standard scores can be developed for normal adults, the therapist would do well to utilize scores as before and after measurements, comparing the client with himself, rather than with a normal population. It has been my experience that sensory integrative treatment interventions produce marked changes in body concept as reflected in the person drawings. These can be quantified and turned into a percentage of change figure.

As early as 1939, Fingert, Kagan, and Schilder collected person drawings before, during the course of, and after metrozol shock treatments of schizophrenics.[32] These were scored on the Goodenough scale and showed steady quantitative improvement during and after the course of treatment. They also noted the disappearance of bizarre features in the drawings.

In the 1977 cooperative study in Illinois cited previously, chronic non-paranoid schizophrenics in long term care facilities were divided into experimental and control groups and administered a variety of pre- and post-tests. The Nurses Observational Scale for Inpatient Evaluation (NOSIE-30) was used as the measurement of psychiatric status. The experimental group which received sensory-integrative treatment showed an improvement of 26.5% on the NOSIE-30 at the end of six months, and an improvement of 26% on the person drawing. The control group improved just under 2% on the NOSIE-30, and lost 1.9% on the person drawing.*

These results suggest that there is a good correlation between clinical improvement and improvement of body concept as measured by the Goodenough-Harris rating scale. Replication of this study, and initiation of other studies is necessary before final conclusions are warranted.

Several other studies have compared before and after person drawings as a part of evaluative procedures connected with gross motor treatment approaches with schizophrenic clients. The earliest study which has come to my attention was McCarthy's "Use of the Draw-a-Person Test to Evaluate a Dance Therapy Program."[3] McCarthy's client group consisted of eight acute reactive clients who did person drawings after each weekly one-hour dance therapy session. The first and last drawings of each client were then assessed by four judges who were to decide 1) whether they could match the two drawings done by each client; 2) if they could tell which one of each pair was done last. They were also to 3) rate the drawings as to most improved, least improved, etc.

The judges were three masters degree psychologists and one masters degree physical education instructor. McCarthy points out that the physical education instructor correctly matched all eight pairs of drawings, "which perhaps reflects her attention to the body concept qualities of the drawings rather than their intrapsychic projections."

Before and after status of pairs were judged correctly 72% of the time, representing a level of significance beyond the .005 level of confidence for a one-tailed test. McCarthy concludes that before and after measures of body concept were significantly different.

I rated McCarthy's illustrated drawings according to the Goodenough-Harris scale and found that the greatest gains in scores (from 18 to 36, and from 7 to 20) were made by the two clients the judges uniformly had rated as most improved.

McCarthy's study assumes added significance for the occupational therapist because he based part of the rationale for his work on Ayres' theories.

The techniques of movement and drama therapy used in the British study by Nitsun, Stapleton, and Bender were similar to McCarthy's dance therapy modalities.[34] The British study also used the person drawing as an evaluative measure before and after treatment. In this study also, changes for the better in body concept were noted by the investigators and described in terms of increased verbalization, improvements in posture, grooming, and socialization. This study differed from McCarthy's in that the client group was chronic rather than acute. I also scored the British drawings on the Goodenough-Harris scale and found higher scores on the post-test drawings.

Levine, O'Conner, and Stacey conducted a pilot study in Montreal with chronic schizophrenics at the Douglas Hospital.[35] Their study was noteworthy in that they were able to control the variable of medication, which remained the same throughout the six weeks of the study. Their clients were all process non-paranoid schizophrenics and had a mean length of hospitalization of 24 years. Since this was a pilot study for a larger project, the "n" was small—3 males and 3 females.

The two sets of drawings included in the paper show substantial improvements. The subjects improved on the other tests also—four sub-tests of the Southern California Sensory-integration test battery.

*This study was partially funded by HEW Grant #RO-V-526-77.

Rider's study of a small group of clients in a Veteran's Administration Hospital also utilized the person drawing test.[36] The "n" was small, the group quite heterogenous, and results inconclusive.

The most recent study to utilize the person drawing is reported by Crist who used the Goodenough-Harris scale to arrive at a quantifiable score.[37] Crist's figures confirm that chronic schizophrenics score less than half the points of normal subjects. Her normative group of 24 scored higher means than the group I studied (52.16 for the drawing of a male; 51.16 for the drawing of a female). The means of scores for the three patient groups ranged from a low of 17.5 to a high of 27.85.

Group I, treated with sensory integration modalities, improved its mean scores on the person drawing. Group II, treated with fine motor sedentary activities, did not do as well on the post-test as on the pre-test. Their pre-test scores were lower than Group I. Group II had a 91 year old member and the mean age for this group was 65.2 versus 37.6 for Group I. Evaluation of results must take this difference into account. Crist confirms the satisfactory inter-rater reliability which can be obtained on the Goodenough-Harris scale. The phi coefficient was .77 and chi-square analysis yielded a .001 level of significance. The significance of improved scores on the person drawing is more apparent when those scores can be correlated with improvement on a psychiatric status evaluation. Credibility is increased by the use of a well-known, reliable, and validated test like the NOSIE-30.

Conclusion

The major purpose of this discussion has been to outline the possible uses of the person symbol in assessing the treatment needs and treatment progress of the psychiatric client. Emphasis was placed on the usefulness of the person symbol as a reflector of both neurological and psychological organization. The central importance of body concept to praxis was also stressed, since motor planning influences the success of therapeutic activities in a wide spectrum of treatment situations. Finally, a method of quantifying the person symbol (the Goodenough-Harris Rating Scale) was discussed, and a standard procedure presented for adminstering the person symbol test.

No therapeutic, evaluative, or educational method is any better than the professional skills and judgment of the person using it. This is most certainly true of the person symbol test. It cannot be emphasized too strongly that it should be used as a basis for asking questions. Care should be exercised in making statements. It is most valuable when used in connection with astute and acute clinical observation and sensitive attention to the client's communication—both verbal and non-verbal. In gauging progress, it is most useful in comparing the client with himself.

The person symbol cannot reveal everything, but when used by a skilled and sensitive therapist, it can be very useful. As Machover concludes, "Finally, although the drawing of a person is not expected to tell all invariably—it does, invariably, tell something, and in many instances, a great deal."[3]

References

1. Jernigan AJ: Judging whether a person is white or black by his draw-a-person test. J Person Assess, 34:503-506, 1970.
2. Cohn R: The Person Symbol in Clinical Medicine. Springfield, IL, Charles C Thomas, 1960, p 44.
3. Machover K: Personality Projection in the Drawing of the Human Figure. Springfield, IL, Charles C Thomas, 1949, p 6.
4. Goodenough F: Measurement of Intelligence by Drawing. Yonkers, World Book Company, 1926.

5. Harris DB: Children's Drawings as a Measure of Mental Maturity. New York, Harcourt, 1963.
6. Hammer E: Projective drawing. In Rabin AI(ed): Projective Technique in Personality Assessment, New York, Springer Pub Co, 1968.
7. Johnson JH: Upper left hand placement of human figure drawings as an indicator of anxiety. J Person Assess, 35:336-7, 1971.
8. Stewart L: The expression of personality in drawings and paintings. Genet Psychol Monogr, 5:45-103, 1955.
9. Buck J, Jolles I: House-Tree-Person Projective Technique. Los Angeles, Western Psychological Services, 1966.
10. Margolf S, Kirchner J: Characteristics of house-tree-person drawings of college men and women. J Person Assess, 34:138-45, 1970.
11. Egal C, Lindgren HC: The house-tree-person test as a measure of intelligence and creativity. Percep Motor Skills, 44:359-62, 1977.
12. Sundberg ND: The practice of psychological testing in clinical services in the United States. Am Psychologist, 16:79-83, 1961.
13. Wade TC, Baker TB: Opinion and use of psychological test: a survey of clinical psychologists. Am Psychologist, 32:874-82, 1977.
14. Schilder P: The Image and Appearance of the Human Body. New York, International Universities Press, 1950.
15. Reznikoff M, Tomblen D: The use of human figure drawing in the diagnosis of organic pathology. J Consult Psychol 20:467-70, 1956.
16. Ayres AJ: Sensory Integration and Learning Disorders. Los Angeles, Western Psychological Services, 1972.
17. Semans S: The Bobath concept in treatment of neurological disorders, neurodevelopmental treatment. Am J Phys Med, 46:1, 1967.
18. Ayres AJ: Development of body scheme in children. A J Occu Ther XV:3, 1961.
19. Mosey AC: Treatment of pathological distortion of body image. A J Occu Ther XXIII:5, 1969.
20. Stein J: (ed): The Random House Dictionary of the English Language, Unabridged. New York, Random House, 1966.
21. Luquet GH: Les Dessin d'un Enfant (The drawing of a child). Paris, T Alcan, 1913.
22. Berman S, Laffal J: Body type and figure drawing. J Clin Psychol, 9:368-70, 1953.
23. Nathan S: Body image in chronically obese children as reflected in figure drawings. J Person Assess, 37:456, 1973,
24. Jordan S: Projective drawings in a cerebellar disorder due to chicken pox encephalitis. J Person Assess, 34:256-8, 1970.
25. McDonald J: An investigation of body scheme in adults with cerebral vascular accidents. A J Occu Ther XV:75-79, 1960.
26. Levy J: in Bellak L, Abt LE (eds): Projective Psychology, Clinical Approaches to the Total Personality. New York, Knopf, 1950.
27. Mainord F: A note on the use of figure drawing in the diagnosis of sexual inversion. J Clin Psychol, 9:188-9, 1953.
28. Fawzi SD: First drawn pictures: a cross cultural investigation. J Person Assess, 40:4, 376-7, 1976.
29. Hassell J, Smith EWL: Female homosexuals: Concepts of self, men and women. J Person Assess 39:2, 154-59, 1975.
30. Edwards B: Drawing on the Right Side of the Brain. Los Angeles, JP Tarcher—St Martins, 1979.
31. King LJ: Theory and Application of Sensory Integrative Treatment for Residents of Long Term Care Facilities with Histories of Chronic Schizophrenia. Scottsdale, AZ, Greenroom Publications, 1978.
32. Fingert H, Kagan J, Schilder P: The Goodenough test in insulin and metrazol treatment of schizophrenia. J Gen Psychol 21:349-65, 1939.
33. McCarthy H: Use of the draw-a-person test to evaluate a dance therapy program. J Music Ther X:141-155, 1973.
34. Nitsun M, Stapleton J, Bender MP: Movement and drama therapy with long stay schizophrenics. Br J Med Psychol 47:101, 1974.
35. Levine I, O'Connor H, Stacey B: Sensory integration with chronic schizophrenics: A pilot study. Canad J Occu Ther, March, 1977.
36. Rider B: Sensorimotor treatment of chronic schizophrenics. A J Occu Ther 32:451-55, 1978.
37. Crist P: Body changes in chronic, nonparanoid schizophrenics. Canad J Occu Ther 46(2):61-65, 1979.

The Person Symbol

Acknowledgments

Grateful acknowledgment is made of the contributions of Betty Snow, R.N., whose expertise in the interpretation of the person symbol first drew my attention to this test. The late Matilda M. Landry, O.T.R., diligently collected clinical data and tirelessly contributed to research in this field.

Thanks are due to the students and members of the Center for Neurodevelopmental Studies for scoring drawings, to Richard Grisard, O.T.R., for the contribution of clinical material, and to John Ludwig for photography.

Lorna Jean King

12
The Activity Laboratory: A Structure For Observing And Assessing Perceptual, Integrative, And Behavioral Strategies

Gail S. Fidler, O.T.R., F.A.O.T.A.

History and Development

In 1959-60, after many years of using a variety of activity observations to assess individual clients, an attempt was made to organize and structure the process. This effort resulted in a "Diagnostic Battery" that consisted of presenting to a client, in sequence, three activities (drawing, finger painting, and clay) and asking the client to comment on each after it was completed. The productions and the responses of the client were interpreted and incorporated in the treatment and team planning. This Diagnostic Battery was published in the Proceedings of the American Occupational Therapy Association Object Relations Institute, in 1964.

During this same time, the need to teach students something about the meaning of activities was resulting in the gradual development of an experiental activity laboratory. Comparison of this laboratory with the more limited focus of the Diagnostic Battery and recognition of the increasing need to service a greater number of clients led to the refinement and development of an activity laboratory that could be used with a group, and was applicable to both student learning needs and the assessment of client performance behaviors.

Since 1965, the Activity Laboratory has been used as an assessment process with hundreds of clients in a variety of settings and with a variety of diagnoses. In addition, it has been employed as a teaching-learning experience with hundreds of students across the country, as well as with a variety of interdisciplinary staffs in many settings. The use of a single instrument with both client and nonclient groups made it possible to compare and contrast responses, describe typical and atypical behaviors in relation to a given activity experience or task element, clarify differences in the characteristics of activities, and discern the relationships among experiences and responses.

Over the years, changes were made to improve constancy of process and to reduce the number of variables. Activity experiences were refined in that some were added, some deleted and/or altered in terms of process or placement in the sequence, in order to most succinctly tap important areas of skill components and performance. A constant effort was made to more clearly identify which behaviors could most obviously be elicited by which activity, in what sequence and by what structure or process. The final format was determined by the desire to cover relevant variables with minimal repetitions in a sequence of activities that could be administered in a relatively brief period of time. The 10 or more years of experience with this process has provided empirical evidence that: a given activity in this laboratory does, more consistently than not, elicit a describable set or class of behaviors; that there is a discernable relationship between the characteristics of an activity, its sequence in the laboratory, and the set or class of behavioral responses elicited (eg, sensory-motor integrative skills, cognitive skills, ego skills). Experience also suggests a high correlation between the information gathered from the laboratory and an individual's characteristic style of adapting, and his or her performance skill strengths and/or deficits.

The Activity Laboratory is a structured process for obtaining initial information. It is not an indepth evaluative procedure, nor *the* single instrument on which treatment planning should be based. It is intended for use during the early stages of data gathering and is useful in obtaining an initial, tentative behavioral profile. The extent to which behavioral responses are characteristic of an individual's typical style, skills, and/or deficits can be confirmed only when the profile of behaviors is compared, contrasted, and put into perspective with other information and data about the person. How data from the Activity Laboratory is interpreted and used will, of course, be decided by one's frame of reference, what are defined as intervention priorities, and what is perceived as dysfunction. The Laboratory has not been designed to delineate or describe psychopathology or to determine what is pathologic about responses or behaviors. Its development has been focused on obtaining a perspective about ways of responding to and managing different kinds of tasks and task environments. Such perspectives can be useful in helping to determine which components of performance should be attended to as well as how strengths and characteristic styles of organizing and responding can be capitalized in both the what and how of intervention.

The fact that there are many different determinants of human behavior means that different observers will value components in different ways. Therefore, a solid theoretical background is essential to the use of the Laboratory along with continuous practice, critique, and feedback.

Administration

The Activity Laboratory is composed of five activities offered in sequence and preferably within a single span of time. If an uninterrupted block of time is not possible, the break should occur between the third and fourth activity. The time required for the complete laboratory depends on the number of clients in the group. For example, a group of 12 requires a maximum of 5½ hours. Size of group must be determined by the skill and experience of the therapist. Experience has shown that a novice therapist can manage between three to five clients, and that this number can be increased as experience is gained. If fewer than five clients are involved, the fifth activity is deleted.

The activity experiences can be offered as single units; however, the value of a continuous sequence in a developing group context is lost. Carry-over of one experience to the next is a useful variable in comparing and contrasting responses.

This Activity Laboratory is an inappropriate assessment process for the severely regressed schizophrenic patient. It is understood that the laboratory experiences are offered in an area where no other activities are going on and where no persons are present except the laboratory staff and client group.

Sequence is planned so that there is progression from a highly structured experience with no demands for independent action, social relatedness, or physical activity, to increasing requests for decision-making, more complex problem solving, social, and physical activity.

The first activity offered in the laboratory is a stencil cutout and crayon. Two drawings (Figures 12.1 and 12.2), each centered on an 8½ x 5½ inch sheet of white bond paper, are provided along with a blank sheet of 8½ x 11 inch white bond paper,

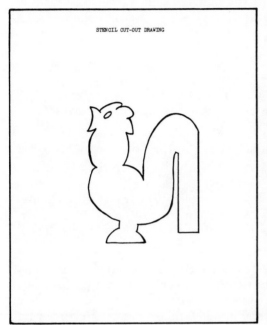

STENCIL CUT-OUT DRAWING

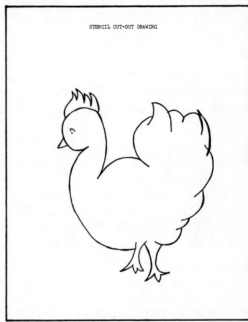

STENCIL CUT-OUT DRAWING

Fig. 12.1.   **Fig. 12.2.**

a small pair of scissors, and two crayons, one of a dark color and one of a light color. The client is asked to choose one of the two drawings, cut out the drawing, reproduce it on the blank sheet of paper, and then color in the form and background. To reinforce structure and external control, the laboratory setting should be prepared and set up for this activity *before* the group arrives. Both drawings are placed evenly on top of one another and then on top of the blank paper. These are placed vertically on the table in the center of each seating arrangement. The small pair of scissors and the dark and light crayons are placed horizontally at the top center of the papers.

The second activity is finger painting. Large finger painting paper, approximately 24 x 18 inches, is provided. Red, blue, green, yellow, black, and brown colors are placed along the center of the table. Containers of water are placed around the table. This activity is offered without structure, and the clients are asked to simply take a piece of paper and work with the paints on that paper.

The third activity is a collage. Large sheets (approximately 24 x 18 inches) of different colors of construction paper are provided, along with several containers of glue or paste, scissors, and a large and varied assortment of materials and objects. It is important that materials and objects for the collage be as varied and in as large a quantity as possible. Both the variety of stimuli and options are critical factors in this activity. These materials should be placed on a table other than the one used for working.

The fourth activity in the sequence is the obstacle course. This activity requires a room or gym area large enough to accommodate a group with free, unobstructed space. Equipment includes a balance beam (which can be made by placing two secured 4 x 8s on the floor), six automobile tires, two or more volley balls, soft balls, whiffle ball sets, and one-foot square targets that can be marked or placed on a wall. The walking, jogging, and hopping activity is done together as a group. Two or more persons can simultaneously engage in the Bat Ball and Target Ball tasks.

The tasks are offered in the following order:

1. Slow walk—50 feet.
2. Fast walk—50 feet
3. Jog—50 feet
4. Hop on right foot, 10 times, or as long as possible
5. Hop on left foot, 10 times, or as long as possible
6. Balance beam—walk across, turn, walk back
7. Tire walk—as rapidly as possible, walk forward in the holes of the tires
8. Bat Ball—toss the whiffle ball in the air, and hit the ball with the plastic bat (three times)
9. Target Ball—with a volley ball, from a distance of 15 feet, hit a 1-foot square target, marked on the wall at 3 feet from the floor (three times)—with a soft ball, from a distance of 15 feet, hit a 1 foot square target, marked on the wall at 3 feet from the floor (three times)

Medication does affect performance. A re-test may be indicated after dosage has been stabilized. Regardless, performance must be considered in relation to drug regimen and prior history of coordination skill level.

The fifth activity consists of a circle ball tag game. One person volunteers or is chosen to be in the center of the circle. Those in the circle throw the ball across the circle, and the person in the center attempts to intercept and catch the ball. When the ball is caught, the person who has thrown the ball must move into the circle, replacing the person in the middle who has caught the ball. The game is played until everyone has been in the center position. If this happens before the allotted time has elapsed, the game should be continued. This offers the group an opportunity to adjust the rules or process to accommodate to their skills and/or interests. Frequently, an individual will have great difficulty catching the ball and getting out of the center position. It is important that the therapist not intervene before the group or one of its members has made attempts at rescue.

At the completion of the final or fifth activity, each person is asked to complete the *Activity Laboratory Questionnaire* (Appendix V). If a client has difficulty reading or otherwise managing this questionnaire, the therapist should read the questions and record responses.

Structure and Format

In any evaluative process, consistency in presentation is critical. The rules or process must be presented and explained in the same way each time the Laboratory is offered. Likewise, the therapist must guard against contaminating responses by intervening, commenting on, or otherwise becoming involved in the process. Requests for clarification, assistance, and/or verification should be handled by either repeating the instructions, or silence, whichever is more appropriate at the time. This is not to suggest that stern aloofness is the preferred behavior. The therapist's manner should reflect comfort, ease, and acceptance. Experience has shown that clients do enjoy the laboratory experiences if the atmosphere is a relaxed one.

The *format* for presenting and managing the activities is as follows:

1. *Stencil Cut-out and Crayon.* The room is set up as described earlier. Clients are asked to go directly to a seat around the table. When everyone has been seated, the therapist will explain:

    "On the table in front of you are two drawings and a blank piece of paper. Choose one of the drawings. Cut out the drawing you have chosen. Trace the outline of the drawing on the blank sheet of paper that is in front of you. Then, use the dark colored crayon to color in the drawing. Use the light colored crayon to color in the background."

    Repeat the exact instructions one more time.

    Ask, "Are there questions?" If there are questions, repeat that part of the instructions, eg, "Choose one of the drawings."

    State, "You will have 30 minutes to complete the activity."

    Five minutes before time has elapsed, a time warning is given. At the end of 30 minutes, the group is asked to stop working. The questions listed in the guides for observing and interpreting responses are asked.

2. *Finger Paint.* See earlier description for setup. The therapist should explain:

    "This is a paint-with-your-fingers activity. You may use any or all of the colors that are available on the table. You are free to do whatever you wish with the paint on the paper. Work on the glossy side of the paper and moisten the paper well with water before you begin. The more water you use, the more the paint will flow."

    Repeat the instructions. Then ask, "Are there questions?"

    Handle questions by repeating the instructions. State, "You will have 30 minutes." Call time as specified in the previous activity. Ask those questions contained in the guide for observing and interpreting responses.

3. *Collage.* The therapist says, "This activity is one in which you may make any kind of picture or design that you wish.

    "There are many different materials and objects on this table for making your picture or design. You may use as many of these as you wish. Please select a sheet of colored paper for the background of your picture or design. Glue is provided so that you can paste your picture or design onto the paper."

    Repeat instructions, then ask, "Are there questions?" Repeat instructions as necessary. State, "You will have 40 minutes." Call time as previously specified. Ask those questions contained in the guide for observing and interpreting responses.

    When the collage is used as a group task activitiy, the group is asked to discuss among themselves what theme for a picture or design they would like to choose, come to an agreement, and complete their project. The other directions for process are then given.

4. *Obstacle Course.* The therapist says, "In this activity you will be doing some physical and recreational activities. I will explain each of these as we go along."

    Note: Tasks are to be presented in the sequence outlined earlier on p 198. Directions for each task are self-evident in the description of the tasks contained in that section.

5. *Circle Ball Tag.* The therapist says, "This is a circle ball game—please form a circle. Keep a distance of about one foot between each of you. The rules of the game are: 1) one person stands in the center of the circle; 2) those around the circle throw the ball across the circle to one another; 3) the person in the center is to try to catch the ball; 4) when the person in the center catches the ball, he leaves the center position, and the person who has thrown the caught ball then goes into the center; 5) those around the circle are to try to keep the person in the center from catching the ball. Let's try it one time for practice." (The therapist demonstrates with the group how the game is played.)

   The therapist then asks, "Who will volunteer to begin in the center?" If after a reasonable time, no one volunteers, the therapist makes a choice of someone who can be expected to manage this position. If no volunteer or choice is possible, the therapist initiates the activity by taking the center position and then moving out of the game at an appropriate time.

   Call time as previously specified. Ask questions contained in the guide for observing and interpreting responses.

6. *Activity Laboratory Questionnaire.* Each client is given the questionnaire (Appendix V). The group is reminded that they have participated in five activities, each of them different, that the therapist would like to know what they felt about these experiences, and would like them to answer the questions on the sheets of paper.

Interpretations of Behaviors Assessed
Stencil Cut-out and Crayon

This is a task that realistically and symbolically contains a high degree of external limits and controls. Outcome expectations are clear and predictable, and processes are sequentially ordered and controlled by pattern, materials, and directions. The only explicit free choice opportunity is the instruction to select one of the two forms for reproduction. The nature of the task, the structure of the setting in which it occurs, the materials used, and its placement as the first activity in the laboratory experience, are most reminiscent of early school years and of child-to-authority social relationships.

The task requires a moderate degree of fine motor skills. The social-interpersonal field requires no interdependent collaborative behavior. It is one of parallel activity with implied expectations that each participant function independently without influence on or from another. Since this is the first experience in the laboratory, participants are unknown to one another.

This activity can therefore most readily provide information about styles and patterns of responding to and managing clearly established external limits and controls; cause and effect predictability; sequential ordering; restrictions on free choice; individuality; risk taking and chance; inferred limitations and task expectations; moderately fine motor skill requirements; time limitations; the interpersonal/social expectations and constraints inherent in this task; and setting.

Observations would thus include such behaviors as:

Verbalized concern for getting instructions clear.

Checking to be certain that directions are accurately followed by:

   —Re-asking the therapist for clarification and/or confirmation.

Gail S. Fidler

—Asking other participants for clarification or validation.
—Checking by looks at how others are proceeding.
—Correcting, advising or "reporting on" others.

Not verifying or checking.

Positioning of form on paper.

Use of both forms.

Altering and/or embellishing form.

Turning the papers horizontally or on an angle.

Reproducing the form more than once on the paper.

Adding to the background, ie, border, flowers, sun.

Trading crayons or taking a preferred color from someone else.

Complaining about restrictions but not acting.

Initiating alterations or changes in the basic pattern or process.

Following another's initiative.

Handling detail with precision and concern for accuracy.

Encouraging others to test limits.

Silent attention to and preoccupation with task.

Joking, introducing, or responding to extraneous task.

Other responses to actual and/or inferred limitations and expectations.

Hearing, retaining, and following through on verbal instructions.

Fine motor skills, visual-motor integration, spatial relationships.

Management of time.

Attention span.

Task focus.

Interpersonally focused behaviors, ie, responses to and/or initiative contact with others, including the therapist.

Outstanding characteristics of completed project, ie, neatness and clarity of outline, exact reproduction, embellishments, similarity with and difference from others.

Additional information is obtained at the completion of the activity by asking each participant:

What did you like about this activity?

What did you dislike about it?

Why did you choose Figure 12.1 and not Figure 12.2?

Finger Painting

This is an activity that realistically and symbolically contains a high degree of freedom in terms of process and outcomes. External limits and controls are virtually non-existent, except in an inferred manner by the size of the paper. There are no rules or patterns to govern process, control decisions, define outcomes or to act as an organizing, task initiating force. Freedom from external limits and control is reinforced by the fluid nature of the paint and water and the smooth surface of the paper. These support the quality of unpredictability and the element of chance. The lack of structure coupled with the fluid nature of the materials and the direct hand contact with the paint, establishes the self as the initiation—the cause and effect agent. Color, texture, smell, and hand-arm movement with the paint are sensory and affective stimuli that re-state the free, self expressive nature of the activity. Permanency of an end product is a matter of free choice. Color most frequently reflects affect while form more usually relates to ideation. Finger painting is most frequently associated with childhood experiences, free expression, and play.

The task does not require fine motor skills. The social-interpersonal field does not require inter-dependent, collaborative behavior.

This activity can therefore most readily provide data about styles and manner of responding to and managing unstructured tasks and settings; the freedom from external controls and limits; risk, chanciness, and change; sensory and affective stimuli; expectations regarding self expression, initiative, individuality, and spontaneity; time limitations; and the interpersonal, social expectations within such an environment.

Observations would include such behaviors as:

Time delay in beginning activity
Choice of color(s)—manner of selecting color(s)
Quantity of color used
Consistency of paint/water mixture
Experimentations with forms, shapes, designs
Experimentations with movement
Experimentations with color, ie, blending, mixing
Number of colors used
Use of finger(s) or whole hand(s)
Request for or use of implement to substitute for hand
Frequency of erasures
Organizing a picture, scene, or design
Using borders, boundaries, or color separations
Absence of forms, shapes, themes, or designs
Handling the boundary of the paper
Relating color to forms, designs, and/or movement patterns
Interrupting activity, frequency of stops or inactivity
Preoccupation with task
Joking, laughing, singing, talking, other spontaneous behaviors
Silent attention to task
Encouraging/cautioning others about expressiveness, experimentation
Frequency of hand washing and/or cleaning of work area
Early termination or continuation of activity
Handling of clean-up at end of activity
Interpersonally focused behaviors, ie, responses to and/or initiative contacts with others—peers and therapist
Outstanding charcteristics of completed work

Responses to:
What did you like about this activity?
What did you not like about it?
What part of the activity most influenced what you did, for example:
—the colors?
—the feel and movement?

Gail S. Fidler

—an idea you had for a picture or design before you began?
What title might you give your painting?

Collage

This activity requires a moderate degree of cognitive organization. The numerous and varied materials and objects available for use and the specifications for the end product comprise a task that requires organization of sensory stimuli and thought. There is an absence of external organizing factors such as a pattern, guidelines, or process directions. The process involves perceiving the number of possible alternatives, ie, what resources are available, what end-product ideas might be possible; assessing the applicability of resources (objects, materials, personal skills, and time) in relation to possible ideas; making a choice; organizing and planning in accordance with that choice; adapting, altering, reassessing the plan, materials, etc; following through the implementing the plan, ie, being goal directed; and inhibiting other alternatives and stimuli that are extraneous or counter-productive to the chosen plan.

The materials and objects used in this activity all have a history and thus, a consensually validated use and purpose in everyday life, eg, buttons, twine, fabric, ads, greeting cards, public communication. The activity requires a degree of abstraction, the envisioning and use of materials and objects out of context of their traditional uses or purposes.

As an individual task, the activity requires interpersonal skills only to the degree of being able to share scissors, glue, and the common stockpile of materials. It is a parallel activity with the implied expectation of independence without influence on or from others.

When the collage is used as a small group task, it taps group member role behaviors—collaborative, interdependent relationship skills.

No significant degree of fine motor skill is required. A moderate ability to manage spatial relationships and three dimension perspectives is necessary. This activity can therefore provide information about styles and patterns of responding to and/or managing multiple, varied, and simultaneous sensory and ideational stimuli; sequential problem solving that involves identifying options, assessing alternatives, organizing and planning without external structure for process or end-product; reassessing, altering, and compromising ideas and plans; implementation and follow-through on a self designed plan; organization, initiation, abstraction, and reality testing; time management; and interpersonal and social expectations inherent in such a task and environment.

Observations would include such behaviors as:

Manner of beginning the activity.
  Time taken in selecting background paper
  Combining or using more than one background paper
  Time spent in scanning or looking through the available materials or objects
  Manner of assessing resources, eg, visual scanning, sorting through and handling materials, single focus.

Variety of materials and objects initially selected.
Experimentation with objects, materials, eg, arranging, altering.
Time between experimentation and choice of materials.
Frequency and kind of alterations made of materials and/or objects chosen.

Frequency of re-looking at stockpile, discard of and new choices of materials or objects.

Effect of such changes, eg, better organization, loss of organization, change in/enhancement of theme or design.

Variety and kind of objects or materials actually used.

Use of space.

Handling of border.

Interpersonally focused behaviors, ie, frequency and kind of responses to and/or initiative contact with others.

Primary characteristics of end-product:

Discernable order and design, random placement, representational, abstract, human, non-human objects, use of words, textures, colors, three dimensions.

Responses to:

What did you like about this activity?

What did you dislike about it?

What title might you give your product?

When used as a group task, observations would include behaviors such as:

Group member role skills and styles; eg, initiator, clarifier, helper, doer, encourager, director.

Compromising, collaborating without negating own interests or ideas.

Mediating, coping with conflict, different ideas, and process styles.

Listening, responding to others.

How the group theme was chosen.

Obstacle Course

This activity consists of a series of individual tasks requiring a variety of basic gross motor coordination skills. The levels and complexity of coordination are evident in each of the tasks described earlier.

Observations will include behaviors and skills relative to:

Gait and posture.

Body balance.

Coordination of body in movement, agility.

Visual-motor coordination.

Muscle control.

Endurance.

Interest in physical activity.

Attention span.

Motivation.

Responses to and management of success, failure, competition, achievement, expectations.

Hearing, responding to, and retaining verbal directions.

Interpersonally focused behaviors.

These are individual tasks and the social-interpersonal field requires no interdependent collaborative behaviors. However, this is the fourth experience in the laboratory and thus there is increasing familiarity among participants.

Gail S. Fidler

Observations within this context should include the frequency and kind of responses to others, initiative contact with others, and comparison of these with the social/interpersonal behaviors in earlier activities when the other participants were unknown.

What were the clients' responses to such questions as:

What did you like about these activities?
What did you disklike about them?

Circle Ball Tag

This activity requires a moderate degree of gross motor coordination and physical assertion. The game is one of competition and cooperative play. It requires attentiveness to the behavior and activity of others, anticipation and judgment about the movement of another, motor planning, and execution. Competition involves the one-against-one, and group-against-one test of gross motor planning and agility. The structure, process, and purpose of the game allows for individual choice of one-to-one and/or an alliance with others to compete against or help the person in the center of the circle. In this context, the shaping or alteration of the basic ground rules is neither prohibited nor explicitly expected. The development of a consensus with regard to helping out or making it more difficult for the one in the center position requires initiating behavior, responsiveness to cues from others, and an incentive to join one or another alliance. The center of the circle position involves coordination of the body in movement, physical assertiveness, second guessing others, motor planning, agility, and competitiveness.

This activity can therefore provide information about styles and patterns of responding to and/or managing: gross motor skills; balance, control, and coordination in movement; physical assertion and forcefulness; motor planning, altertness, and agility; competition, success, failure, frustration; cooperative, responsive expectations; the skills, limitations, and feelings of others; scapegoat, aggressor, mediator, helper roles; group identification; and collaborative expectations.

Observations would include such behaviors as:

Volunteering for center position.
Force of ball toss.
Accuracy of toss or pass.
Tossing across or around the circle.
Accuracy of timing.
Use of one or both arms.
Throwing consistently in one direction.
Throwing consistently to one person.
Developing alliance between two or more persons.
Encouraging competitive/responsive behavior in others.
Tossing/bouncing ball so that it is easily caught.
Tossing/bouncing ball to trick others.
Tossing/bouncing ball so that it is difficult to catch.
Verbal encouragement to person in center.
Verbal disparagement of others.

Rescuing/helping person in center.

Behaving so as to avoid the center position.

Behaving so that being in the center is inevitable.

Alertness.

Attention span.

Responsiveness, following behavior.

Energy level.

Adherence to the rules.

Asking for clarifications.

Asking for intervention by the therapist or others.

Leaving the circle.

Laughing at/with others.

Verbal/non-verbal expression of frustration, pleasure, anger.

Periods of non-participation, unresponsiveness.

Productive/non-productive teasing, tricking.

Center position behaviors, such as skill, balance, speed, agility, motor planning.

Future Research

Some of the questions that should be raised and researched are:

1. Does a given task or activity elicit certain behaviors?
2. Does a given task or activity elicit certain behaviors more readily than another, dissimilar activity?
3. What are the key elements of a given task or activity that are most frequently related to certain responses?
4. Are behavioral responses to certain tasks or activities able to be generalized to key tasks and activities of daily living?
5. Is there a relationship between the character trait profile of an individual and the profile describing the characteristics of an activity?
6. Is a relationship discernible in choice, pleasure, investment and quality of performance?

Such investigations would clarify the elements used in the Laboratory, as well as give a tested basis for treatment planning in clinical occupational therapy.

Conclusion

The Activity Laboratory provides a structure for observing and assessing certain perceptual, integrative, and behavioral strategies. Information gathered from observations and feedback from the participant makes it possible to at least describe the most salient sensory, motor, cognitive, psychological, and social behaviors that are evident in responses to certain circumstances and task expectations. Assumptions can then be developed and tested with regard to what may be the client's most characteristic ways of managing and coping with the demands of everyday living, and what kinds and levels of remedial experiences may be indicated.

The value of the Laboratory is that its structure and process make it possible to compare and contrast different responses of a participant in different situations. Such comparative observations are critical to understanding responses and generalizing these for a comprehensive view of behavior. The amount of information that can be obtained and used to formulate a behavioral description will depend upon the skill and experience of the therapist. The novice therapist will find it useful to limit observations to a few key factors in each activity unit of the Laboratory rather than attempt to cope with the many behavioral strategies that are manifested. With experience, the number of factors that can be identified, compared, and understood will increase. When observations are the key means of data gathering, the risk of subjectivity is always a concern. Therefore, a firm theoretical background must be emphasized as essential to the use of the Laboratory. Continual critique, practice, and feedback from others is critical—especially for the inexperienced therapist.

Difficulties with accuracy of recall can occur in summarizing and generalizing observations and data if a format for noting key observations is not developed. If additional staff or students are available as observers and assigned responsibility for recording key responses of specific clients, the task of keeping track of responses is considerably easier. Such a process is an excellent teaching-learning experience for staff and students, and has the added value of providing several perspectives and increasing the probability of objectivity. Nevertheless, those key factors that are chosen for observation in each activity unit should be listed on a recording sheet. Brief notations, such as key words or symbols can then be jotted on these sheets and used as references in preparing a summary. In the three activities that include an end product (stencil, finger painting, collage), the participants should be asked to sign their names to their product, record the title they have given to the production, and turn these in to the therapist.

PART 4
QUESTIONNAIRES, OBSERVATIONS, AND PERFORMANCE SCALES

13
The Comprehensive Occupational Therapy Evaluation

Sara J. Brayman, M.S., O.T.R.
Thomas Kirby, Ph.D.

The Comprehensive Occupational Therapy Evaluation (COTE) scale was developed to identify behaviors in an acute adult psychiatric setting, enhance observation of clients, reduce the subjectivity in reporting observations, eliminate the inherent problems in the narrative note, facilitate efficient communication of the client's progress, and aid in planning treatment. The COTE enables the therapist to report a large volume of comprehensive and pertinent information quickly in a consistent format with defined terminology. This instrument has been invaluable in defining the scope of occupational therapy in the acute adult psychiatric facility.

The development of the COTE has been, in part, a reflection on the current state of the profession of occupational therapy, which is a rapidly growing, changing profession. Inherent with this are problems with its identification as a profession, the development of a body of knowledge, accountability, and the lack of effective measurement tools. Identification as a profession seems less of a problem, with the general agreement that occupational therapy deals with "...activity or occupation that is purposeful, meaningful, and structured to accomplish specific therapeutic objectives."[1]

With this general agreement, development of a body of knowledge, evaluation, and accountability need to be addressed. These problems are due, at least in part, to the lack of effective measurement instruments. Thus, a major task facing occupational therapists is the development of good measurement instruments.

The need for good measurement instruments and for the information they would provide has often been voiced. In 1949, Beals wrote,

> Occupational therapy as a science demands a universal and valid expression acceptable to all. Yet professional writings and research are often misunderstood by others than the author because of lack of general yardstick, or of resistance among the profession to face a completely new evaluation of characterstics.[2]

Literature Review

Rationale

Fidler and Fidler, in referencing the work of Azima, point out that,

> The use of occupational therapy as a process for measuring and predicting change and for evaluating psychotherapeutic progress has been neglected. Such lack of development reflects the need for increased concomitant skills in this area and for increased research and study.[3]

In the special session of the Representative Assembly in November, 1978, West stated that the bases of occupational therapy "rest in the knowledge we [borrow] from the biological, psychological, and social sciences."[4]

The researcher further suggested that, "our research directions are unlimited in the sense that validation of practice is needed in every aspect of our service to patients with physical and psychosocial dysfunction."[1]

Fidler states, "We should also be equally aware of the limited energy and resources we have directed to the development and refinement of knowledge and education as compared with many of our colleagues in the health care system."[4] West selects the need for evaluation instruments as a major issue, and emphatically states, "There is a need for evaluation instruments developed by and for occupational therapists."[1]

However, occupational therapists have been active in developing evaluative tools. West found in her 100-issue review of *The American Journal Of Occupational Therapy*, "16 articles reporting specific assessments, evaluations, and scales developed by occupational therapists."[3] Other research suggests a "moratorium on development of more therapist-made evaluations until those currently in use are validated." However, reviews of certain areas of occupational therapy reveal a dearth of evaluative instruments, and indicate the need for significant attention. One of these areas has been evaluation instruments for the acutely ill patient in a short term psychiatric facility.

Fidler and Fidler note that one of the common difficulties in recording occupational therapy evaluative measures is that information often gets lost or diluted in progress notes.[5] Wolff states that, "various rating scales now in use have proven to be invaluable in evaluation of the effectiveness of therapies for the determination of clients' readiness to leave the hospital."[6]

Because of the need for evaluative instruments and their value to the therapist, numerous rating scales have been developed. In 1954, Ayres developed a rating scale to evaluate work behavior.[7] The scale that resulted was one consisting of 25 items with ratings of 0 through 4 and a score range of 0 to 100. The researcher points out the need to correlate the results of the scale with the client's behavior in an actual work situation. In 1955, Ayres also developed an evaluation of work habits.[5] A form was constructed to rate trainees on 10 different work habits. In 1961 Wolff developed a rating scale for use in occupational therapy with clients in state mental hospitals.[8] The researcher selected 15 behaviors and completed reliability and validity studies on the scale. An item analysis was done to determine the extent of each scale's contribution to the total score. In one of the items of behavior it is found that there were actually two "ends" to it, and thus an A and B category for the item was developed. Alard describes the development of a scale for ranking activities used in occupational therapy with mentally ill clients. The researcher concludes that the scale gave "credence to the judgments an occupational therapist makes when using activity characteristics as a measuring device in client evaluation and treatment."[2] Beals also developed a scale that would "afford a reasonably accurate and comparative recording of the reaction and response of the psychiatric client in the occupational therapy situation."[8] Beals points out that the results of the measurements are graphically displayed, and gives the busy psychiatrist a quick resume of the client's performance as observed by the occupational therapist.

In addition, Clark, Koch, and Nichols developed a scale for rating psychiatric clients in occupational therapy. The scale was developed "to fill a gap left by existing instruments which, while applicable to occupational therapy, did not

Sara J. Brayman and Thomas Kirby

assess some of the unique characteristics of the area."[9] Through factor analysis, the authors arrived at a 21 item scale which measured five factors.

Esser speaks to the broad appeal of rating scales. Pointing out that "generally speaking, they are easy to use, and require a minimum expenditure of staff time and energy. However, in addition to being easy to use, rating scales should also provide the user with accurate information about the individual being rated."[10] The researcher further notes that rating scales "...may be a useful tool for sharing information and facilitating communication."[9]

Thus, it can be easily seen that there are many needs for rating scales and many reasons for developing them. Often occupational therapists find themselves in a situation where there is no appropriate instrument available for use in that particular setting. We found ourselves in a similar situation, which led to the development of the COTE scale.

Several objectives guided the development of the scale. The first was to identify behaviors that occurred in and were particularly relevant to the practice of occupational therapy. Most of the behaviors identified are those that are usually evaluated by occupational therapists and then reported in an evaluation or in progress notes.

The second objective was to define the identified behaviors in such a mannner that they could be reliably observed and rated by two or more therapists. Numerous revisions were required in the definitions, some of which are still ongoing.

A third objective was to direct the information on the scale primarily to the busy referring psychiatrist. A short, one page form without definitions was first selected. After several months of use, it was decided that the scale would be more useful if the definitions were printed on the back of the form. Also, the scale was designed to provide a record of client progress of each behavior since sufficient rating blocks were provided to cover the average length of stay for most patients. Thus, the scale provides the doctor with effects of the total treatment process on each of the behaviors evaluated by occupational therapy, and shows daily progress from the baseline evaluation.

A fourth objective was to provide an efficient method for data retrieval, to assist in treatment planning, and evaluation of treatment results. All behaviors can be identified by numbers, and progress or lack of progress can easily be seen, and comparisons made between admission and discharge behaviors.

The understanding of the role of occupational therapy in the overall psychiatric therapeutic milieu is becoming increasingly important. The trend in all areas of health care is toward greater accountability. Third party payers often do not pay for services that are not measured or defined.

Typically, occupational therapists have used the narrative note to both describe behaviors and progress of clients. However, many occupational therapists and other health care professionals have found that the narrative note is inadequate in communicating the process and results of occupational therapy.

Numerous problems are associated with narrative notes. Although informative, they are time consuming for the therapist to write and for the reader to read. Too often, narrative notes are expressed in vague generalities, are inconsistent, and provide very limited information. For the therapist, notewriting is often tedious, and is postponed until the end of the day or squeezed into an already overloaded schedule. Good notes take time to write and should be done immediately after a therapy session. Even then it is often difficult for the therapist to find just the right word or phrase to accurately and concisely describe what occurred during the session. It is easy to confuse the behavior of one client with that of another. Even when time is scheduled for the actual writing of the notes, the charts may be unavailable, or there may be other conflicts that cause delays in the timely entry of information into the client's chart. The notes may be further delayed if they are dictated, because of the time required for typing. The end result is that notes are not available on a timely basis, and information from the therapist is not utilized by other members of the treatment team.

Another problem with narrative notes is that reporting styles differ from therapist to therapist. Each therapist develops his own phrases and descriptive terminology with his own unique meanings. This often makes notes varied, and relay little information. The statement, "Patient seems better today," tells the reader very little. To determine the meaning of this statement, the reader must refer to previous notes which are often buried deep within the chart.

The occupational therapy process provides the therapist with the unique opportunity to observe many behaviors. It is unlikely that these observations would all be recorded on the patient's record in a narrative note and if they were, few staff could or would take the time to read them. Reports tend to concentrate on the most outstanding or exteme behaviors. Other behaviors which may be significant are over-shadowed or may even be omitted. The psychiatrist monitoring the effects of a new medication may be more interested in a client's fine motor performance on an occupational therapy project than in the extremes of affect that are so often reported.

Research

The COTE Scale was developed at Marshall I. Pickens Hospital, a 50 bed acute care, community based adult psychiatric facility that is a part of a comprehensive community mental health center. Seventy percent of the clients come from the county in which the hospital is located, and the remaining 30% come from three surrounding counties. The county served had a population of approximately 240,000 when the scale was developed.

The client population was primarily Caucasian (97%) and female (68%). Over half the clients (57%) were diagnosed as depressive neurosis. The second most frequent diagnosis was involutional depression (9%). Eight percent were schizopherenic, 5% were manic-depressive, 3% were anxiety neurosis, and 3% were organic brain syndrome. Other diagnoses included suicidal, chronic pain, psychosis, and adjustment reaction of adolescence.

Weekly incomes were as follows: Twenty-seven percent were under $100, 16% were $100 to $149, 12% were $150 to $199, 15% were $200 to $299, 12% were $300 or over. In 18% the income was unknown. In education, 26.5% had completed grade school, 50% had completed high school, and 22% had at least a year or more of college.

As noted earlier, the majority of these clients came from the local community and returned to their community. Average length of stay was approximately 11 days and the clients did not require further or more intensive hospitalization. Most of the clients were quite capable of handling basic self-care tasks.

Upon admission, clients are assigned to a nursing station and are given a schedule which indicates their nursing station and their assigned activities for each day. After the first day or two, when clients are given assistance in following the schedule, they are expected to be independent.

The admitting psychiatrists are in private practice and there are no house staff to

Sara J. Brayman and Thomas Kirby

direct hospital treatment teams. Therefore, the OT Department is faced with a variety of philosophies and treatment approaches which require a great degree of flexibility. Each psychiatrist monitors the treatment program of his clients. As a group, the psychiatrists provide differing degrees of direction to the different therapies. The result is the psychiatrists require different types of information from the therapists. This factor was the prime reason for the development of the COTE Scale; it provides a format for conveying consistent information to these psychiatrists, who then choose the information required for their treatment approaches.

Administration

Twenty-five behaviors identified as being observable in occupational therapy are listed down the left margin of the scale (Appendix W). Following the behaviors are a grid which provides space for successively recording the scores of each behavior. Scores on the scale range from 0 to 4, with 0 meaning normal, and 4 indicating extreme behavior. Behavior ratings are totaled after each session and recorded on the scale—immediately indicating any changes in behavior. Space is provided beneath the grid for listing treatment goals and for noting unusual occurrences.

The format utilized in the COTE provides the therapist with an efficient mechanism for reporting observations made in occupational therapy. The therapist merely assigns a single numerical score for each of the 25 behaviors. Scoring of all behaviors takes less than two minutes. The grid permits the therapist to record each day's observation on the same sheet, thus providing a mechanism for comparing one session's behavior with that observed in previous sessions. This, too, saves time, as the therapist does not have to search through the chart to see what was recorded earlier. The grid provides space to record observed behaviors for 16 days, usually adequate for the entire hospitalization period in the setting where the COTE Scale was developed, which has an average length of stay of 11 to 12 days.

The qualities that make reporting easier for the writer also make for easier reading. All of the information is located on one page, so there is no need to sift through the chart. If there is any question about terminology, the definitions for each rating, are stated in technical terms, and printed on the back of the form (Appendix X).

The COTE Scale imposes a structure for reporting observations made during the occupational therapy process. Use of this format eliminates the need for vague, narrative statements such as, "seems better today". The problem of unique definitions is also eliminated, in that any person using or reading the scale can refer directly to the definitions.

Behaviors Assessed

The 25 behaviors are divided into three areas: 1) General Behavior, 2) Interpersonal, and 3) Task Behaviors. The seven behaviors listed in Part One, although not uniquely observable in occupational therapy, provide valuable information about the client's overall functioning. The six behaviors listed in Part Two involve interpersonal skills which can be evaluated in other therapies as well as occupational therapy. Part Three of the COTE Scale consists of 12 behaviors that are related to task performance, which are unique to occupational therapy. This weighting toward task performance emphasizes the importance of the role of purposeful activity in the occupational therapy process.

Behaviors in Part One provide for an evaluation of the client's general level of functioning. While these behaviors are observed and reported by other health professionals, the occurrence and performance during the occupational therapy process provides an additional perspective of the patient's overall behavior. The five possible scores for each of the six behaviors appear in Appendix Y.

Behavior 1A, *appearance*, tells how the client is caring for himself. The six factors were selected because they are within the control of the client in the hospital. Appearance is rated according to the number of factors involved.

Behavior 1B, *nonproductive behavior*, includes such things as rocking, playing with hands, and talking to oneself. These behaviors prevent the client from becoming involved in day-to-day experiences. Excessive socialization can also be considered nonproductive behavior. When these behaviors interfere with performance of an activity or establishment of a relationship, they are considered to be nonproductive and are measured on the COTE Scale by the amount of treatment time involved.

Behavior 1C, *activity level*, may be two directional. A normal level of activity is balanced midway between hyperactivity and hypoactivity. When the level of activity is so high or low as to attract the attention of others, disrupt performance, or prevent participation, it is a problem. Activity level is rated according to its effect on participation.

Behavior 1D, *expression*, includes many of the elements that make up expression, any of which may provide an indication of a client's feelings. Some of these elements are: body language, volume and tone of voice, facial expression, posture and bearing, and the degree of animation displayed. Expression is rated according to its appropriateness to the situation.

Behavior 1E, *responsibility*, is a measure of the client's accountability for his actions. This behavior is reflected in such areas as attendance patterns, adherance to known rules, care of equipment and supplies, keeping appointments, and in fulfilling behavioral contracts. Responsibility is measured according to the degree it is assumed.

Behavior 1F, *punctuality*, is a behavior that reflects a client's responsibility, commitment, motivation, and reliability. This behavior is applicable to the setting in which the COTE scale was developed, because clients are responsible for attending therapy sessions independently. The rating is based on the number of minutes a patient is late for occupational therapy.

Behavior 1G, *reality orientation*, shows how aware the client is of himself, place, time, and situation. It is rated according to the number of factors of which the patient is unaware.

Interpersonal relationships affect performance in all social activities. Effective performance of tasks in daily living often are dependent upon effective social interaction. Occupational therapy provides a structured situation for these relationships to occur, and thus, is a good setting for observing them (Appendix Y).

Behavior 2A, *independence*, tells how independently the client can function in occupational therapy. While occupational therapy may include structured activity, opportunities exist in each session for a client to demonstrate independent actions. These actions are qualifiable and are rated accordingly.

Behavior 2C, *self-assertion*, is divided in a manner similar to activity level. Normal assertion lies approximately midway between very passive and compliant behavior and totally dominating behavior. This behavior is rated according to the amount of time the patient is either passive and compliant, or dominating.

Behavior 2D, *sociability*, is a measure of how well the client socializes with the staff and other patients during the therapy session. This behavior is rated according to whether or not the client can participate, initiate, or respond to social interaction.

Behavior 2E, *attention-getting behavior*, reflects how much time the client spends in this type of behavior. Examples include: repeated questions, frequent requests for assistance, overt requests for approval, or doing nothing in order to get attention.

Behavior 2F, *negative response from others*, is an indicator of the client's effect on the therapists and other clients. This behavior includes asking or demanding special privileges from staff, or interactions with fellow clients that result in negative responses, and is rated according to the number of negative responses evoked from other people.

Behaviors in Part Three of the COTE (Appendix Y) reflect occupational therapy's emphasis on task performance. The therapy session provides the opportunity to observe actual task performance in situations that can be related to the client's daily life.

When observing behavior, the occupational therapist can use numerous types of activities. Sample ratings of task performances using various activities are included to clarify these 13 behaviors. However, in therapy sessions, only one activity would be used to evaluate all 13 behaviors.

Behavior 3A, *engagement*, indicates motivation toward work or activity. Since no task can be completed unless it is begun, this task behavior is significant. The client's willingness to participate in a magazine collage activity can illustrate the degree of engagement displayed and would be scored as follows:

0: After receiving directions, the client chooses a magazine, gathers scissors and glue, and begins to select items for his collage. He then cuts out the desired items, arranges, and glues them as directed.
1: The client is able to perform as above but requires gentle encouragement to begin.
2. The client participates in the activity but needs to be encouraged by name to begin, and then encouraged to continue at each step of the activity.
3. The client needs a great deal of encouragement at each step of the activity and can participate only with constant encouragement and support from the therapist.
4. The client is unable to participate in the activity.

Behavior 3B, *concentration or attention span*, is an important factor in the ability to perform life tasks, and is measured quantitatively in terms of the amount of time spent attending to the activity. Tooling copper foil as a treatment modality, a client's performance would be rated as follows:

0: The client is able to attend to the tooling of the metal foil that is secured to a plastic template, working on it throughout the session; he is able to resume it even after interruption.
1: The client has difficulty resuming the activity after interruption. He exhibits some nonproductive behaviors.
2: The client is able to participate in the task only one half of the session and is unable to resume the activity after interruption without intervention from the therapist.
3: The client is able to concentrate on the tooling activity less than one fourth of

the session, and needs the therapist's reminders to resume the activity. He is easily distracted by others around him.

4: The client loses concentration in less than one minute, and lapses into nonproductive behaviors.

Behavior 3C, *coordination,* can serve as a measurable monitor of the side effects of medication, and indicates how well the body and brain are functioning as a unit. Glazing a ceramic stein is an activity in which coordination can easily be observed, and would be scored as follows:

0: The client is able to apply underglaze or stain and can conform to the outlines of the mold in very fine detail.
1: The client is able to glaze or stain the project and is able to stay within the lines except in very precise areas.
2: The client has some difficulty but can glaze neatly in large areas.
3: The client is able to manage a one color overglaze only. His hand is unsteady but he can complete the task.
4: The client is unable to manipulate the brush; hand and upper extremity are unsteady.

Behavior 3D, *following directions,* is an important aspect of all daily life skills. The occupational therapist may use games such as charades to demonstrate the client's ability to follow directions. This behavior would be scored as follows:

0: The client is able to play charades and can respond to and give standard symbols once he has been taught them. He is able to utilize them without reinforcement.
1: The client needs minimal assistance. He can remember most of the rules but may forget some of the common symbols or rules of the game.
2: The client needs assistance and reinforcement regarding the procedure. He may forget several rules, and needs to be reminded each time he has a turn.
3: The client is able to participate only with the therapist providing guidance at each step of the activity.
4: The client is unable to participate in the activity.

Behavior 3E (a-b), *activity neatness or attention to detail,* are listed as opposites on the COTE scale, and one or the other is rated. These behaviors relate to how well a client can accomplish a task, and to the quality of his work. Either of them can be readily observed while the client is doing a tile trivet activity. These behaviors are scored as follows:

(a) *activity neatness*

0: Given directions, a large box of assorted tile, a trivet and glue, the client is able to create a pleasing design, select, place, and glue tiles neatly to the trivet within a 30 minute session.
1: The client's design is somewhat sloppy and he may use too much glue and get it on the surface of the tiles. However, the activity can be completed within the allotted time.
2: The client's design may be haphazard and the surface of the tiles may be sloppy and marked.
3: The client spills glue or is very sloppy with it, and may get it on his hands and work surface. The titles may be scattered and glued at random. Many are not upright.

Sara J. Brayman and Thomas Kirby

4: The therapist has to intervene during this activity as the client is apt to pour large quantities of glue onto the trivet and then dump the tiles into it.

(b) *attention to detail*

0: Given directions, a large box of assorted tiles, a trivet, and glue, the client is able to create a pleasing design, select, place and glue tiles neatly to the trivet within a 30 minute session.

1: The client has some difficulty selecting tiles and some preciseness is noted when the patient places them on the trivet. The client takes a full 60 minutes to accomplish the entire task.

2: The client takes excessive time to decide on the design or to select tiles. However, once these steps are accomplished, he can complete this phase of the task within 60 minutes.

3. It takes the client at least two hours to complete the activity. Each tile is very precisely placed and the client may even use the tools to assure proper placement.

4. The client takes many sessions to complete the task, if it is completed at all. He seems to select the tiniest tiles available and may use calipers to set and space them.

Behavior 3F, *problem solving*, can be observed in many situations. For example, in a group activity such as puzzle completion, this behavior can be easily observed. The clients are given packages containing all but one of a simple jigsaw puzzle plus one odd piece belonging to another puzzle. The clients are directed to assemble them. The behavior would be scored as follows:

0: Given instructions, the client quickly assembles his puzzle. He is able to determine that he has an odd piece and approaches other clients seeking to trade for his missing puzzle piece and to donate his odd puzzle piece to the client in need of it.

1: The client is able to assemble his puzzle systematically but realizes that he has an odd puzzle piece and that he lacks a necessary piece to complete his puzzle. He seeks advice from the therapist.

2: The client utilizes trial and error assembly. Once he realizes that he lacks a puzzle piece he goes from table to table and tries all odd pieces, finally able to complete his puzzle by trial and error. He is unable to recognize his needed piece without trying to fit it into the puzzle.

3: The client is able to put together his puzzle with effort. He tries repeatedly to fit the odd piece into the puzzle and does not recognize that it is foreign.

4. The client is unable to assemble the puzzle.

Behavior 3G, *complexity and organization of tasks*, can be rated using multilevel activities such as leather lacing. Each style of lacing carries its own level of complexity. This behavior is scored as follows:

0: Given instructions, the client is able to accomplish the double buttonhole stitch, and can splice the lacing and begin and end it without difficulty.

1: The client can do the lacing but cannot figure out how to splice, begin, or end it, even with detailed instructions.

2: The client can do the double stitch with difficulty. He has trouble keeping the twist out of the lace and does one stitch at a time rather than organizing a method or developing a rhythm.

The COTE Scale   219

3: The client can only do simple stitching such as the running stitch or the whip stitch, and needs reinforcement from the therapist.

4. The client cannot manage the task.

Behavior 3H, *initial learning*, can be demonstrated by activities that are unfamiliar to the client and would require instruction. Assembling a leather link belt may provide an excellent media in which to observe this behavior and would be scored as follows:

0: The client is able to follow all written or verbal instructions and begins the belt, even the double wide variety, without assistance from the therapist.

1: The client is able to learn the activity during the session but needs reinforcement from the therapist to begin. After the therapist starts the activity, the client is able to continue independently.

2: The client is unable to do double wide links but can accomplish a single wide variety with minimal assistance from the therapist. However, as above, the therapist must begin the belt.

3: The client is unable to assemble the link belt without occasional assistance from the therapist throughout the activity.

4: The client is unable to put together even the most elementary belt with full support and instruction from the therapist.

Behavior 3I, *interest in activity*, illustrates the client's willingness to try new or different things. This behavior can be observed during a gross motor activity using the parachute. This behavior is scored as follows:

0: The client participates with enthusiasm.

1: The client is willing to participate and does, though somewhat guarded at first. After 10 or 15 minutes, he enthusiastically participates.

2: The client participates by being there, otherwise demonstrating no commitment to the task.

3: The client may join in the activity for the first five minutes, but then stands outside the circle and watches the others participate.

4: The client does not participate and is unwilling to be a spectator.

Behavior 3J, *interest in accomplishment*, indicates whether the client can set goals and work toward them by taking the steps necessary. Craft activities such as decoupage require many steps, and a commitment to complete it. This behavior is scored below:

0: The client carefully selects his design or article to be decoupaged, prepares the wooden surface appropriately, and sands between coats. He expresses concern that everything is done correctly and desires his end product to be pleasing.

1: The client wants to do the activity and initially makes the investment, although his interest wanes before it is completed. Very often the first parts of the activity are done with care and the last steps are hastily accomplished.

2: The client seems to want to get the activity done as quickly as possible and demonstrates no real investment. However, he does express the desire to complete the task.

3. The client does the activity only because the therapist encourages him. He demonstrates no investment or commitment to complete the activity.

4. The client demonstrates no interest or pleasure in the activity. He does not complete it and discards or abandons it when he leaves occupational therapy.

Sara J. Brayman and Thomas Kirby

Behavior 3K, *decision-making*, is an integral part of daily living, and may depend on the number and kinds of choices and the degree of support available. The process of selecting an activity to do during occupational therapy can illustrate this behavior and would be measured as follows:

0: After discussion with the therapist regarding the goals for treatment, the client is able to choose an activity from those available and proceed independently.
1: After discussion with the therapist regarding the goals for treatment, the client selects an appropriate activity but occasionally seeks the therapist's approval.
2: The client makes decisions about his activity but often seeks the therapist's approval.
3: The client is able to select an activity when given two alternatives.
4: The client is unable or refuses to make any decisions.

Behavior 3L, *frustration tolerance*, can be an indicator of the client's ability to persevere in activities when each phase does not come easily. This behavior can be observed when patients are asked to assemble wooden kits.

0: The client is able to assemble the wooden pieces of a tool rack. He carefully plans the assembly and is able to continue, surmounting minor problems.
1: The client often becomes frustrated when assembly is not smooth, but can handle simple tasks.
2: The client often becomes frustrated with more than one step tasks, but he is able to accomplish them.
3: The client becomes frustrated with all aspects of assembly, but tries to continue the activity.
4: The client becomes so frustrated with a simple task that he refuses or is unable to continue.

Case Study

The format of the COTE is helpful in developing a treatment plan. It graphically displays areas of strengths and weaknesses and can help the therapist to establish priorities for treatment. For example, a 49 year old female client with a diagnosis of depressive neurosis was evaluated using the COTE scale. This client was escorted to occupational therapy by a mental health technician. After being introduced to the occupational therapy area by the therapist, she sat quietly at the table, seemingly unaware of the activities about her. She responded when approached and answered inquiries, but did not volunteer information or initiate conversation. The therapist directed the client to sit in a chair at a table with two other clients, and introduced them to each other. To assess task behavior, the therapist selected a tile trivet activity. The client was directed to select tiles of any three colors, place a small amount of glue on the back of each and glue them to the trivet in any pattern or design desired.

The client needed to be encouraged three times to begin selecting tiles. She was unable to determine a design or pattern for the tiles and began gluing only after the therapist had suggested a design. She was able to manipulate the tiles and the glue bottle. The tiles were all placed upright but were glued somewhat haphazardly. She was unable to complete the task, and demonstrated no interest in the activity or in the activities about her.

After recording this client's performance on the COTE scale, treatment planning was already somewhat defined. The client's major difficulties seemed to be in the areas of independence, self-assertion, sociability, and concentration. After looking at her profile and reviewing her performance in occupational therapy, the therapist determined that these difficulties were interdependent (Figure 13.1). Based on this profile, the therapist developed an outline for treatment with goals to increase independence, socialization, self-assertion, and self-esteem.

The COTE scale has also been helpful when auditing medical records. Since entries on the COTE are numerical, outcome criteria can be expressed numerically. For example, discharge criteria for a client diagnosed as depressive neurosis may be: 1) able to socialize with more than one person at a time, 2) follows three step directions, and 3) functions independently in occupational therapy. The retriever would be directed to look for scores of 0 to 1 in behaviors 2A (independence), 2D (sociability), and 3D (follow directions) entered on the last day of hospitalization. If the scores are higher, then the treatment objectives of occupational therapy were not met. The deficiency must then be explained by the therapist to the reviewing body.

Research Studies

Reliability

Reliability was determined by computing percentage agreement between the ratings of two therapists with five different therapists involved. Ratings within one degree of each other were considered acceptable and the percent agreements for 55 patients ranged from 76% to 100% and averaged 95%. Percent agreements for exact agreements ranged from 36% to 84% and averaged 63%.

In personal correspondence from the director of occupational therapy of a large general hospital with a 13 bed psychiatric unit, reliability data were reported on seven patients. Two therapists and one aide had completed the ratings. Percent agreements for ratings within one degree of each other ranged from 96% to 100% and averaged 98%. Thus, reliability data from two different settings were very comparable.

Validity

Validity was determined by randomly selecting the charts of five discharged patients from a group of 400. Total scores for the first and last days in occupational therapy were compared. The scores averaged 31 and 17, respectively, and the drop in score agreed with the observation of other professionals in the acute hospital setting. Similar results have been reported by therapists from other hospitals.

In a study conducted by an occupational therapy student in the psychiatric unit of a medical university hospital, it was observed that a client's total scores decreased from the first to the last day in occupational therapy.* To insure validity of each day's ratings, the student scored the clients on a new scale each day to avoid the influence of the score from the previous day. The average score for the first day of occupational therapy was 20 with a range of 0 to 62. The average score on the last day was eight, with a range of 0 to 28. The average decrease in scores was 11 points, with a range of 0 to 57. Again, similar results in a different setting support the validity of the instrument.

Further Research

The COTE scale is still in the developmental stage. A great deal of research is needed in order to complete its development and to determine its overall value.

One of the first studies needed is a factor analysis of the scale, similar to that

---

*Cook, P. L.: A Study: The Comprehensive Occupational Therapy Evaluation Scale, 1977.

     Sara J. Brayman and Thomas Kirby

FIGURE 13.1

COTE PROFILE OF A 49 YEAR OLD FEMALE WITH DEPRESSIVE NEUROSIS

Date   9/6

I. GENERAL BEHAVIOR

A. Appearance	1
B. Non-Productive Behavior	2
C. Activity Level (a or b)	3a
D. Expression	1
E. Responsibility	1
F. Punctuality	1
G. Reality Orientation	1
Sub-Total	10

II. INTERPERSONAL BEHAVIOR

A. Independence	3
B. Cooperation	0
C. Self Assertion (a or b)	3a
D. Sociability	3
E. Attention Getting Behavior	0
F. Negative Response From Others	0
Sub-Total	9

III. TASK BEHAVIOR

A. Engagement	2
B. Concentration	2
C. Coordination	1
D. Follow Directions	1
E. Activity Neatness or Attention to Detail	1a
F. Problem Solving	2
G. Complexity and Organization of Task	2
H. Initial Learning	2
I. Interest in Activity	3
J. Interest in Accomplishment	2
K. Decision Making	2
L. Frustration Tolerance	2
Sub-Total	22
TOTAL	41

SCALE: 0 — NORMAL, 1 — MINIMAL, 2 — MILD, 3 — MODERATE 4 — SEVERE

The COTE Scale

reported by Clark, Koch, and Nichols. Such a study is needed to determine if the 25 behaviors presently used are all necessary, and whether or not additional or more significant behaviors should be added to the scale.

Once this study is completed, further research is needed with regard to the reliabilty of the scale. Such a study should include the replication of the approach used for determining the initial reliability of the scale in other settings than those reported. Other reliability studies could include comparisons between experienced occupational therapists and students in occupational therapy, and comparison between occupational therapists and other professionals who are trained in the observation of behavior.

Other validity studies are also needed. These studies should include a comparison of the COTE to other scales that are used in occupational therapy. Studies could also include comparisons of the COTE with scales used by other therapists in the treatment of the mentally ill. This would include scales used by recreational therapists, social workers, nurses, etc. The purpose of this study would be to determine whether or not the same type of behavior is observed in other situations as is observed in the typical occupational therapy sessions.

Upon completion of the above studies, revisions should be made, and the necessary research conducted to establish the validity and reliability of the revised scale. Studies should then be conducted in order to determine the possibiity of profile analysis of diagnosis; studies should also be done to determine any that occur in a typical course of treatment in the institution. Such research may provide predictable cycles which would, in turn, be a valuable aid to therapists and the physician, and would also serve to alert these persons in the event of deviation from the cycle. Another area of study is standardization to determine the level of scores demonstrated by the normal population. It should be shown that the scale differentiates between the normal population and the mentally ill. Some informal work has been done in this area, in that the normal group scores averaged seven to eight, which supported differentiation.

Finally, to determine the generalization of the scale, studies should be conducted with psychiatric populations in other settings. This would include private settings that have a similar treatment program as that of Marshall I. Pickens Hospital, as well as state institutions where long term care is provided. Such a study should probably include the more severe mentally ill population that is frequently not found in the Marshall I. Pickens setting.

Conclusion

While still in its developmental stages, the COTE has proven to be a useful tool for organizing the reporting observations made during the occupational therapy process. It identifies and defines the parameters of 25 behaviors usually observable in OT, and provides the therapist with a structured format for reporting them. In so doing, the COTE overcomes many of the shortcomings of the narrative note alone. It communicates clearly to the reader, since the same definitions are readily available to all. The COTE also supplies a comprehensive numerical profile which can be easily compared to previous performances.

In performing the above function, the COTE appears to have good potential as a measurement tool. Thus, it may help provide and broaden the field of knowledge in Occupational Therapy. It has met the objectives which guided the development of the scale, and definitely provides better information than, "Seems better today."

Daily use of the COTE has been effective for charting on most of the clients seen

Sara J. Brayman and Thomas Kirby

in the Occupational Therapy Department for which it was designed. However, when a client's behavior is so extreme as to prevent participation, the defined behavior parameters are inadequate. It is probable that although marked changes in behavior are evident, no change in score would be reflected. The COTE scale is ineffective in this situation and the narrative note is better used. As the client's behavior falls within the parameters of the COTE, the rating scale can then be utilized.

Behavior problems that are very subtle are difficult to rate on the COTE. For example, a client whose behavior is very controlled and precise may demonstrate significant changes and the numerical score remain in the 0-1 range. In this instance, the narrative note should again be employed.

From correspondence we have received, the COTE has been very effective in departments similar to the one where it was developed. Many therapists indicated that they were using it in its original form and that it has become a part of the permanent medical record. Some therapists have shared modifications made for their facility and the COTE format can be readily adapted to a variety of settings. For example, one therapist suggested adding to the definition of punctuality because in that facility how the client gets to OT is a consideration. Although the original intent was for daily reporting, expanding the interval could be effective in longer term facilities.

Therapists working in a rehabilitation setting have found that the COTE Scale is useful with clients who are learning to cope with altered life styles caused by pain or chronic disability. In addition, therapists often have to address the behaviors concomitant to the physical restoration programs. Using the structure of the COTE Scale, a functional evaluation has been drafted for use in a rehabilitation facility. (Appendixes Z, AA). This functional evaluation replaces neither the narrative note nor a specific evaluation, but does impose a mechanism for relaying a large quantity of general information at regularly scheduled intervals to supplement the progress note.

Therapists employing rating scales such as the COTE, have a responsibility to teach the reader how to retrieve data from the instrument. Inservices to Social Services, the other therapies, Nursing, and the Medical Staff, are essential prerequisites to the utilization of all the information. Rating scales can be seen as a shortcut to complete professional reporting and it is very easy to limit reports to simple numerals on a scale. However, rating scales such as the COTE which are designed to convey a great deal of information concisely can in no way be the only organ of the therapies.

References

1. West W: Historical Perspectives: In Occupational Therapy: 2001 AD. Rockville, MD, American Occupational Therapy Association, 1979, p 10, 12, 33.
2. Beals RG. Measurable Factor in Psychiatric Occupational Therapy. A J Occu Ther 3:297, 1949.
3. Fidler GS, Fidler JW: Occupational Therapy: A Communication Process in Psychiatry. New York, The MacMillen Co, 1963, pp 19, 102-103.
4. Fidler GS: Professional or Nonprofessional. In Occupational Therapy: 2001 AD. Rockville, MD, American Occupational Therapy Association, 1979, p 33.
5. Wolff RJ: A behavior rating scale. A J Occu Ther 15:13-16, 1961.
6. Ayres AJ: A form used to evaluate the work behavior of patients: A Preliminary Report. A J Occu Ther 8:73-74, 1954.
7. Ayres AJ: A pilot study on the relationship between work habits and workshop production. A J Occu Ther 9:264-297, 1955.
8. Alard I: Our professional judgement: Sound or haphazard? A J Occu Ther 18:107, 1964.

The COTE Scale

9. Clark JR, Koch BA, Nichols RC: A Factor Analytically Derived Scale: For Rating Psychiatric Patients in Occupational Therapy: Part I. Development A J Occu Ther 9:14, 1965.
10. Esser TJ: Client Rating Instruments for Use in Vocational Rehabilitation Agencies. Menomonie, Stout Vocational Rehabilitation Institute, University of Wisconsin, 1975, p 1,2.

Bibliography

Jantzen, A: The Current Profile of Occupational Therapy and the Future—Professional or Vocational. Occupational Therapy: 2001 AD Rockville, MD, American Occupational Therapy Association, 1979, pp 71-75.
Mosey A: Three Frames of Reference for Mental health. Thorofare, NJ, Charles B Slack, 1970, pp 104-105.

Acknowledgement

The authors wish to acknowledge the contributions of Marvin J. Short, M.D., former Medical Director of Marshall I. Pickens Hospital. His interest and continual support of Occupational Therapy fostered the search for a more efficient, effective means of conveying information to the treatment team. The contributions and support of the occupational therapy staff continue to be invaluable.

Sara J. Brayman and Thomas Kirby

14
The Adult Psychiatric Sensory Integration Evaluation

Carolyn Van Schroeder, O.T.R.
Marjorie Papke Block, O.T.R.
Elizabeth Campbell Trottier, O.T.R.
Mary Savage Stowell, M.S., O.T.R.

The Schroeder Block Campbell Adult Psychiatric Sensory Integration Evaluation (SBC) was developed to meet the need for a comprehensive assessment tool for use by psychiatric occupational therapists. The evaluation covers areas such as: sensory and motor responses including abnormal movements resulting from disease process or medications; developmental history; and various neurologic soft signs.

The purpose of the ongoing research project is to establish validity, inter-rater reliability, and norms on a collection of measures familiar to psychiatric occupational therapists; this will create a scoring system which reflects physical and neurological function and dysfunction and will be beneficial to the psychiatric treatment team, as well as the client.

Through the use of the SBC in the future, it will be possible to compile a data base with norms that will aid in quantifying the physical abilities and disabilities of psychiatric clients.

For too long, psychiatric occupational therapists have relied on an intuitive body of knowledge, developing various theoretical frameworks and using various untested evaluation measures on a trial and error basis. Objective and reliable measures of function are needed, and without them one cannot profess that treatments have been instrumental in physical, behavioral, and/or emotional change. The unique perspective of occupational therapy needs to be a part of the research body of knowledge presently being created.

At this point, no formalized sensory integration assessment procedure has been developed, tested, and normed for adult psychiatric clients. Various evaluation procedures or parts of evaluations normed for children are used informally by clinicians for adult clients with brain damage. Our experience is that neurologists and psychiatrists are finding themselves in the same dilemma when attempting to find statistically reliable, and fully tested measures needed to report clinical data.

Thus far, the low rate of instrument development has slowed the systematic development of research in this field, and has contributed to the relative lack of studies produced. The studies completed by most researchers from varied professional backgrounds can be said to have problems in the following areas: smallness of sample, diversity of outcome criteria, lack of replication, utilization of inappropriate statistics, and the use of inadequate control groups and instrumentation.[1] Control for type and duration of illness, medications, other treatments, socioeconomic status, ethnic heritage, sex, and age were considered as part of the SBC development. The use of a small homogenous sample versus a large heterogeneous sample has been explored. These issues have been examined carefully throughout the past development, and will be in the future development of the SBC as a research and clinical measure.

Historical Development

The original pilot work for the Schroeder Block Campbell Adult Psychiatric Integration Evaluation was completed at the San Diego Veteran's Administration Medical Center on 15 clients with the diagnosis of chronic schizophrenia, paranoid schizophrenia, and hyperkinetic adult syndrome. Some of these subjects were tested both off and on medications. All subjects were given the SBC evaluation, and 11 subtests from the Southern California Sensory Integration Tests by Ayres.[2] This original pilot work was undertaken with the full knowledge that the Ayres tests were normed for children only. We were interested in the distribution of dysfunction across both tests while still in the pilot stage of design. This original testing implicated dysfunction in a variety of areas that led us, and other medical colleagues to specific questions about the role of medications, neurologic soft signs, abnormal developmental history, and the specific disease processes found within a psychiatric setting. The result was the development of the current experimental edition of the SBC.[3]

Rationale

Measures chosen for the SBC are from a review of the functional abilities necessary for an adult to perform daily life tasks. The items were selected with the hope of being able to report the most valuable and representative picture of an individual's physical functioning. Issues of objectivity, judgment, staff time, energy, cost, and patient tolerance were all considered in the measurement selection procedure.

The potential benefits of the SBC are considerable. By establishing reliability, validity, and norms for a group of measures which have long been part of neurologic and psychiatric evaluations, it would be possible to have an objective numerical score of a patient's ability to perform at any given point in time. This would be a great benefit, since the classical method of scoring these measures has been by clinical description only. When reliability, validity, and norms are established, it is possible to objectively evaluate: an individual client over time; the effects of medication or other forms of treatment, both acutely and over time; and groups of clients by diagnosis or by other criteria. This representation is a great step forward in quantifying often observed clinical phenomenon.

The benefits to the client are at least three-fold: The physician and treatment team have a better understanding of their client's physical ability to interact with his environment, the client himself better understands his physical abilities and disabilities, and an increased understanding of the neurologic components of psychiatric illness is provided. A further benefit to the client is the documentation at a point in time of the ability to perform on the evaluation. Any changes over time can then be compared to an objective numerical score so that changes in ability and

CV Schroeder, MP Block, EC Trottier, MS Stowell

disability are clear. The physical influence of medication changes and medication over time can also be carefully evaluated. The SBC provides a scheme for looking at and summarizing multiple scoring categories, and will ultimately relate overall functional behavior to diagnosis and current medical concerns.

Literature Review

There is extensive literature documenting perceptual and motor disturbances in psychiatric illness—most notably in schizophrenia. Much of this literature reports specific sensory or motor problems in the context of the development of a theory about the etiology of schizophrenia. In other words, evidence of disease process is presented as part of "proof" of a theory. Evidence or data still needs to be collected in as complete and objective a manner as possible. Any investigator would state that preconceptions can hopelessly bias the observer and alter the objectivity. Occupational therapists have the unique opportunity of working with psychiatric clients in sensory, motor, and task oriented situations. The therapist is able to see pieces of evidence in the form of behaviors which indicate difficulty with such things as crossing the midline, standing balance, slowed reaction time, etc. Occupational therapists are trained to observe these behaviors, and are also aware of the role of perception in providing a sense of environmental stability, giving meaning to stimulus input, and facilitating integration of input so that experience can be categorized and responded to in order of priority. The perceptual changes experienced by schizophrenic clients can disrupt any or all of these functions. Until now there has been *no* way to accurately measure these perceptual changes and to quantify the behaviors at any point in time.

The changes seen in schizophrenia have been studied the most because they are so striking; however, we feel that it is important to look at other areas such as minimal brain dysfunction, adult hyperactivity, and depression. The review of the literature, therefore, will focus primarily on measurable perceptual and motor changes in schizophrenia.

This literature is large and unwieldy; there are many methodological and technical flaws in the reported results. As with any work with the perceptual system, there is an overflow of information categories. It is, for example, almost impossible to separate peripheral stimulus response from central processing response. It is difficult to discern if schizophrenics do have reduced cutaneous sensitivity or if they have such a fluctuation of levels of arousal that reduced cutaneous sensitivity is just an artifact. In short, any research on perception is as complicated as the perceptual response itself. We have some ideas about which tracts and which structures are involved in a given perception, but any perceptual response takes place in the context of the body and brain as a whole.

Our review of the literature focuses on the following eight areas: neurochemistry, the vestibular system, psychomotor speed, body image, anatomical changes, laterality, abnormal movements, and neurological dysfunction.

Neurochemistry

It is important to remember that disorders of neurochemical transmission may not only play a part in schizophrenia, but also a role in syndromes such as learning disabilities, the affective disorders, borderline syndromes, and hyperkinetic adults. The neuro-regulators are thought to be primarily under genetic control but responsive to stress. Given enough of a specific stress, the neurochemical mechanisms are altered, initiating changes in perception and behavioral responses which are then labeled as a psychiatric disorder. It should be acknowledged at the onset that any investigation of neurochemistry is enormously complex. This is a field which is just beginning to be understood. It is quite probable that many of the functions of neurotransmitters are as yet undiscovered. Known neurotransmitter systems currently being studied are: serotinergic, antiserotinergic, dopaminergic, antidopaminergic, cholinergic, anticholinergic, and gabaergic. This discussion will focus on only a few of them.

The preliminary evidence is very interesting. All of the known anti-psychotic medications which are effective in the treatment of schizophrenia have, to a greater or lesser degree, a dopamine blocking effect. Their therapeutic potency is almost perfectly correlated with their ability to block dopamine agonists in an in vitro solution. This is thought to parallel dopamine blockage in vivo. Dopamine is known to be a neurotransmitter active in: 1) the nigrostriatal pathways from the midbrain substantia nigra to be neostriatum caudate and putmen, 2) the meso-limbic projections through the lateral hypothalamus to limbic structures including the septal nuclei and olfactory tubercle, and 3) mesocortical projections from the midbrain substantia nigra to be neostriatum caudate and putamen, 2) the meso-a tubero infundibular system within the hypothalamus which effects the pituitary and 5) a retinal dopamine pathway. Dopamine transmission is then active in areas of the brain involved in the regulation of levels of arousal, intensity of stimuli, gateing of stimuli, emotion, olfaction, regulation of impulse, smooth eye pursuits, and the behavioral expressions of hunger, thirst, and sexual affect.[4-7] This is an indication of some functions which are probably directly affected by dopamine. Occupational therapists have seen clients who show one or more disorders in the areas mentioned above.

Eighty percent of the dopamine in the brain is found in the basal ganglia. Clinical syndromes associated with pathology of the basal ganglia include chorea, ballism, athetosis, dystonia, and, Parkinson's disease.[4] All these are movement disorders, and have been seen in psychiatric clients—both unmedicated clients and clients who have been treated with antipsychotic medications.[8] With the exception of two antipsychotic agents, thoridazine and clozapine, the antipsychotic *potency* of a drug also appears to directly parallel its extrapyramidal *toxicity*. That is, a drug such as haloperidol has a much higher potency and a much higher incidence of extrapyramidal side effects than chlorpromazine. It is important, however, to remember that correlation does not indicate causation. There is no proof to date that dopamine is directly involved in schizophrenia. These same medications are effective antipsychotics for many different types of psychiatric disorders. Efforts to directly test the dopamine hypothesis have so far revealed mixed results.[9] Most of the evidence for abnormally overactive dopamine transmission has been based on drug responses, and these are only indirect relationships. There are several excellent discussions of the role of dopamine in schizophrenia,[10,11] including a summary by Baldessarini,[9] which appeared in the November 1977 issue of the *New England Journal of Medicine.*

In addition to the evidence of disordered dopamine transmission in schizophrenia, many other neurochemical findings have been reported. Many times an interesting finding is reported in the literature, but the study is never replicated. The findings, however, may be supported later when more sophisticated technologies are available. One finding which awaits further investigation is a report of lowered MAO platelet activity in schizophrenics, and a correspondingly low

CV Schroeder, MP Block, EC Trottier, MS Stowell

platelet activity in first degree relatives. There is also a reported correlation between lowered Monomine Oxidase Inhibitors, platelet activity, increased incidence of abnormal electroencephalogram, and presence of auditory hallucinations. Plotkin has reported a significant difference in the level of MAO in the platelets between schizophrenics and normals and between schizophrenics with paranoid features and those without.[12]

An area which is just beginning to be explored is the role of endorphins in schizophrenia. Endorphin literally means, "morphine within", and is found in the pituitary and the brain, particularly the limbic structures. Endorphins are a sort of natural opiate which is thought to mediate perception of pain, and to have extensive interactions with the catecholamines. Preliminary work with the endorphins and schizophrenia has focused on the theory that schizophrenics have a high level of endorphins, and that opiate antagonists or blockers such a naloxone might reduce symptoms. There is considerable controversy over whether this is true, and several well-done studies have failed to replicate the initial claim that schizophrenic hallucinations decreased with administration of naloxone.[13]

The report of an exciting finding and then difficulty in replicating the results has plagued schizophrenia research. It is quite possible that all the scattered bits of neurochemical evidence will fit into a meaningful pattern as more is learned about the roles of neurotransmitters and neuroregulators. Until the time that the mechanisms are understood, it is important to carefully document findings relevant to the clinician's expertise.

Vestibular System

The vestibular system is another area that has often been mentioned in connection with schizophrenia. Many studies have been done on vestibular functioning in schizophrenia. Leach did a study of 75 schizophrenic patients and compared them to 96 non-institutionalized males.[14] The author found that the schizophrenic groups showed diminished reactivity, with the greatest deficits occuring under conditions of weak stimulation, and were relatively more normal with increased stimulation. Myers, Caldwell, and Purcell studied both caloric and rotational nystagmus with a group of 10 severely ill, chronic, drug free, schizophrenic patients. Myers, *et al,* found deficits in vestibular reactivity and significant differences as the stimulus conditions became more intense.[15]

In general, studies of vestibular responses have shown a great variety of findings. Some studies report transitory hyperreactivity which corresponds to various stages of catatonia.[16] Sporadic vestibular abnormalities are reported in both catatonic and noncatatonic clients associated with deteriorating clinical condition. Repeat testing shows a correlation between normal levels of vestibular reactivity and improved clinical status.[17,18] Many studies report random or inconsistent vestibular abnormalities, and use varying methods of stimulation to elicit the vestibular response. In some studies, acute and chronic schizophrenic clients demonstrate normal vestibular responses. What is the meaning of all these contradictory findings? Probably several things, including the variability of individual response, the need for clearer diagnostic criteria, the need for valid and reliable measures of nystagmus response, and the need for more sophisticated monitoring of levels of arousal while nystagmus is being tested.

Levy, Holtzman, and Proctor used caloric stimulation to test nystagmus in 84 psychiatric patients, 39 of their relatives, and 35 non-patient controls.[19] While no difference was found between the schizophrenic group and the control group, the schizophrenic group showed a significantly greater dysrhythmic response. Since these studies were done using electronystagmography, it is felt that previous reports of vestibular dysfunction might actually represent undetected dysrhythmias. The findings indicate that schizophrenic responses may actually reflect disturbances in the level of alertness. Holtzman and his colleagues have observed eye tracking dysfunctions in schizophrenic patients and their relatives, and found a statistically significant difference between a schizophrenic group and a control group showing deviant eye tracking.[20-22] The relationship between poor eye tracking and schizophrenia is stronger when psychologic test evidence of thought disorder is used to operationally classify patients.

A 1908 study done by Diefendorf and Dodge reported difficulty with smooth ocular pursuit in patients with dementia parecox.[23] Holtzman, *et al*, refer to the phenomena reported in 1908 as being consistent with their observations in 1974, although the researchers did not discuss any association between the eye tracking dysfunctions observed and the literature on vestibular changes in schizophrenia. Certain abnormal vestibular responses are correlated with a number of disorders thought to represent a deficit in central processing. The work of Ayres[24] and deQuiros[25] with vestibular function and learning disabilities are outstanding examples.

Huddleston has reported the ability to distinguish between process and reactive schizophrenic patients based on vestibular reactivity.[26] To induce vestibular response, a technique modeled after Ayres was used, measuring reactivity by timing the duration of nystagmus which can be observed by the examiner. Huddleston does not address the issues of rater reliability or discuss the effects of antipsychotic medications on vestibular response. In his article, *The Psychotropic Drugs, Considerations Relative to the Vestibular Pathways, and Testing*,[27] Shuster discusses concerns about which psychiatric occupational therapists should be aware, whether they are reusing sensory integration or not.

An article by Nancy Keating entitled, *A Comparison of Duration of Nystagmus as Measured by the Southern California Postrotary Nystagmus Test and Electronystagmography*,[28] discusses the methodologic problems of measuring nystagmus. Keating found a significant correlation between electronystagmography reading of nystagmus and the Southern California Postrotary Nystagmus Test for female adults, but did not find a significant correlation between the two techniques in measuring duration or excursion in a small group of learning disabled girls. However, the learning disabled population in general is a more difficult group to test, and is often distractible due to a short attention span and difficulty in following directions.[28] This is also true of many schizophrenic clients. Keating's excellent study serves as a caveat to aspiring researchers and clinicians that evaluation tools must themselves be carefully studied before their value can be determined.

To summarize, the vestibular system plays an integral role in perception, and is intricately interconnected to many brain structures, some of which are known to be affected by dopamine. Many researchers have reported various abnormalities in the vestibular responses of schizophrenics. Antipsychotic medications have some effect on the vestibular system which may be in part why they are helpful to patients. More research needs to be done to clarify which sub-types, if any, of schizophrenic clients show vestibular involvement.

Psychomotility

Change in psychomotor speed is a clinical observation that has long been associated with psychiatric illness, including schizophrenia, affective disorders, and minimal brain dysfunction. Psychomotility is a complex phenomena which involves processing information and responding to stimulation. It is likely that all the aspects of pathology related to neurochemistry and the vestibular system play a role in determining psychomotility. There are many ways to assess psychomotility. H.E. King is an articulate supporter of the use of measures of psychomotility to detect clinical changes.[29] King reports from various studies that psychomotor measures are found at times to be more sensitive than clinical judgment, because trends can be detected before an overall behavior change is documented. Another study by Weaver and Brooks reports that psychomotor changes parallel the course of clinical improvement, and clients responding favorably to tranquilizing drugs do significantly better on psychomotor tests before and after drug administration.[30] Weaver and Brooks report a high association between good or poor psychomotor performance and release from the hospital, with or without rehabilitation.[29,31] In a sample that included 1,000 schizoprhenic, manic depressive, chronic brain syndrome, personality disordered, and mentally deficient clients, a 75% accurate prediction of patient outcome was made based on psychomotor speed.[31] The overall conclusion shows that improved speed is found to accompany improved psychiatric status, whether the improved status is brought about by drugs, electroconvulsive therapy,or natural remission.

What about the effects of medication? King reports that the use of antipsychotic medications is associated with increased reaction time, and with improved dexterity. In cases where there was significant interference from Parkinsonian side effects, psychomotor speed improved almost immediately after administration of the appropriate anti-Parkinsonian medication.[29]

There are many ways to measure psychomotility, but the simplest methods measure psychomotor speed. It is an extremely simple task, and performance is not affected by level of education, culture, or intelligence (above an IQ of 60).[29] Tapping speed meets the above criteria, and was chosen to measure psychomotor speed in the SBC.

Body Image

Body image is integrally related to perceptual and motor functions, and particularly to the vestibular system. Ayres discusses it extensively, and Leach prefaces his paper on nystagmus with a statement about distortions of body image in psychopathology, and the relationship to proprioceptive mechanisms. Body image can be inferred from many situations, but remains an elusive phenomena to measure.[32] Almost all reports of body image refer to figure drawings. There is no lack of imaginative reports in the literature, including changes in body image after the administration of lysergic acid diethylamide,[33] and the drawings of sex offenders.[34] The problem has been to establish research criteria to measure responses which are valid and reliable.[32] The striking visual differences in the drawings of before-and-after therapy are part of the continual lure to find a valid and reliable way to measure body image. We, as authors of the SBC, worked hard to find criteria which provides a valid measure of body image. Body image is included in the data gathered because it tells so much about the quality of the client's perception of himself.

Disturbances in body image are only to be expected, given the disturbances in vestibular function, central processing of data, and psychomotor speed reported in schizophrenia. The following discussions of anatomical changes, laterality, neurologic soft signs, and abnormal movements, point out further reasons to observe body image disturbance in schizophrenia.

Anatomical Changes

The role of anatomical changes in psychopathology is emerging as one of the most exciting areas of knowledge and understanding. Cerebral atrophy and cognitive impairment observed via encephalography in chronic schizophrenics is reported by Marsden.[35] Marsden questions whether or not the findings are attributable to current treatment modes employing neuroleptic drugs and their tendency to produce extrapyramidal side effects. Another study by Johnstone, et al,[36] looks at cerebral ventricular size and cognitive impairment in chronic schizophrenia. Johnstone matched the age of the controls and 17 institutionalized schizophrenic clients. Through axial computerized tomography the results show that schizophrenics have increased cerebral ventricular space, and Johnstone, *et al*, concluded that ventricular size is highly significant in relation to cognitive impairment. A conflicting opinion voiced by Crow and Johnstone states that cerebral changes are due to an unidentified pathological process, and are not necessarily secondary to neuroleptic medications.[37] The examination of six clients was unable to replicate the preceding results. Crow and Johnstone felt that institutional neglect, dietary deficiency, and endemic encephalitis were negative factors that needed future study. In addition, they thought that the beneficial roles of vitamin B_{12} and hemoglobin should be further investigated.

Interesting findings regarding anatomical changes and schizophrenics' musculature have been reported. These include: motor end plate alterations or branching and sprouting of nerve twigs, abnormal electromyograms, increased electrical activity of skeletal muscles at rest, and reports of increased incidence of morphological abnormalities of skeletal muscles.[38,39]

Laterality

Issues relative to laterality are regaining prominence in current psychiatric literature. In a study by Gur, 200 schizophrenics and 200 normal subjects were examined for eye, hand, and foot dominance. Schizophrenics showed more left sidedness on laterality scores. This leftward tendency may be manifested in cognitive, as well as conative functions and may relate schizophrenia to left hemisphere dysfunction.[40] Other researchers have found less eye and hand congruence in schizophrenics than normals, although others feel that congruence is of pathologic importance. Some researchers have reported lateralization changes during drug related psychotic episodes.[41] It is also interesting to note that increased left handedness has been reported in populations with presumed central nervous system impairment such as epileptic and dyslexics. Flor-Henry reports increased EEG foci in the left temporal lobe of schizophrenics, which would further point to left hemispheric function.[42]

Abnormal Movements

When considering abnormal movements in psychiatry, it is important to be aware of the fact that some abnormality of movement exists across most diagnostic labels. Movement disorders are seen in Parkinsonism, drug induced conditions, alcoholism, nutritional deficiencies, central nervous system dysfunction, old age, and psychosis.

CV Schroeder, MP Block, EC Trottier, MS Stowell

Abnormal movements are seen in conditions ranging from mania and hyperkinesia, to catatonia and psychomotor retardation. Movement disorders in schizophrenia have been reported before the advent of drugs, and include stereotypic mannerisms, hypo and hyperkinesia, and are observed in all ages and in clients institutionalized less than a year. There is evidence of abnormal movements in abnormal spinal reflex activity and poor performance in neuromuscular coordination tasks.

Abnormal movements also involve involuntary ocular movements, specifically in schizophrenia. These include deviant eye tracking, gaze disturbance, altered blink rates, eye deviation, abnormal saccadic movements, and failure to converge.[10,43]

Movement disorders can occur from side effects of neuroleptic medications due to toxicity, hypersensitivity, and long term use. The drug induced reactions can take the form of dystonic reactions, akathesias, or as Parkinson-like reactions (akathesia, tremor, and tardive dyskinesia). Movement disorders seem to be affected by a subject's anxiety, by interpersonal contact, and by physical contact with persons or objects. Dyskinesias are frequent in occurrence and often irreversible. Tardive dyskinesias are involuntary movements and are thought to occur in older psychotic patients in whom long term treatment with the anti-psychotic drugs of phenothiazine and butyrophenone groups has occurred. Current thinking is that all clients risk the development of neurologic syndrome, regardless of age.

Withdrawal symptoms can follow abrupt disuse of antipsychotic medication in a form of tardive dyskinesia called "covert dyskinesia". This condition becomes clinically detectable after discontinuation or reduction in dosage, and usually disappears spontaneously within six to 12 weeks.

The benefits of drug treatment have been variable. The importance of attempting early recognition of dyskinesias and reduction in drug dosages when possible cannot be stressed strongly enough in order to minimize the risk of permanent neurologic disorder.[44] We can only hope that research will produce a choice of antipsychotic agents for clients without disabling side effects.

Neurologic Soft Signs

Conventional neurologic studies of adult psychiatric clients show varied results, but if the criteria of soft or minor neurologic signs are used, there is evidence of neurologic dysfunction in adult schizophrenics and other diagnostic categories.[45,46]

Neurologic soft signs can refer to any neurologic deviations: motor, sensory, or integrative, which does not localize the site of a putative central nervous system lesion. Soft signs are chronic, and non-life threatening. The cause is usually unclear. Among possible causes are intrauterine or perinatal injury or anoxia. The following manifestations of soft signs can be seen in cognitive and integrative dysfunction: delay in reaching developmental milestones, difficulty in acquiring simple athletic skills, learning problems, and organic indicators on mental status exams.

Schizophrenic patients of mixed subgroups on medication show an increased number of soft signs compared to those not receiving medication. Clients showing a greater preponderance of soft signs also show evidence of intellectual impairments that have not been previously associated with cognitive disturbance.[47]

Various researchers have discussed evidence of minimal brain dysfunction across diagnostic categories, indicating a relationship between minimal brain dysfunction characteristics in childhood and psychiatric pathology in later life.[48,52]

Bach-y-Rita, studying violent clients showing episodic dyscontrol but no dysfunction on conventional neurologic examinations, found histories of childhood hyperactivity, psychosomatic illness, enuresis to age five, pyromania, cruelty to animals, and EEG abnormalities, as well as possible incidents of brain injury.[54]

Behaviors Assessed

The purpose of this section is to describe the individual test items used in the SBC. The scoring for the SBC is based on zero to three scale—zero as normal, one, two, and three showing the degrees of divergence from normal. The SBC is an evaluation tool consisting of definite procedures, observations, scoring, work sheets, and summary sheets. The following is intended as a description of the measure only. The technical information needed for administering and scoring the measure is found in the manual.

The individual test items are listed below in the order in which they are presented. This is the same order in which the evaluation is administered (Table 14.1).

Dominance is the first item in the SBC. Eye, hand, and foot dominance are each evaluated. The preliminary concern for evaluating dominance is looking for dominance switches from one side to the other. For example, if at the beginning of the testing, the right eye is dominant, does the dominance switch to the left eye? This type of switching in dominance within a session is called *mixed* or *confused* dominance, and has been seen in many of the subjects who have been tested. The SBC is not concerned with cross-dominance, where, for example, the right eye is dominant along with the left hand. While studies do not show any clear reason for concern with cross-dominance, mixed or confused dominance is specifically mentioned in the literature on laterality problems in schizophrenics.

The SBC tests eye dominance in three ways. In the first test the subject is asked to look through a paper tube at an object on the wall. The examiner notes: 1) which hand the subject uses to hold the tube, and 2) to which eye the subject holds up the tube. The second and third tests utilize the same basic procedure and evaluation; however, in the second test, the paper tube is replaced by a piece of cardboard which has a ¼ inch hole in its center, and the third test uses a key ring. To insure accurate evaluation of dominance, the test objects for each of the individual tests must be placed before the subject at his midline.

The test for hand dominance utilizes a blank piece of paper and a pencil. The subject is asked to write his name at the top of the paper. The key observations for hand dominance are then: 1) with which hand does the subject pick up the pencil, and 2) with which hand does he write his name? The paper is kept to be used later when testing body image.

To test for foot dominance, the subject is asked to hop on one foot three times. The foot used for hopping is considered the preferred foot. Dominance is tested a second time by placing a ball in front of the subject, and asking him to kick it softly.

The next three test items in the SBC are *posture, neck rotation*, and *gait*. Included in each section are tests designed specifically to further evaluate observations made by Lorna Jean King, and reported by others. These observations include: a pronounced "S" curve from head to toe, a shuffling gait, the arms and legs flexed, adducted, and internally rotated while standing. A lack of head rotation and a lack of the ability to roll the head forward, backward, and to the side are also observed.[55]

To evaluate *posture*, the subject is asked to stand in a relaxed position while the therapist looks at his posture from all sides. Loose fitting clothing inhibits clear observation of posture. Observation of posture is aided by running the fingers down

TABLE 14.1

A LIST OF TEST ITEMS USED IN THE SBC IN NUMERICAL ORDER

1. Dominance	14. Stability—Trunk
2. Posture	15. Classical Romberg
3. Neck Rotation	16. Sharpened Romberg
4. Gait	17. Overflow Movements
5. Hand Observation	18. Neck Righting
6. Grip Strength	19. Rolling
7. Fine Motor Control	20. Asymmetrical Tonic Neck Reflex
8. Diadochokinesis	21. Symmetrical Tonic Neck Reflex
9. Finger-Thumb Opposition	22. Tonic Labyrinthine Reflex
10. Visual Pursuits	23. Protective Extension
11. Bilateral Coordination— Upper Extremity	24. Seated Equilibrium
	25. Body Image
12. Crossing the Midline	26. Abnormal Movements
13. Stability—Upper Extremity	27. Self-Reported Childhood History

the client's spine, and can help identify if any of the following conditions are present: lordosis, kyphosis, scoliosis, asymmetrical posture, or inward rotation of the shoulders.

To test for *neck rotation,* the subject is asked to rotate his head first clockwise, then counter-clockwise. The important observations are whether the neck movements are smooth or jerky, and whether the subject uses his full range of motion.

The test for neck rotation is followed by the test for *gait.* The subject is simply asked to walk away from the therapist and to return. Observations are made for any lack of associated arm movements and for shuffling of the feet.

In performing *hand observations,* the therapist asks the subject to first place his hands palms down on the table, and then to turn them palms up. In hand observation, the therapist should look for any change from normal hand structure, including an adducted thumb, atrophy of thenar eminance, or ulnar deviation of the wrist.[55] If the subject seems to have some ulnar deviation, further measurements can be made with a goniometer.

A dynamometer is used to test *grip strength.* The subject is given three trials with the dynamometer, and the best of the three is recorded and compared with the norms.[56]

The test for *fine motor control* requires the use of a tapping board. The subject is instructed to tap as fast as he can, using his index finger. This procedure is repeated three times with both his dominant and non-dominant hands. The average of the three trials is recorded for each hand.

The next two items included in the SBC are observations for neurologic soft signs, which indicate the subject's ability to synchronize bilateral movements. They are diadochokinesis and finger-thumb opposition.

To test for *diadochokinesis,* the subject is asked to alternately pronate and supinate both hands simultaneously for ten seconds. Observations are made for both smoothness and synchronization of movement. Normally, the non-dominant hand is a little slower and slightly less coordinated.[57]

Finger-thumb opposition is used by the SBC to test the smooth coordination of the hands and fingers. The subject is asked to touch each finger of one hand to the thumb, beginning with the index finger, then following with the middle finger, the ring finger, the little finger, and then in reverse order. Each hand is done separately, and then together. The evaluation is based on smoothness of movement, speed, coordination, and the ability to perform without visual clues.

To test for *visual pursuits*, the subject is asked to visually track a penlight without moving the head. The subject may overshoot, lag behind, or lose the target. There may be an attempt to move the head instead of the eyes, squint, blink repeatedly, or have trouble changing directions. In addition, a sign of a disorder in postural and bilateral integration is difficulty in tracking the target across the midline.[58] Holtzman reported abnormal visual pursuits in schizophrenics.[22]

Bilateral coordination—upper extremity is tested by having the subject draw two circles simultaneously on a blackboard, one with each hand. The subject is asked to draw the two circles starting from the top, and is then asked to draw two more circles in the opposite direction. By comparing the size of both sets of circles and the synchronization of the subject's movements, evaluation can be made of his eye-hand coordination, and his ability to coordinate the motor use of both upper extremities. Deficits in this area may correlate with deficits in other tasks requiring bilateral coordination.

The next test items evaluate the subject's ability to *cross the midline*. The syndrome affecting postural and bilateral integration causes failure to establish a strong unilateral dominance.[58] In a pilot study for the SBC, many subjects who seemed to have trouble with bilateral integration had trouble crossing the midline. In testing the subject's ability to cross the midline, the subject draws a line from his left to his right on the blackboard, and then retraces it. Assessment is based on whether the subject crosses, or avoids crossing, the midline, and whether the line is irregular where the subject crossed the midline. The subject might avoid crossing the midline by moving his body or by switching hands.

The next two areas of the SBC, *stability of the upper extremity*, and *stability of the trunk*, are evaluated on the basis of the subject's ability to co-contract various muscle groups. The ability of a muscle group to exert its maximum strength is based on the patterning of movements governed by the nervous system, and not only the contraction of isolated muscle groups.[57] Co-contraction is necessary to provide a stable base for the performance of the trunk and upper extremity.

To test the stability of the upper extremity, the subject is asked to clasp his hands in front of his chest. The therapist places one hand above and one hand below the subject's hands, then pushes and pulls. The amount of resistance which the subject gives, and whether he can keep his hands within eight inches of his chest, are the key observations to be made for upper extremity stability. Notice that this section is not concerned with the subject's balance.

In testing trunk stability, the subject is asked to stand and hold his body still. The examiner stands to the back of the subject to avoid visual input. The examiner first pushes the subject forward, then to each side, and finally pulls him backwards. Assessment is made of the subject's ability to co-contract his trunk muscles, whether or not he has to take a step to avoid losing his balance, and whether the subject demonstrates excessive fluidity.

The SBC uses the *classical Romberg* to test for balance. This test puts a greater strain on the subject's ability to compensate for changes in posture, by requiring the subject to walk on a narrow base. The subject is asked to walk a line on the floor without looking at the line, then to retrace his steps backwards. The main observations are: 1) is the performance smooth or awkward; and 2) is the subject able

CV Schroeder, MP Block, EC Trottier, MS Stowell

to maintain his balance while walking forward and backward?

Following classical Romberg, *sharpened Romberg* is used to assess the subject's ability to maintain an upright posture while standing. Maintaining an upright position assesses the subject's ability to quickly and accurately adapt proprioceptive information—adjusting for changes in position and for the amount and direction of deviation—in order to overcome the threatened loss of balance.[57]

To test for balance, the subject is asked to cross his arms over his chest and place his feet in the tandem walking position. The subject is to hold this position for 30 seconds with eyes open, then for 30 seconds with eyes closed. Evaluation can then be based on how well the subject held his balance with and without visual cues. If the subject opens his eyes during the test, it is stopped, and the time recorded. Also, comparison can be made between the test performed with and without visual input.

The next item is the test for *overflow movements*. The subject is asked to stand with both arms extended at shoulder height with fingers extended and slightly apart. With his eyes closed, he is asked to hold this position for 30 seconds. Slight movements of the fingers and hand, or the arms, and/or the arms drifting up or down, inwards, or outwards exceeding three inches, are all key observations. Commonly seen with motor disorders, overflow movements are neurological soft signs. They may be seen in medicated and unmedicated subjects.

The position used to test *neck righting* is the same as used to test overflow movements. However, for neck righting the examiner first rotates the subject's head to the right, then to the left, observing whether the arms or the trunk show a tendency to align with the head. Neck righting assesses a midbrain reflex which brings the head into a normal spacial relationship with the shoulders. It is seen from birth until six months, and is affected by the normal distribution of tone and active righting movements.[59] During a preliminary study of the SBC, many subjects showed a residual neck righting reflex similar to those reported by Bender for schizophrenic children.[60]

Rolling, the next item, evaluates the subject's ability to rotate his trunk. The subject is asked to roll on a mat to his left, then to his right. Key observations include whether the subject is able to roll segmentally, whether he rolls without one part of his body leading (log-roll), and the amount of difficulty the subject has with the task of rolling.

The SBC tests lower brain stem reflexes in the sections on *asymmetrical tonic neck reflex*, *symmetrical tonic neck reflex*, and *tonic labyrinthine reflex*. Changes in postural muscle tone can effect one or more sections of the body, and, in some cases, can be evidence of lower brain stem reflexes.[59]

To test for *asymmetrical tonic neck reflex*, the subject assumes the quadruped position, making sure that his elbows are clearly visible. The examiner places one hand behind the subject's neck, and the other hand under the chin. The head is turned to the right, held for five seconds, then turned to the left, and held for five more seconds. Indications include change in tone, contralateral limb flexion less than 45°, contralateral limb flexion greater than 45°, and slight or marked unilateral limb flexion.

The test for *symmetrical tonic neck reflex* is also done while the subject is in the quadruped position. However, for this test the examiner extends the subject's neck, holds it for five seconds, then lowers the head towards the chest and holds it for five more seconds. Observations should indicate any changes in tone, arm flexion and leg extension with the neck ventroflexed, or arm extension and leg flexion with the neck dorsiflexed.

The SBC Evaluation   239

The third of the tonic reflexes, *tonic labryinthine reflex*, should not be done if the subject has a history of back problems. For this test, the examiner demonstrates the pivot prone position. The subject is then asked to assume the position, and to hold it for 30 seconds. The examiner observes for tremors in the upper or lower extremity, and/or for the subject's ability to assume and hold the proper position.

In the test for *protective extension*, the subject is asked to kneel upright in the center of the mat. The examiner upsets his balance by pushing him to the front and to the sides, and by pulling him backwards. Included in the observations for this test are the quality of the protective extension used by the subject to catch himself, and whether the reaction was adequate, slow, or absent.

The test for *seated equilibrium* requires two therapists. To begin this test, the subject is asked to wear a safety belt, to straddle an inflatable, and to rock side to side without holding on to the inflatable. If necessary, the examiner should demonstrate for the subject. There are three areas for evaluation of seated equilibrium: 1) the subject's ability to right his head and trunk when rocking; 2) the ease with which the subject does the task (eg, does the subject do the task without holding on); and 3) the subject's ability to balance on the inflatable. Note any lack of full compensatory body movements.

In order to test for *body image,* the examiner gives the subject the piece of paper used during the test for hand dominance. The subject is asked to draw a complete picture of a person. Although there may be many ways to interpret this type of test, the SBC focuses on how sensory and motor disturbances may be reflected in body image. The specific categories evaluated attempt to reflect the subject's interaction with the environment. The two main categories used are: 1) the size of the drawing, which examines the relationship of the drawing to the paper itself, whether large or small; and 2) anatomy indicators, which include specific emphasis on individual body parts.

In the section on *abnormal movements,* two types of abnormal movements are evaluated—those that show up upon activation, and those that show spontaneously. Observations are made for stereotyping, mannerisms, psychomotor retardation, blocking, automatic obedience, mitgehen, cooperation, and extrapyramidal signs such as akinesia, tremor or pseudoparkinsonism, akathesia, acute dyskinesia, and tardive dyskinesia. Three areas specifically tested are: 1) automatic obedience, 2) cogwheel rigidity, and 3) tongue protrusion. To test for automatic obedience, the examiner extends the subject's arm over his head, holding it for 30 seconds. Assessment is made of the length of time the hand remains in the position after the examiner has said "OK, thank you." Cogwheel rigidity, a sign of acute dyskinesia, is tested by flexing the subject's arm and feeling for intermittent contraction of either the biceps or triceps. To test for tongue protrusion, a symptom of tardive dyskinesia, the examiner first demonstrates, then asks the subject to protrude his tongue, timing it for 30 seconds. Observations for all three areas should include the difference between the movements seen at rest, and those observed during the testing.

Abnormal movements may be caused by either disease process, or by medications. Medications may change the abnormal movements being observed. In addition, abnormal movements may be observed in areas other than those specifically tested in the SBC. Other abnormal movements that are observed and documented, but not specifically tested are listed in Table 14.2.

The last area of the SBC is the *self-reported childhood history*. The examiner reads aloud the list of questions to the subject, and checks off whichever items the subject indicates apply to him. The developmental history is taken to see if the subject has had any indication of sensory motor problems as a child. Specific areas noted are: delayed development, neurological soft signs, and childhood hyper-activity.

Case Study

The purpose of this case study is to focus on the SBC as a comprehensive evaluation tool using as an example the assessment of sensory and motor dysfunction in a chronic schizophrenic before medication, and after a four week trial on haloperidol.

The results reflect changes in the subject's functional ability, most noticeably in areas of equilibrium and balance, body image, and abnormal movements. Scoring refers to the SBC 0-3 scale.

Background

The subject was a 28 year old single male with a previous diagnosis of chronic schizophrenia. He had a six year history of hallucinations and paranoid delusions. On his first hospital admission he was described as dull, manneristic, vague, and circumstantial. He was discharged after six months on 100 mg/day chlorproma-zine. Two years later he was hospitalized for one week following an increase in withdrawn behavior and inability to continue school. His records describe him as being unable to comprehend, respond, or relate to his peers. He was residing at home with his mother, who was also described as withdrawn. The subject stated that he had stopped taking chlorpromazine because it was making him "too

---

TABLE 14.2

Abnormal Movements that are observed and documented, but are not specifically tested.

A. Hyperkinesia
    1. Stereotypy
    2. Mannerisms

B. Hypokinesia
    1. Psychomotor Retardation
    2. Blocking
    3. Automatic Obedience
    4. Mitgehen
    5. Cooperation
C. Extrapyramidal Symptoms
    1. Pseudoparkinsonism
        a. Akinesia
        b. Tremor
    2. Akathesia
    3. Acute Dyskinesia
    4. Tardive Dyskinesia
        a. Facial or Oral Movements
        b. Extremity Movements
        c. Trunk Movements

---

drowsy." The subject was discharged the second time on thiothixene, 5 mg, three times a day, along with multi-vitamins.

He was admitted four years later after a period of increasingly withdrawn behavior, decreased activity, and reduced spontaneity. At this time the subject had psychomotor retardation described as verging on catatonia. His mood was anxious, suspicious, and he showed no insight. Prior to this last admission, he had a history of sudden and unprovoked acts of violence. The subject had a tendency to be noncompliant and was reported to have not taken medication for five years since the last hospitalization. One week after admission the subject was started on haloperidol 25 mg/day.

Method

The SBC was first administered to the client on the second day after admission. At that time be had been completely free from all psychotropic medication for at least five years. The subject was admitted to the locked ward due to his inability to care for himself and the severity of his withdrawn behavior. The SBC evaluation was completed in the dayroom of the locked unit. All necessary equipment was taken to the unit. There was a minimum of distraction during the evaluation, as all the other patients were out of the room. The SBC was administered according to the procedure manual.

Four weeks after the first evaluation, the subject was evaluated with the SBC for a second time. The subject had been stabilized on haloperidol for three weeks. At this time the subject was on an open unit and was able to come to the occupational therapy clinic for the evaluation.

Results

The results of both testing sessions are presented in Table 14.3, showing the off-medication findings in Column 1 and the on-medication findings in Column 2. Column 3 shows changes in pathological responses for each test item. After medication, the subject improved in 12 of 29 areas of functional ability. In two areas, the subject's functional responses decreased. The remainder of the test items showed no change.

The patient exhibited clear eye, hand, and foot dominance in session 1; however, he demonstrated mixed dominance during session 2.

Asymmetrical posture was noted during session 1 and was not evident in session 2. In both testing sessions, full rotation of the head was restricted due to limited range of motion and rigidity.

Gait observation revealed a lack of associated arm movement and a shuffling gait in both sessions.

Hand observation in session 1 revealed ulnar deviation of both wrists, which decreased in session 2.

Grip strength for both sessions was below normal for age related males. His strength decreased seven pounds in session 2.

In fine motor control, the right side remained constant and within normal limits for both sessions 1 and 2. The left side showed an increase in function in session 2.

Diadochokinesis showed moderate dysfunction in both session 1 and 2 with slow, awkward and unsynchronized movements. During session 1 of finger-thumb opposition, the client needed visual and verbal clues to complete the procedure. Movement was slow, awkward, and unsynchronized. Session 2 showed a slight improvement in synchronization; however, the subject's movements continued to be slow and awkward.

TABLE 14.3

DATA SUMMARY—SBC ADULT PSYCHIATRIC SENSORY INTEGRATION EVALUATION

	A Test Session #1	B Test Session #2	C Improvement
Dominance	0	1	−1
Posture	0	0	—
Neck Rotation	0	0	—
Gait	2	2	—
Hand (Ulnar Deviation)	1	0	+1
Grip (right)	1	1	—
(left)	2	2	—
Fine Motor Control (right)	0	0	—
(left)	2	1	+1
Diacochokinesis	2	2	—
Finger Thumb Opposition	2	1	+1
Visual Pursuits	2	0	+2
Bilateral Coordination-UE	2	2	—
Crossing Midline	3	3	—
Stability-UE	2	2	—
Stability-Trunk	2	0	+2
Classical Romberg	3	1	+2
Sharpened Romberg (EO)	0	0	—
(EC)	3	0	+3
Overflow Movements	1	0	+1
Neck Righting	3	0	+3
Rolling	2	3	−1
ATNR	1	1	—
STNR	2	1	+1
TLR	3	1	+2
Protective Extension	1	1	—
Seated Equilibrium	2	2	—
Body Image	3	2	+1
Total	47	29	18
Abnormal Movements Total	6	2	+4

Key: 0 = No problem
  1 = Slight
  2 = Moderate
  3 = Severe

Visual pursuits during both sessions revealed the subject's general ability to track an object across the midline; however there was excessive blinking and jerkiness as the midline was approached in session 1. In session 2 no dysfunction was evident.

Bilateral coordination of the upper extremities showed evidence of impairment during both sessions. The subject was unable to complete the task adequately, and demonstrated unsynchronized movement. The subject was unable to cross his midline, and avoided doing so by moving his entire body.

In testing upper extremity stability, the client showed difficulty with co-contraction and was not able to offer adequate muscle resistance during either session.

Trunk stability in session 1 showed excessive fluidity and lack of balance. In session 2, the subject exhibited no dysfucntion.

Classical Romberg testing revealed the subject's inability to maintain balance and walk backwards in session 1. The subject improved in session 2, although his performance was rated as awkward.

Sharpened Romberg was normal with eyes open in sessions 1 and 2. With eyes closed the subject was unable to maintain the desired position in session 1, but his performance was normal in session 2. Throughout the second testing session, the patient was observed to have cogwheeling in some of the large muscle groups.

Observation of overflow movements revealed some digital movements of the upper extremity and slight arm drift of less than three inches during session 1. Improvement was seen in session 2 with no overflow movements observed.

During neck righting, the subject was observed to align his trunk and head as it was rotated in session 1. No dysfunction was seen in session 2. During the initial evaluation of rolling, the subject was able to initiate part of a segmental roll. In session 2 the subject showed a more pathological response by attempting a simultaneous log-roll with extreme difficulty.

Asymmetrical tonic neck reflex demonstrated only a change in muscle tone during both sessions 1 and 2. Symmetrical tonic neck reflex testing revealed a dysfunctional response in session 1. Slight arm extension and leg flexion was noted during dorsiflexion of the head. In test session 2 the subject displayed less dysfunction; however, he still had evidence of changes in muscle tone. In testing the tonic labyrinthine reflex, the subject initially was unable to assume and hold the proper position. In session 2, the client was able to assume the correct position and to hold it for 30 seconds.

Protective extension was slowed and delayed in both sessions 1 and 2. There was no apparent change between sessions 1 and 2 for seated equilibrium: the subject held the inflatable continuously throughout the test and demonstrated inflexible muscle tone.

Body image testing showed severe dysfunctional responses in the initial sessions, with omission of the following: ears, arms, hands, fingers, legs and feet. Also evident were extra mouth details and special neck size. Session 2 showed an improvement; however, the subject still omitted ears, fingers, and one foot. There was also special emphasis on biceps (Figs. 14.1 and 14.2).

Some abnormal movements were observed during session 1. Hypokinesia was present, as evidenced by automatic obedience along with general psycho-motor retardation and blocking. Acute dyskinesia in the form of cogwheeling was also evident throughout much of the session. Other extrapyramidal symptoms included akinesia, and rigidity in the upper extremities. During the second session akinesia and cogwheeling were still present, and hypokinesia was not observed.

The self-reported childhood history was non-contributory, partly due to the severity of the subject's symptoms and his inability to recall or relate this kind of information.

Interpretation of the Results

Comparative evaluations using the SBC documented a marked change of this subject's functional response in many of the areas tested. Specifically, coordination

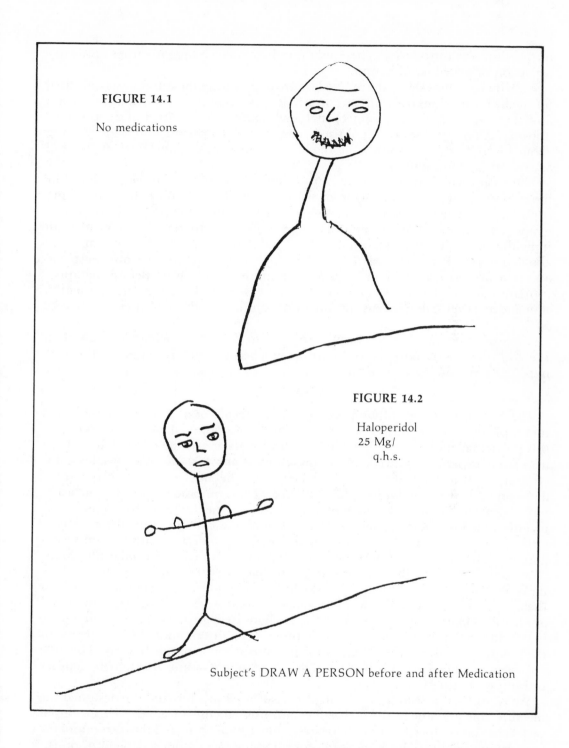

FIGURE 14.1

No medications

FIGURE 14.2

Haloperidol
25 Mg/
q.h.s.

Subject's DRAW A PERSON before and after Medication

and equilibrium responses were improved after the introduction of neuroleptic medication over the short period of three weeks. Changes were apparent in primitive postural reflexes (neck righting, asymmetrical and symmetrical tonic neck reflexes, and the tonic labyrinthine reflex). Improvement was noted in two of these areas—symmetrical tonic neck reflexes and the tonic labrinthine reflex—after

The SBC Evaluation

medication was introduced. There was no observable change in either protective extension or seated equilibrium.

Body image scores showed a marked improvement after the subject was stabilized on medication. A decrease in the bizarreness is evident in the subject's second drawing (Figure 14.2). The subject included many items omitted in the previous drawing. A projective drawing of this type represents a person's subjective feeling about himself and offers a few more clues in this complex and intricate field of assessment and evaluation.

The scores which reflect the amount of abnormal movement were reduced by more than half, after medication was introduced. It must be taken into consideration whether there was actual improvement, or if the medication had temporarily masked the symptoms. It is always important to consider an individual's sensitivity to a particular drug and to have an awareness of individual absorbtion rate. Periodic assessment is extremely important to determine progress, and is a necessary part of the treatment planning procedure. Before therapists intitiate the use of sensory integrative treatment with the psychiatric patient, a standardized evaluation, assessing functional abilities and disabilities, needs to be administered.

A sensory integration evaluation is integral to the total psychiatric assessment. We feel it is as important as monitoring clients' drug response, orthostatic hypertension, and ward behavior.

Research

The SBC is a new evaluation tool. We have been working on the sensory and motor problems of schizophrenics for the last six years, and have been working on this particular measure the last four. Professionals across the country have been using the experimental version of the SBC. Thus far, the use has been for clinical application and to gather data to test the inter-rater reliability, validate, and further standardize the measure. The components of this measure have been chosen both because of the review of the literature on sensory integration, neurologic dysfunction, and schizophrenia, and the clinical experiences with psychiatric clients. Components of the SBC are derived either from Occupational Therapy evaluation procedures and/or from neurologicaal evaluations. The significant contribution this measure makes is the gathering of all these measures into one comprehensive tool which can be administered by occupational therapists, and which will result in a standard total score to reflect the functional ability of a client at any one point in time. There are many reports in the literature which address problems in one sensory integrative area or another, but almost all the reports use different techniques for measuring these problem areas. The SBC has been designed to fulfill a need for a standard adult psychiatric sensory integration evaluation.

We completed a search of the literature, devised a pilot study, redesigned the measure, and are now in the phase of examining whether or not the definitions of each behavior are specific enough to be reliable. Establishing reliability is one of the first criteria necessary for a measure, for all subsequent studies depend upon it.

There are several ways to determine the reliability of a measure. The method used differs depending upon the type of measure. Reliability is often assessed by what is known as inter-rater reliability. High inter-rater reliability means that the instrument has been written in a way that is clear and unambiguous. Thus, different therapists evaluating the same client will rate the client the same. For the

CV Schroeder, MP Block, EC Trottier, MS Stowell

SBC, inter-rater reliability is an important factor to be established. Inter-rater reliability was initially assessed by having one occupational therapist and two students evaluate a total of 29 clients. The results are discussed below.

Although inter-rater reliability can be assessed by having a number of viewers rate the behaviors recorded on a film made of an evaluation session, the SBC does not lend itself well to this method. In performing the SBC, the therapist has to observe the whole client, noting such subtleties as changes in muscle tone, which are hard enough to detect in the flesh, and would be very difficult to catch on film.

A second form of reliability is *intra*-rater reliability, where the same rater evaluates the same client twice or more. This type of assessment is valid if the measure being used is not subject to a learning effect and if the behaviors being measured do not change over time. The possible learning effect in the SBC is currently being assessed. Because some of the tasks involved in the SBC are often incorporated into therapeutic activities, it is assumed that there will be minimal effect. A further problem with intra-rater reliability is that some of the items measured might fluctuate as a factor of changes in psychiatric status and medications. The literature on both vestibular reactivity and psychomotor response have noted this phenomenon.

Inter-rater Reliability Findings

The findings for the inter-rater reliability studies completed with the experimental edition of the SBC are very encouraging. A percentage of agreement was computed for each of the three measures which were scored on the SBC. Because there were three raters for each client, statistical tests were restricted. A high percentage of agreement means that the criteria for scoring the measures were clear (Table 14.4).

The scores show that over half of the measures have a percentage agreement of 80% or more. The two scores that fall below the 70% level of agreement were *abnormal movements* and *rolling*. The scoring criteria for these measures were clarified in the second experimental edition of the SBC.

The data were also examined to see if the scores were affected by any one rater's tendency to score in a particular way. A Friedman two-way analysis of variance by rank was performed, and the correlation between rater and tendency to occupy a particular rank was not significant ($p > 0.05$). There was a slight trend in this direction however, which will be looked at further as the measure is developed.

The goal of the reliability testing is to make the scoring specific and behavioral enough to permit occupational therapists to administer and score the measure without special training, and to provide an objectively reliable evaluation of a client.

Suggested Research

Validity is the second important element of any measure. It is especially important to look at the validity in terms of any claims the measure makes about the conclusions that can be drawn from it. Validity refers to what is being measured. Different types of validity include criterion related content validity, construct, and predictive, or concurrent validation. Content validity refers to whether the instrument covers a representative sampling of the behaviors being assessed. In other words, there would be little content validity if a measure claimed to measure sensory and motor responses and only asked the subject to draw a picture and hop on one foot. In order for a measure to have content validity, it must include in a balanced way each

TABLE 14.4

RELIABILITY SCORES OF SBC BASED ON THREE RATERS

Percentage Agreement (3 raters)

Test Number	Test Name	10%	20%	30%	40%	50%	60%	70%	80%	90%	100%
1.	Dominance	Not Scored									
2.	Posture	Not Scored									
3.	Neck Rotation									(88%)	
4.	Gait									(90%)	
5.	Hand Observation										(96%)
6.	Grip Strength										(100%)
7.	Fine Motor Control										(100%)
8.	Diadochokinesis								(73%)		
9.	Finger Thumb Opposition								(75%)		
10.	Visual Pursuit								(79%)		
11.	Bilateral Coordination								(87%)		
12.	Crossing the Midline								(88%)		
13.	Stability, Upper Extremity							(71%)			
14.	Stability, Trunk								(88%)		
15.	Classical Romberg								(81%)		
16.	Sharpened Romberg									(96%)	
17.	Overflow Movements								(87%)		
18.	Neck Righting							(73%)			
19.	Rolling						(62%)				
20.	Asymmetrical Tonic Neck							(72%)			
21.	Symmetrical Tonic Neck Reflex							(72%)			
22.	Tonic Labyrinthine Reflex							(75%)			
23.	Protective Extension								(85%)		
24.	Seated Equilibrium										(98%)
25.	Body Image							(70%)			
26.	Abnormal Movements							(67%)			
27.	Childhood History										(100%)

CV Schroeder, MP Block, EC Trottier, MS Stowell

behavior it proports to measure, giving approximately equal weight to equal portions. By sampling a wide range of behaviors, the SBC has taken the first steps toward establishing content validity.

Construct validity refers to the meaning of the instrument, to the reasons why different individuals may score differently on the measures, and to whether those differences reflect what is supposedly being measured. A familiar example of this concept is the controversy over whether IQ tests measure intelligence, or whether they measure social class and upbringing. Construct validity becomes more of a concern the further the measure gets away from what is actually measured to what meaning is imputed to the results.

In evaluating a new measure for construct validity, the measure should correlate somewhat with other measures which claim to rate a similar phenomenon. On the other hand, if the measures correlate exactly, then the measure under question would not be rating anything new. In a pilot study using sections of the Southern California Sensory Integration Tests with the SBC, some correlation was found. The correlations were not subjected to full statistical analysis since we were in the process of revising the SBC, and since the Southern California Sensory Integration Test was designed and normed for children. Future work on the SBC should include convergent and divergent correlational studies with other established measures in order to establish construct validation.

Predictive and concurrent validation both refer to whether it is possible to predict from the results of the measure to an outside criteria. Although often very difficult to do, the ability to refer to an outside criteria is an indication of the value of the measure. An example of predictive and concurrent validation cited above in the literature review was the attempt by Weaver and Brooks to predict discharge from the hospital based on psychomotor performance.[31] The SBC does not at this point make any claims about the predictive value of any scores. However, once content and construct validity, intra-rater reliability, and norms have been established, predictive and concurrent validation will be an interesting aspect to explore. It will be at that point that the SBC can be used to work on such problems as whether certain diagnoses do indeed have greater or lesser difficulty with sensory and motor performance, and how these difficulties are correlated with clinical state.

The issue of collecting norms for the SBC is quite complex. It will be necessary to test a large sample of clients in different geographical and physical settings. Data, such as level of medications, diagnosis, age, sex, and other parameters, must be gathered and diagnostic criteria established. The question of diagnosis has been the subject of innumerable journal articles. The use of the DSM III may provide the consistency needed for valid diagnostic research.

The effective use of the SBC on an appropriate population requires detailed norms on a wide variety of psychiatric clients, and is a major research focus. In this way, it would be possible to determine whether there is or is not a reliable difference in the sensory and motor abilities of different types of clients. It would be valuable to the medical and scientific community if a measure such as the SBC aided in determining subtypes, causes, and course of schizophrenia, or any of the other major psychiatric illnesses. It may be possible to gain a greater understanding of such diagnoses as borderline schizophrenia, adult hyperactive syndrome, and character disorders through the use of the SBC. Some of the preliminary research reporting neurological soft signs in these groups may lead to a better understanding of the disorders and to more effective therapies.

In addition to gathering data for norms based on a wide range of psychiatric clients, it will be important to gather normative data on normals and other institutionalized, nonpsychiatric subjects. Just as it is impossible to know whether the sensory motor problems attributed to chronic non-paranoid schizophrenics are a factor of medications without comparing them to another group of subjects similarly medicated, so it is impossible to know if the problems attributed to chronicity are a factor of institutionalization, without a reference group. Some researchers claim that it is not valid to make any statements about psychotic subtypes based on defense style without comparing them to neurotics and others with similar defense styles. These researchers argue that the qualities attributed to paranoid schizophrenia, to use one example, might actually be qualities held in common by all people using a paranoid style defense.

In addition to the problems of accurate diagnosis, there is the role of medication. It is quite possible that medications will improve performance on some aspects of the SBC and make other aspects appear more pathological. It would be a great luxury to be able to evaluate unmedicated patients and then assess the effects of medications, but in most cases this is not possible. Even though it is often acknowleged that the present antipsychotic medications are far from ideal, these medications are almost a part of the illness, even if, in some respects, they contribute to the pathology. It is the occupational therapist's responsibility to go ahead and treat the whole person, medications included, and to document as carefully as possible any changes in sensory and motor integration which are observed. The potentials for future research in this area are vast. The initial data on inter-rater reliability indicate that very few changes were needed in the measure before collecting data for norms. Once normative data are collected, there are a number of valuable ways that this measure could be used.

Conclusion

Occupational therapists are trained as rehabilitation therapists to work with clients to facilitate the most adaptive response. By using a measure such as the SBC, the ability to evaluate a client's sensory and motor problems and prescribe remedial treatments is valuable to the total treatment. In addition to knowing which specific areas to treat, psychiatric occupational therapists will have an objective measure to document changes in clients which result from therapeutic intervention. In this era of increased emphasis on accountability, objective documentation is clearly needed for occupational therapy.

We do not see this measure being limited to occupational therapy evaluations and treatment. There are several implications for the occupational therapist's ability to provide an evaluation of a client's sensory and motor responses. There is an increasing awareness in the medical community that antipsychotic medications can cause long term and irreversible movement disorders. There is also an increasing interest in the SBC on the part of physicians and other professionals for evaluating clients. The capability of the measure to provide an evaluation of client functioning, which can be repeated after a medication change, is very appealing. It is important to have a way to report in a quantifiable form the observations that occupational therapists have been making for years. Occupational therapists are the professionals on the treatment team who have the expertise to observe and evaluate these behavioral changes.

Many researchers have mentioned the role of physiologic changes in psychosis, and many have speculated that there are several different subtypes of schizophrenia which may be identified by physiologic responses. The problem is that to date there has not been a measure which assesses a representative range of behaviors used on a large population. It is our hope that such subtypes will be clarified by the use of the SBC. Having a measure which occupational therapists can use in a variety of settings will make it possible to gather data on such diverse groups as normal men and women, prisoners, psychiatric clients, retarded persons, learning disabled persons, or any other groups of interest. We feel the SBC is an appropriate measure to use for such assessments.

References

1. Fisher L, Jones FH: Planning for the next generation of risk studies. Schiz Bull 4(2):223-235, 1978.
2. Ayres AJ: Southern California Sensory Integration Tests Manual, Los Angeles, Western Psychological Services, 1972.
3. Schroeder CV, Block MP, Campbell ET, Stowell M: SBC Adult Psychiatric Sensory Integration Evaluation. San Diego, 1979, (2nd experimental edition).
4. Patton HD, Sundsten JW, Crill WE, et al: Introduction to Basic Neurology. Philadelphia, WB Saunders, 1976.
5. Noback CR: The Human Nervous System. New York, McGraw-Hill, 1967.
6. Fischer R, Ristine LP, Wisecup P: Increase in gustatory, acuity, and hyperarousal in schizophrenia. Biol Psychiatry 1:209-218, 1969.
7. Fish B: Visual-motor disorders in infants at risk for schizophrenia. Arch Gen Psychiatry 27:594-598, 1972.
8. Stevens, JR: An anatomy of schizophrenia. Arch Gen Psychiatry 29:177-189, 1973.
9. Baldessarin RJ: Schizophrenia. New Eng J Med 297:988-995, 1977.
10. Stevens JR: Neurologic Aspects of Schizophrenia. NIMH Research Unit, St. Elizabeth's Hospital, Washington, DC.
11. Meltzer HY, Stahl SM: The dopamine hypothesis of schizophrenia: a review. Schiz Bull 2:19-76, 1976.
12. Plotkin SG, Cannon HE, Murphy DL, et al: Are paranoid schizophrenics biologically different from other schizophrenics? N Eng J Med 198-61-66, 1978.
13. Watson SJ, Akil H, Berger PA, et al: Some observations on the opiate peptides and schizophrenia. Arch Gen Psychiatry 36:35-41, 1979.
14. Leach WW: Nystagmus: An integrative neural deficit in schizophrenia. J Abnorm Psychol 60:305-309, 1960.
15. Myers S, Caldwell D, Purcell G: Vestibular dysfunction in schizophrenia. Biol Psychiatry 7:255-261, 1973.
16. Claude H, Baruk H, Aubry M: Contribution a l'etude de al demence precoce catatonique: Inexcitabilite labyrinthique au cors de la catatonie. Rev Neurol 1:96, 1927.
17. Angyal A, Blackman W: Vestibular reactivity in schizophrenia. Arch Neurol Psychiatry 44:611-620, 1940.
18. Fitzgerald G, Stengal E: Vestibular reactivity to caloric stimulation in schizophrenia. J Ment Sci 9:93-100, 1945.
19. Levy DL, Holzman PS, Proctor LE: Vestibular responses in schizophrenia. Arch Gen Psychiatry 35:972-981, 1978.
20. Holtzman PS, Proctor LR, Levy DL, et al: Eye tracking dysfunction in schizophrenia patients and their relatives. Arch Gen Psychiatry 32:143-151, 1974.
21. Holtzman PS, Levy DL, Proctor LR: Smooth pursuit eye movements, attention, and schizophrenia. Arch Gen Psychiatry 33(12): 1415-1420, 1976.
22. Holtzman PS, Kringlen E, Levy DL, et al: Abnormal pursuit eye movements in schizophrenia: evidence for a genetic factor. Arch Gen Psychiatry 34(7):802-805, 1977.
23. Diefendorf AR, Dodge R: An experimental study of the ocular reactions of the insane from photographic records. Brain 31:451-489, 1908.
24. Ayres AJ: Learning disabilities and the vestibular system. J Learning Disabilities 11(1), January, 1978.
25. deQuiros JB, Schranger OL: Neuropsychological Fundamentals in Learning Disabilities. San Rafael, Academic Therapy Publications, 1978.
26. Huddleston CI: Differentiation between process and reactive schizophrenia based on vestibular

reactivity, grasp stength, and posture. A J Occu Ther 32(7):438-444, 1978.

27. Shuster AR: The psychotropic drugs: considerations relative to the vestibular pathways and testing. Laryngoscope 75(5):707-749, 1965.

28. Keating NR: A comparison of duration of nystagmus as measured by the Southern California Post Rotary Nystagmus Test and electronystagmography. A J Occu Ther 2:92-97, 1979.

29. King HE: Psychomotility: A Dimension of Behavior Disorder. In Subin, Shagass (ed): Neurobiological Aspects of Psychopathology, New York, Grune and Stratton, 1969.

30. Weaver L, Brooks G: The use of psychomotor tests in predicting the potential of chronic schizophrenics. J Neuropsychiat 5:170-180, 1964.

31. Weaver L, Brooks G: The prediction of release from a mental hospital from psychomotor test performance. J Gen Psychol 76:207-229, 1967.

32. Maloney MP, Payne LE: Validity of the Draw-A-Person Test as a measure of body image. Percept Mot Skills 29:119-122, 1969.

33. Silverstein AB, Klee GD: A psychopharmacological test of the body image hypothesis. J Nerv Ment Dis 127:323-329, 1958.

34. Hammer E: The Clinical Application of Projective Drawings. Springfield, IL, Charles C Thomas, 1971.

35. Marsden CD: Cerebral atrophy and cognitive impariment in chronic schizophrenics. Lancet II:1079, 1976.

36. Johnstone EC, Frith CD, Crow TK, et al: Cerebral ventricular size and cognitive impairment in chronic schizophrenia. Lancet II:924-926, 1976.

37. Crow TJ, Johnstone EC: Cerebral atrophy and cognitive impairment in chronic schizophrenia. Lancet I(8007):357 1977.

38. Crayton JE: Motor endplate alterations in schizophrenic patients. Nature 264(5581):658-659, 1976.

39. Crayton JW: Smith RC, Klass D, et al: Electrophysical (H Reflex) studies of patients with tardive dyskinesia. Am J Psychiat 134:775-780, 1977.

40. Gur RE: Motoric laterality imbalance in schizophrenia. Arch Gen Psychiat 34:33-37, 1977.

41. Wexler BE, Heninger GR: Alterations in cerebral laterality during acute psychotic illness. Arch Gen Psychiat 36:278-284, 1979.

42. Flor-Henry P: Lateralized temporal-limbic dysfunction and psychopathology. Ann NY Acad Sci 280:777-797, 1976.

43. Stevens JR: Eye blink and schizophrenia. Psychosis or tardive dyskinesia. Am J Psychiat 135(2):223-226, 1978.

44. Crane GE: The prevention of tardive dyskinesia. Am J Psychiat 134:756-758, 1977.

45. Quitkin F, Klein DF: Two behavioral syndromes in young adults related to possible minimal brain dysfunction. J Psychiatr Res 7:131-142, 1969.

46. Quitkin F, Rifkin A, Klein DF: Neurologic soft signs in schizophrenia and character disorders. Arch Gen Psychiat 33:845-853, 1976.

47. Tucker G, Campion E, Silberfarb P: Sensorimotor functions and cognitive disturbances in psychiatric patients. Am J Psychiat 132:17-21, 1975.

48. Wender PH: Minimal Brain Dysfunction in Children. New York, Wiley Interscience, 1971.

49. Halperin KM, Heringer C, David PS, et al: Validation of the Schizophrenia-organicity scale with brain damaged and non brain-damaged schizophrenics. J Consult Clin Psychol 45:949-950, 1977.

50. Pollack M, Krieger EP: Oculomotor and postural patterns in schizophrenic children. AMA Arch Neurol Psychol 79:720-726, 1958.

51. Goldstein C, Halperin KM: Neuropsychological differences among subtypes of schizophrenia. J Abnorm Psychol 86:34-40, 1977.

52. Fish B, Shapiro T, Halpern F, et al: The prediction of schizophrenia in infancy: III. A ten year follow-up report of neurological and psychological development. Am J Psychiat 121:768-775, 1965.

53. Bach-y-Rita G, Lion JR, Climent CE, et al: Episodic dyscontrol: A study of 130 violent patients. Am J Psychiat 127:1473-1478, 1971.

54. Wood E, Reimherr FW, Wender PH, et al: Diagnosis and treatment of minimal brain dysfunction in adults. Arch Gen Psychiat 33:1453-1460, 1976.

55. King LJ: A sensory integrative approach to schizophrenia. A J Occu Ther 9:529-536, 1974.

56. Kellor M, Frost J, Silberberg N, et al: Hand strength and dexterity. A J Occu Ther 25:77-83, 1971.

57. Van Allen MW: Pictoral Manual of the Neurologic Tests. Chicago, Year Book Medical Publishers, Inc, 1969.

CV Schroeder, MP Block, EC Trottier, MS Stowell

58. Ayres AJ: Sensory Integration and Learning Disorders. Los Angeles, Western Psychological Services, 1974.
59. Trombly C, Scott AD: Occupational Therapy for Physical Dysfunction. Baltimore, Williams and Wilkins, 1977.
60. Bender L: Childhood schizophrenia: Clinical study of one hundred schizophrenic children. Am J Orthopsychiat 17:40-56, 1947.

Bibliography

Ayres AJ: Southern California Sensory Integration Test Manual. Western Psychological Services, 1972.

Ethridge D, McSweeney M: Research in Occupational Therapy. Rockville, MD, American Occupational Therapy Association, 1971.

Kerlinger FN: Foundations of Behavioral Research. New York, Holt, Rinehart & Winston, 1964.

Phillips JS, Thompson RF: Statistics for Nurses. New York, MacMillan, 1967.

Roscoe JT: Fundamental Research Statistics for the Behavioral Sciences. San Francisco, Holt, Rinehart, & Winston, 1975.

15
The Bay Area Functional Performance Evaluation

Judith Bloomer, M.S.W., O.T.R.
Susan Williams, M.A., O.T.R., A.T.R.

The Bay Area Functional Performance Evaluation (BaFPE) is designed to assess in a consistent and measurable way, some of the functions that people must be able to perform in general activities of daily living. This evaluation consists of two subtests: the Task Oriented Assessment (TOA) measures general ability to act on the environment in specific goal-oriented ways; the Social Interaction Scale (SIS) assesses general ability to relate appropriately to other people within the environment. The combined results of these two assessments are used as indicators of overall functional performance, and provide information about the person's cognitive, affective, and perceptual motor characteristics.

The BaFPE was developed at Langley Porter Psychiatric Institute, part of the University of California in San Francisco. The development of the BaFPE constitutes the first phase of a potential three phased project in which the impact of occupational therapy on functional performance could be assessed (phase 2), and the ability of the BaFPE to predict community functioning could be evaluated (phase 3). Widespread field testing of the BaFPE began with dissemination of the adminstration manual in April, 1979 to facilitate further validation of the instrument, and to elicit feedback from test users in order to refine the BaFPE in a future revised edition.

The following chapter will introduce the broad concept of functional assessment, discuss the theoretical frames of references utilized in the development, and the design of the BaFPE, and review the general content, standardization, and research implications of two subtests. Specific administration protocol is included in the BaFPE manual. This manual is available through Consulting Psychologists Press. See page 304 for more information.

The Concept of Functional Assessment

The broad concept of functioning is felt to be of interest to any professional group working in the field of rehabilitation, and concerned with the assessment of functional performance in a client population. We believe, however, that occupational therapists are more accustomed to assessing a person's functional performance, or ability "to do," than many other disciplines. As the construct of functional ability has been considered from different points of view, the following definition of function is presented as the main construct of our study:

> *Function:* A dynamic, active process, a "bodily or mental action, behavior, or performance, a contribution of an element to the consistency or equilibrium of a culture, or an organizational unit performing a group of related acts and processes: activity."[1] Function is stressed as productive; ie, a "useful activity such as the function of maintaining balance."[2]

Functioning, then, is defined as employing useful activity to achieve an active mode of adaptation to the environment. This process or activity would include the ability to satisfy physiological and psychological needs through interaction with both people and objects in the environment. The term *functional*, as used in the study, pertains to this definition of functioning, and is a descriptive adjective connoting purposeful activity and active adaptation to the environment.

Purposeful activity can be classified into three functional areas: self care, work, and leisure. We view *functional skill* as the foundation of everyday performance in each of these three areas, integrating the following performance components: 1) motoric; 2) social; 3) cognitive; 4) psychological; and 5) sensory integrative. The term, *functional* is also used to pertain to the "development or maintenance of a larger whole,"[1] or to an individual who is able to perform, synthesizing the components listed above. The conceptualization of functional performance is an integrative construct incorporating these components.

Literature Review

The intent of studying functional performance is not new, although the subject has not been well-developed in the theoretical literature of various mental health fields. The terminology of functionalism was coined as early as the late 1800s, and refers to a general psychological approach that views behavior in terms of active adaptation to the environment. John Dewey, the noted educator, philosopher, and psychologist, contributed heavily to the development of the functionalist point of view. This frame of reference defines psychology as the study of the adaptation process. This is an expansion of the then current definition which limited psychology to the dissection of states of consciousness. It emphasizes the coordinated activity of the total organism and the use of the mind as an instrument in meeting the practical problems of life.[3] Functionalism emphasizes action and utility, and in stressing the practical, is closely aligned with the philosophy of pragmatism. This functionalist school of psychology is not interested in the operation of mental processes by themselves, but rather, in mental activity that is part of a larger system of biological forces which are continuously at work. Functionalists stress the process of accommodation, both the interaction of the human being with the environment, and the working relationship of the physical and mental portions of the organism. Functionalism advanced psychology into a relationship with the well-established field of biology. It also spurred investigations of the physiological as well as the psychological processes which underlie behavior.

Functionalism was the precursor of the behaviorist point of view. John Watson, the originator of behaviorism, started out as a functionalist. Watson followed the teachings of Angell, a functionalist, who stated that all mental processes which involve accommodation eventuate in motor phenomena.[4] Watson developed behaviorism as a school of psychology that is a purely objective experimental

Judith Bloomer and Susan Williams

branch of natural science. He believed that introspection and the interpretation of conscious and unconscious acts are not important. What is important is the manifestation of the organism's psychological processes in observable behavior.

Another theoretical frame of reference stemming from the late 1800s that looks at the area of functioning is that of act psychology. This theory focuses on psychic acts or mental processes rather than psychic content, stressing the interpretation of psychological processes in terms of activity.[3] Act psychology, however, seemed to emphasize these mental, or more cognitive, processes more than what many clinicians now stress in a holistic approach to the interaction of the mind *and* body relative to activity.

In current times, most people who look at the individual's comprehensive behavior adopt somewhat of a functionalist approach. Behavioral psychologists today study components of actual performance, emphasizing stimulus-response theory to explain the behavior being observed. Indeed, behavioralists have developed a body of literature explaining behavioral theory and the experimental analysis of behavior.

Although the disciplines of psychology, psychiatry, social work, nursing, vocational rehabilitation, and other rehabilitation specialties have addressed the topic of functional ability, we want to emphasize the unique philosophical premise that the field of occupational therapy brings to the study of human functioning. This will be discussed at length in the section on theoretical frames of reference relevant to occupational therapy.

Just as the school of functionalism in the early 1900s was associated with American pragmatism, our current emphasis on functional performance reflects an American cultural bias valuing productivity in a work-oriented society. We acknowledge that parameters of function and dysfunction are determined by American society's correlation of normal functioning with productive, active performance, whether at work or play. The assessment of functional performance within the parameters defined by society seems relevant for many diagnostic groups, even though the initial research on the BaFPE was standardized with a psychiatric population.

Rationale for the Development of the BaFPE

The occupational therapist is frequently in a unique position to undertake, and feel competent in, assessing functional performance because of an inherent professional emphasis on returning the client to his optimal level of functioning within our society. Although occupational therapy programs provide treatment through activity, standardized methods of evaluation on which to base this treatment generally have not been well-developed. Evaluation instruments have generally fallen into four categories:

1. Projective activities or activity batteries;
2. Functional behavior rating scales;
3. Neuropsychological test batteries; and
4. Contingency management schedules.

Although the above evaluations are strong in certain areas, none include all the following criteria that are characteristic of a sound instrument:

1. A clearly defined objective indicating what is to be evaluated;

2. A well defined set of norms, or description of the population to be assessed;
3. A consistent administraton and scoring procedure;
4. A controlled assessment situation; and
5. The establishment of reliability and validity.

The research on the BaPFE was undertaken with the intent to meet these criteria and develop a tool that would allow reliable and valid assessment of functions that people must perform for accomplishment of general activities of daily living. General functioning in the environment involves some degree of the presence of two abilities: 1) the ability to engage in goal directed and task oriented interaction with objects in the environment; and 2) the ability to interact in a socially appropriate way with people in the environment. Evaluation of functioning, then, might involve a combination of assessment in these two areas. The BaFPE assesses the first area, that of goal directed interaction with objects in the environment, through the Task Oriented Assessment (TOA). The second area, that of socially appropriate interaction with people in the environment, is assessed through the Social Interaction Scale (SIS). These two areas were considered essential to the overall assessment of functional performance. The concept of functional performance is that considered from different points of view as outlined in the following discussion of theoretical frames of reference specific to the field of occupational therapy.

Theoretical Frames of Reference

Because of its emphasis on functional performance relative to people and objects in the environment, this evaluation draws from several existing frames of reference utilized by occupational therapists. It may be helpful to mention these frames of reference and the degree to which they relate to the theoretical premises adopted in the development of the BaFPE.

The psychoanalytic frame of reference, for example, emphasizes man's continual struggle with internal conflicts and past experiences. In this model, dysfunction is seen as a breakthrough of unconscious content with a subsequent decline in ability to relate satisfactorily with people or objects in the environment. The BaFPE does not attempt to look at etiology of dysfunction or relate it to unconscious conflicts. Instead, the BaFPE seeks to measure the extent of functional performance regardless of etiology, and therefore, reflects little of a psychoanalytic model.

The developmental frame of reference, which has been most notably addressed by Lela Llorens,[5,6] in contrast to psychoanalytic theory, emphasizes the mastery of various skills and abilities in areas of physical and psychological growth. These abilities are considered interdependent, qualitative, and stage specific. Their acquisition provides the basis for satisfactory coping behavior and adaptive relationships within society. From this point of view, when a person becomes dysfunctional in conjunction with psychological trauma or stress, the resulting clinical picture is evidence of an arrest in the developmental progression, or a regression to an earlier stage of development. During times such as these, the occupational therapist provides activities which can assist in facilitating normal growth, development, and promotion of more adaptive functioning. Certainly this frame of reference acknowledges the importance of the ability to interact satisfactorily with both objects and people in the environment. To this extent it is similar to the theoretical base upon which the BaFPE has been developed. A prinicipal difference, however, is that while we are interested in specific behaviors that may be reflective of developmental mastery, there is no concern with the etiology of those behaviors. The BaFPE does not attempt to align functioning with the acquisition of any specifically defined developmental stages, although it acknowledges our society's expectation of "age/stage" skills acquisition.

Other frames of references have been developed, such as the biopsychosocial model by Anne Cronin Mosey. In this model, the initial goal seems similar to the BaFPE; ie, to identify the level of functioning of clients.[7] However, the ultimate goal in the biopsychosocial model appears to again stress developmental mastery in that the occupational therapist's role, once the level of functioning has been identified, is to assist the client in repeating the necessary developmental stages. Consequently, the theoretical foundation of the BaFPE, while it may have some areas in common with the above frames of reference, is not exclusively reflective of the psychoanalytic, developmental, or biopsychosocial models.

Two frames of reference that are in keeping with our approach in the BaFPE, are the acquisitional frame of reference, and the occupational behavior frame of reference. The acquisitional model, one of three outlined by Mosey,[7] focuses on the skills and abilities that, "the individual needs for adequate and satisfying interaction with the environment."[7] Within the framework, the author mentions three subcategories, two of which seem relevant to this study: ego functions and unlabeled behavior. From an ego function point of view, adaptive behaviors—those that are positively reinforced by society—occur when the basic functions of the ego are intact. These functions may include balanced use of defense mechanisms, differentiation, synthesis and organization of perceptions, reality testing and control, investment, expression, and use of libidinal and aggressive drives.[7] In the BaFPE, scores on the functional end of the continuum imply intact ego functioning, including the components listed above.

The unlabeled behavior subcategory of this framework is also relevant to the BaFPE in that it too, identifies as dysfunctional any behavior that interferes with adaptive functionings. However, in this acquisitional model, behavior assessment stresses the individual's specific life tasks. In contrast, the BaFPE attempts to isolate components of functional behavior that are generally assumed to be necessary within society, across various life roles.

Evaluation in the acquisitional frame of reference usually taps the individual's present, rather than past, interaction with the environment. This is the emphasis in the BaFPE as well, although in the BaFPE there is an attempt to take into account the possible influence past personal and/or cultural experience may have played in an individual's response to a specific task. Past information that may be relevant was gathered during the research both during the TOA and on a demographic data sheet which was considered in interpreting the overall results. The principles underlying the BaPFE, like those of the acquisitional frame of reference, imply that functional performance can be measured. We also believe, as is reflected in the second projected phase of the project, that a client may be helped to become more functional through exposure to situations in which more adaptive behavior can essentially be "practiced." This implication draws heavily on learning theory, especially principles of operant conditioning. The principles underlying the acquisitional frame of reference seem close to those on which the BaFPE is based.

The second theoretical model which is reflected in the development of the BaFPE is the occupational behavior (OB) frame of reference. Although much of the teminology used in the OB frame of reference has been coined in the occupational therapy literature in recent years and many old terms have taken on new meanings, the underlying concepts are not new. Much of the theory inherent in the occupational behavior frame of reference comes from the social sciences: sociology, anthropology, social psychology, and economics. General systems theory is also highly reflected in the OB model. Using a systems approach, occupational behavioralists seek to understand environmental factors and relationships, especially affecting choice and behavior. The occupational behavior frame of reference convincingly puts together many of the concepts occupational therapists have been using in practice for years. Occupational therapy has always addressed human performance in its broadest scope, and occupational therapists traditionally, although by history, informally, assess a person's ability to perform in most general areas of daily life tasks. The body of literature encompassing the occupational behavior frame of reference speaks to the necessity of maintaining a balance between the daily life tasks of work, play, rest, and sleep.[8] This frame of reference identifies the nature of adaptation, and stresses the importance of the acquisition of new skills and socialization patterns to support the daily living (or occupational) performance of clients in various life roles.[9] The OB model includes some of the aspects of the developmental and acquisitional frames of references; specifically, the concept of an "age/stage continuum" (or relationship of developmental stage to chronological age), and the acquisition of life roles.

In reviewing the occupational behavior frame of reference, it may be helpful to review a format utilized in teaching theory in occupational therapy education programs developed by Shapiro and Shanahan.[10] The authors reviewed the components of a frame of reference which include: 1) a theory base concerning the relationship of man and his environment; 2) the nature and relationship of function and dysfunction; and 3) the corresponding postulates for change. The occupational behavior frame of reference, as outlined by Reilly,[11,12] has its origins in the psychosocial concept of role theory. The OB frame of reference, like the acquisitional frame of reference, emphasizes the acquisition of roles throughout an individual's life, progressing from infancy to old age.[13] Occupational behavior, as defined by Moorhead[14] is seen as social behavior or active productive behavior which is molded and defined by social institutions in the service of group needs and as a manifestation of an individual's response to the demands of his environment. Occupational behavior stresses balance among the activities of work, play, rest, and sleep. Through these activities, the individual acquires the skills necessary for role performance, and builds these skills into daily habits of behavior. In assessing functional performance in the acquisition of roles, we see role performance or occupational behavior as being functional when it is productive and facilitates adaptation to an environment.

The relation of man to his environment is often conceptualized in terms of role acquisition.[15] Black defines *role* as a position in society that contains a set of expected responsibilities and privileges.[13] Within the boundaries of a role, expectations are formed by both society and the individual assuming the role. Performance is then compared to the expectations of the role. We believe that basic functional performance is evaluated as a prerequisite to the undertaking of any role (unless, of course, the role is that of a nonfunctioning individual in our society). Role theory takes into consideration boundaries, internal and external expectations, feedback, and performance. Both a functional theory and an occupational behavior theory would also consider the boundaries (geographic, socio-cultural, economic, environmental, etc) within which the person is functioning. The internal expectations of the person, as well as the external expectations of the family,

Judith Bloomer and Susan Williams

immediate environment, and society all play a part in the person's performance. Both informal and formal assessments of an individual's functioning are processed in relation to these expectations and boundaries, and are issued as feedback regarding the persons's performance.[15]

Using the Shaprio-Shanahan model of reviewing the nature of the function-dysfunction continuum, we see that in the occupational behavior frame of reference, dysfunction is shown as a lack of identification with occupational role, and the acquisition of skills and habits identified with occupational behavior in any number of roles.[13,14] In fact, the occupational behavior frame of reference tends to avoid focusing on the concept of dysfunction, which it sees as being a perspective based on pathology aligned with a medical science base.[9] In the functional orientation, we see dysfunction as also including the lack, or loss, of skill acquisition demonstrated by non-productive behavior. Additionally, we believe that functional behavior can be considered a prerequisite to the acquisition of occupational behavior.

Intervention, in the occupational behavior frame of reference, is focused on the acquisition of new skills along an age/stage continuum. The goal of the therapist utilizing this model is to create an environment that promotes or facilitates the development of occupational behavior, as it is defined within the OB framework. In the functional orientation, we also stress the development of skills to promote adaptive behavior. Like the occupational behavior frame of reference, the principles of achievement motivation are used.[16] In dealing with a person who is immobilized or dysfunctional, a prime objective would be to motivate that person to mobilize his resources and skills into adaptive action.

There are numerous similarities between the philosophy behind the development of the BaFPE and the occupational behavior frame of reference. Functional behavior is closely related to occupational behavior. We view it essentially as a *precursor* to occupational behavior, as illustrated by a schematic diagram of a behavior continuum:

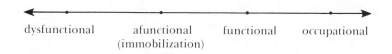

dysfunctional   afunctional   functional   occupational
(immobilization)

We realize that occupational behavior theorists state that occupational behavior is assumed at early stages of development: for example, the preschooler assumes the occupational role of student, or the infant the early role of learner.[17] The major point is to emphasize the continuum from dysfunction to function to the development of occupational behavior.

Additionally, the concept of helping people to mobilize and develop their adaptive skills is discussed by Lorna Jean King[18] in a treatise on the adaptive process. The author describes adaptation as, "an active response evoked by specific environmental demands," much like the functionalist view of adaptation. This theoretical concept is seen as being crucial to a person's overall functional performance and thus, an important consideration behind the development of the BaFPE.

The BaFPE not only reflects the ideas behind the occupational behavior and adaptational theoretical framework, but even more specifically, the theory and application of occupational therapy as delineated in Spencer's chapter on

"Functional Restoration" in the fifth edition of *Williard and Spackman's Occupational Therapy.*[19] In this bible of the occupational therapy discipline, Spencer reiterates that one of the basic theories of occupational therapy, "is the use of performance as feedback to the patient to assist him or her in becoming involved in self-initiated, purposeful activity."[19] Although Spencer relates the treatment principles of functional restoration to the patient with physical and neurological conditions, we believe that the objectives of occupational therapy treatment are applicable to any and all client populations in which there has been a disruption of functional performance. These objectives include: 1) awareness of self; 2) maximum level of self-care independence; 3) restoration of functional ability; 4) exploration of vocational and avocational potentials; and 5) socialization and adjustment to new life patterns.[19]

Spencer sees an occupational therapy program incorporating three major areas: the identification of function through evaluation procedures; the development of function through the use of specific activities to increase function; and the integration of function into the client's routine tasks. The evaluation of function in physical and neurological conditions is achieved through a variety of well-established methods of assessment commonly used in the practice of occupational therapists working in the area of physical dysfunction. These evaluation methods include assessment of the client's range of motion, proprioception, sensory perception, reflex and muscle testing, sensory integrative, and perceptual-motor functioning. Evaluation methods in the area of psychosocial dysfunction (as discussed in the previous section) have not reached the same level of development or sophistication evident in non-psychiatric areas of practice.

In summary, the principles on which the BaFPE have been developed seem most closely allied with the acquisitional, occupational behavior, adaptational, and functional restoration frames of reference. The evaluation procedures are based on the assumption that man needs specific identifiable skills to function in everyday activities. In the research project, the hypothesis is made that the functional components of these skills are measurable through a sampling of task-oriented behavior, and recording observations of interactional behavior. Further research correlating occupational therapy intervention with functional performance, as measured by the BaFPE, is based on the principle that more functional behavior can be attained through provision of an environment in which new skills can be learned[20] and behavior utilizing these skills be practiced.[11,12]

Historical Development of the BaFPE

The development of the content of the BaFPE was influenced by the theoretical emphasis on functional ability. The design of the evaluation was determined by two factors: first, the need for the development of a standardized evaluation within psychiatric occupational therapy mandated a consistent and easily applied protocol. Second, the BaFPE research project at Langley Porter Psychiatric Institute required the development of a formal research design.

The research goals necessitated a two-phased study: one phase was to develop an instrument which could predictably measure functional performance, and another phase which could utilize the instrument to measure the effectiveness of occupational therapy interventions. The BaFPE is the result of phase 1. Phase 2 would utilize an experimental design with a control group to evaluate the impact of occupational therapy intervention on client functioning using the BAFPE as a reliable indicator of functional performance. Although we did not utilize an experimental design for Phase 1, it was important to adhere to a research design which would facilitate the collection of data to standardize the BaFPE.

In order for an evaluation to be methodologically and statistically sound, it must be able to be used with predictable accuracy, and agree with other instruments which measure areas similar to those being investigated in the evaluation (see Standardization, pp 275-277). An evaluation that meets this criteria has probably been developed through the use of comparisons, calculations, and measurements most easily accomplished by computer analysis of data. It is also important to have accurate information about areas which may influence performance on an evaluation like the BaFPE, such as age, cultural factors, educational level, job history, etc. We recorded this information on a Demographic Data Sheet. The collection of data such as this requires facilities and resources not available to many therapists. The time alone required for gathering data and compilation of information is frequently far in excess of that available to most clinical occupational therapists. We were fortunate to have access to facilities and the support of colleagues for research time.

The BaFPE was developed over a three year period at Langley Porter Psychiatric Institute, (LPPI) at the University of California, San Francisco. The statistical validation of the BaFPE took place on two inpatient adult units at LPPI: the Inpatient Treatment and Research Service (ITRS) and the Crisis Intervention Unit (CIU). ITRS is an 18 bed unit which provides psychiatric treatment for adult clients with diagnoses including schizophrenic, affective, and character disorders. The average length of stay on this unit is approximately six to eight weeks. The CIU provides treatment for acutely ill psychiatric clients and is the inpatient facility for one of the five mental health districts in San Francisco. It has a bed capacity of 11, and during the data collection period, an average length of stay of eight days on inpatient status and four days on outpatient status.

Because we wished to develop an assessment tool that would be useful and valid for as broad a population as possible, the criteria for participation in the study was also broad. All clients, regardless of diagnosis, who were 16 years or age or older, were willing to participate, and able to sign a consent form (parents signed if the client was under 18), were included.

Subjects were divided into two groups on the assumption that it would be optimal to sample a wide range of functional performance and that this range would be reflected by assessing functional performance on admission and discharge. One group was tested within four days of admission, and the other was tested on the day prior to discharge. For both groups the following procedures were followed:

1. Pre-assessment Interview:
   a) A consent form was signed by the client.
   b) A demographic data sheet was filled out by the examiner after an interview with the client.

2. The TOA was administered during a 30 to 60 minute session with the examiner. A second rater was included for establishment of inter-rater reliability.

3. The SIS was filled out by a rehabilitation therapist or rehabilitation therapy

student familiar with the client during the same 24 hour period as administration of the TOA.

4. On the same day, or not more than 24 hours before or after the TOA and SIS were completed, the ward nursing staff filled out two rating scales: the Global Assessment Scale (GAS),[21] and the Functional Life Scale (FLS).[22] The GAS is used to rate overall functioning of a subject during a specified time period on a continuum from psychological or psychiatric health to illness. The FLS is also used to rate overall functioning in nine specific areas, such as cognition, socialization, and activities of daily living. Although initially developed for a physically disabled population, it has subsequently been adapted for use with psychiatric populations.[23]

Overview of Administration

Pre-Assessment Interview

Following the recommended guidelines for summarizing the test which are included in the BaFPE administration manual, the therapist explains to the client the general purpose of the evaluation. It has been found that this interview provides time to familiarize the client with the research project and further clarify the consent form if the client has any questions. In most clinical settings, a consent form is not required unless the data is being gathered to supplement a research project specific to their setting. A demographic data sheet which provides a format for the gathering of basic information such as age, race, diagnosis, as well as educational experience, past occupational functioning, and socio-cultural considerations is then filled out. At this time, additional clinical information may be collected to supplement the demographic data and help establish a pre-assessment rapport between the examiner and the subject. For example, the therapist may want to inquire about the client's perception of his own ability to function in such basic living skills as budgeting finances, housekeeping, using public transportation, communication, and socialization, etc. For this purpose, an interview format such as the "Performance Status Examination,"[24] would be a useful supplement to the BaFPE. It is generally recommended that the pre-assessment interview be limited to no more than 15 minutes (or be completed at another time), so as not to fatigue the client prior to the administration of the TOA.

Task Oriented Assessment (TOA)

The TOA is an evaluation instrument consisting of five tasks which can be administered to a subject in approximately 45 minutes. The maximum time allotted for the completion of the tasks is 32 minutes, but in order to allow for preparation, verbalizations between tasks, and collection of demographic data, it is wise to allow approximately 45-60 minutes. For specific administration protocol and instructions, the BaFPE administration manual is required.

We used five tasks in the TOA to rate 10 different functional behaviors. All tasks have been chosen to reflect task oriented behavior, but the structure of each task differs so that there is a graduation from extremely structured to more unstructured. The process of task selection began with consideration of 10 initial tasks which we felt reflected functioning in the areas assessed. We found that five of the tasks could be eliminated without affecting the assessment of each of the relevant functional areas. Although all tasks are able to be rated across the 10 functional components, some tasks appear to tap more directly into certain functional components than others. The actual content of each task was chosen because it was felt that the specific materials and the structure would allow competent evaluation of the functional performance of the subjects across all 10 functional components, as well as providing some specific task observations. The following is a brief description of each task. Specific instructions and materials are described in more detail in the BaFPE administration manual.

Sorting Shells. The subject is requested to sort shells into 10 containers according to size, shape, and color. This task is quite structured and concrete. Verbal instructions clearly imply a right and wrong way to accomplish the task. Shells were selected because they are not sexually biased, are aesthetically appealing, and appear to be intrinsically motivating.

Bank Deposit Slip. The subject is requested to fill out a deposit slip according to clearly defined written instructions. This task utilizes a greater sequence of instructions than the shell sorting task, and includes information regarding orientation (to person and time) as well as cognitive functions such as addition and subtraction. The subject is initially asked whether or not he has had experience with a bank account. If the subject has not, and is under 18 years old, a different set of instructions (Form B) is given to complete the task.

House Floor Plan. The subject is requested to draw a square representing the outside walls of a house and then to draw rooms chosen from a list. The subject is free to choose five rooms from the list of 10 and place them where he chooses inside the square. This task provides some structure, but also allows the subject to make decisions regarding choice and placement of rooms. Although portions of this task emphasize such cognitive functions as measurement and spatial organization, it is clear that projective elements are involved in the subject's explanation of the room selection and placement. In establishing this task, we considered the possiblity of socio-cultural bias in asking subjects to draw a floor plan. In this task the subject's knowledge of a floor plan of a house is ascertained. If no knowledge exists, or if the client is unsure, a sample of a floor plan is shown for not more than three seconds. In our experience, and specifically, in the sample of 62 subjects, no subject was unfamiliar with floor plans. Most subjects recognize the format from exposure to diagrams or blueprints in the media, play experiences, or educational background.

Block Design. The subject is asked to look briefly at nine blocks on which there is a design, and then to duplicate the design after the blocks have been randomly mixed up. If the subject is not able to do this after two minutes, he is shown a cue card on which the design is drawn. The subject is then asked to duplicate the design with the blocks by copying the cue card. This task is very structured, and yields information about memory, and visual and spatial perception as parts of functional performance.

Draw-A-Person. The subject is asked to draw a picture of a person doing something. This is the most projective task on the TOA. It is scored according to task oriented behavior as are the rest of the tasks. However, it may give supplementary content information which has relevance to clinical issues, as might any projective test, regarding defenses, object relations, and self concept.

Each task is timed in order to provide outside limits for the time of test administration, although we have not considered the actual time taken in the statistical data analysis. Again, the length of time may provide information important to clinical issues, but we believe that if a person successfully completes the task within the allotted time, the response can be considered functional. If the subject is not able fo finish the task in the allotted time, the response is recorded as an unfinished task. Time limits for the task are derived from time averages of the normal population samples for each task. Time limits are as follows:

Sorting Shells	5 minutes
Bank Deposit Slip	8 minutes
House Floor Plan	10 minutes
Block Design	2 minutes (4 minutes possible)
Draw-A-Person	5 minutes
Total	32 minutes maximum

Functional Parameters and
Behaviors Assessed on the TOA

As mentioned, these five tasks are rated along 10 functional components. This was done by establishing behavioral guidelines which describe behavior along a continuum of function to dysfunction for each of 10 functional behaviors. A rating guide is used to further clarify certain descriptive phrases of these guidelines. The behavioral guidelines consist of two pages which delineate the 10 functional components. The presence or absence of certain task specific behaviors on a TOA Scoring Sheet is also recorded. The behavioral guidelines and TOA Scoring Sheet are included in total in the BaFPE administration manual. These 10 functions are listed on the behavioral guidelines and have been utilized in accordance with the following definitions:

Paraphrase. This is defined as the restatement of a text or passage in another form or in other words, often to clarify meaning.[25] This functional area tests the ability to comprehend both written and oral instructions. Comprehension of written or verbal instructions involves the ability to obtain information by reading or hearing a passage and understanding relationships and general principles involved. The respondent is frequently required to answer questions about the content.[2] Comprehension in the TOA is measured by the subject's ability to paraphrase the verbal or written instructions. Because the definitions of *general idea* and *essential specifics* needed to rate this functional component are different for each task, they are included and clarified in the Specific Task Instructions in the BaFPE administration manual.

Productive Decision-Making. This functional area measures the ability to formulate a cohesive plan and act on it. Although a decision is defined as the formulation of a course of action with intent to act on it,[2] the TOA takes this definition one step further and looks at the qualitative as well as the quantitative aspects of decision-making. The category of decision-making takes into account both the ability to make a decision as well as the degree to which the decision utilizes good judgment. The process of changing one's mind in the TOA is manifested behaviorally by the interruption of what appears to be a goal directed series of actions and the adoption of a different apparent progression. This different progression may or may not advance the subject toward correctly and appropriately completing the task. This is recorded as the presence or absence of good judgement on the behavioral guidelines. Inability to make a decision may be manifested by verbalizations indicating lack of decision-making skills, such as, "I can't make up my mind," or "I don't know which thing to do," etc.

Motivation. This functional area measures the subject's attitude about working toward the completion of a task. Motivation is frequently connected with drive, and

Judith Bloomer and Susan Williams

may be defined as a reaction to some stimuli which activates a drive and brings into action an organized sequence of actions which persist in a given direction. It is demonstrated that acceptance of a task can create a motivation in and of itself.[26] In the TOA, it is assumed that if a client agrees to participate in the assessment and accepts each task, there will be an inherent drive to complete the task. Fiske also recognizes that the desire to complete the task can be contingent on task acceptance.[27] We believe that motivation is not always clearly manifest behaviorally and so suggest that ratings of motivation consist of both objective and subjective scales. Because of this, subjects should be given a brief checklist (Task Questionnaire) to fill out after the assessment, inquiring about subjective feelings of motivation and frustration tolerance.

Organization of Time and Materials. This functional area measures the ability to organize. It is defined as the ability to arrange parts through foresight and planning so that they work together in a coordinated way.[2] The element of time is included in this function because of a belief that the ability to organize materials will promote efficient use of time. Conversely, poor organization of materials may lead to ineffective use of time. A subject may appear very organized in approach to materials, but still be very slow. It is believed that over-organization of materials can be detrimental if the subject is not able to finish the task in the allotted time. Because the definition of *finishes task* needed to rate this functional component is different for each task, it is included and clarified in the Specific Task Instructions in the BaFPE administration manual.

Mastery and Self-Esteem. This functional area measures the degree to which the subject is able to project his basic sense of self-confidence regarding ability with the specific task and/or self-worth in general. It is felt that although a lack of mastery is frequently displayed behaviorally, for the purposes of clarity and/or rating, feelings of inadequacy are rated only if they are demonstrated verbally.

Frustration Tolerance. This is defined as the ability to accept the blocking of, or interference with, an ongoing goal-directed activity without disruption and disordering of behavior.[2] This functional area measures the ability to accept any portion of the materials or instructions involved in the TOA which might produce feelings of discomfort or anxiety in the subject. As was stated in *Motivation*, it is assumed that the subject's agreement to work on the task produces a need. Rosenzweig defines primary frustration as the "sheer existance of an active need," and secondary frustration as "supervenient obstacles in the path to the goal of the active need."[28] If acceptance of the task generates a need, any obstacle to completing the task might be considered a secondary frustration. In this task, it is assumed that this frustration may come from external (eg, difficulty with materials, hyperactivity due to environmental stimuli) or internal (voices, preoccupying thoughts) sources. Frustration is frequently manifested in many different ways behaviorally: by projection onto the environment; by isolation and withdrawal; by denial, etc. Because behaviors may look different for each of these defenses, the subject is given a brief checklist (Task Questionnaire) to fill out after the assessment, inquiring about subjective feelings of frustration tolerance and motivation.

Attention Span. This functional area measures the ability to concentrate. Concentration is defined as the ability to exclusively and persistently sustain attention to a limited object or aspects of an object.[2] In this assessment, the inability to concentrate may be due to either internal or external stimuli.

Ability to Abstract. This functional area measures the ability to generalize from the specific task to the overall goal of the task as it relates to day-to-day functioning.

The BaFPE   267

Ability to abstract is defined as:

1. The ability to comprehend relationships and react, not merely to concrete objects, but to concepts and abstract symbols.[25]
2. The ability to characterize any quality of something considered apart from the thing itself, or from other qualities with which it is associated.[2]

The abstraction questions used in this assessment are similar for all tasks except the last one, the Draw-A-Person. Because this is more of a projective task rather than related to functioning in everyday activities, the question assessing abstraction ability is worded slightly differently. We feel that similar functions of abstraction ability are measured in both. Because the definition of *generalized goal* of each task is needed to rate this functioning component, but is different for each task, it is included and clarified in the Specific Task Instructions in the BaFPE administration manual.

Verbal or Behavioral Evidence of Thought or Mood Disorder. This functional area measures the degree to which affective and/or psychotic elements interfere with adequate task performance or may effect the task oriented working situation. Scores on this function may affect scores on other functional areas; eg, if the subject is overly hostile, it may affect ratings on motivation and/or frustration tolerance. Affective, or mood, disturbance may be evidenced by the presence of one of the listed qualities (eg, hostile or by related states not mentioned—for example, psychomotor retardation or agitation. Psychotic thought process may be evidenced by delusions, hallucinations, or loose associations. Any of these may be manifested by verbal or behavioral expression.

Ability to Follow Instructions Leading to Correct Task Completion. This functional area measures ability to complete the task correctly according to instructions. Because correct task completion is a crucial area and most important in the TOA, it is weighted doubly to give proper emphasis. Correct task completion measures both quantitative and qualitative areas. Whether the subject does or does not finish the task, the number of errors that are made is recorded. Because the definition of *finishes task* and *number of errors* is needed to rate this functional component, it is different for each task. It is included and further clarified in the Specific Task Instructions in the BaFPE administration manual.

In summary, the preceding functional components were felt to be important in assessing a person's ability to act on objects in the environment. In accordance with our beliefs that these functional components are measurable given a consistent setting, the five tasks mentioned earlier were developed. Although these tasks vary in structure, each one provides information about all of the functional components listed.

Perceptual Motor Observations
on the TOA Scoring Sheet

In addition to the functional components, each task provides information thought to be clinically important, such as observations in perceptual motor and/or cognitive areas. This specific information is recorded on the right side of the TOA Scoring Sheet in a yes-no checklist format. Some of the perceptually related information observed in this section is summarized below.

Perception is defined as "a physiological function which, by means of the sense organs enables the organism to receive and process information on the state of an

Judith Bloomer and Susan Williams

alteration in the environment." It is believed that perception may be distorted when the perceiving individual is in a state of need. Therefore, perception is the result not only of stimulus structure, but also of personality structure and its motivational state.[29] In the TOA, motor observations are used as indicative of the ability to receive and process information.

The observations on the Scoring Sheet are listed below along with the primary perceptual-motor function they are thought to demonstrate. Presence or absence of a number of these is indicative of questionable functioning in perceptual-motor areas and may warrent further testing.

Sorting Shells

1. Sorts shells by size, shape, color: discriminates between size, form, and color.
2. Crosses midline: integrates functions of two sides of the body.[30]
3. Uses both hands at some point: bilateral integration.[30]
4. Movements steady and directional: evidence of motor apraxia: inability to perform certain purposive movements without the loss of motor power, sensation, or coordination.[31]

Bank Deposit Slip

1. Reading acceptable: if no, vision, or literacy; evidence of dyslexia or difficulty in reading due to neurological etiology[31] or illiteracy due to lack of education.
2. Copies numbers correctly: visual perception and motor accuracy.
3. Calculations acceptable: evidence of acalculia or inability to solve simple mathematical problems.[31]
4. Personal information acceptable: if not, note name/address or date: orientation to time and person, evidence of agraphia for any reason.

House Floor Plan

1. Draws six inch square accurately: visual perception, measuring, motor accuracy.
2. Divides rooms with logical proportion: judgment related to spatial relationships.
3. Labels rooms: memory or evidence of agraphia for any reason.
4. Justifies room placement acceptably: judgment and abstraction.

Block Design

1. Duplicates design from memory: short-term memory, ability to perceive and duplicate by manipulation, a three-dimensional design.
2. Copies design from cue card: visual perception, motor accuracy, figure-ground perception.
3. Accurate placement of colors: accurate figure-ground perception and discrimination.
4. Manipulates blocks with ease: evidence of apraxia (see Sorting Shells, number 4).

Draw-A-Person

1. Logical progression in drawing: concept formation.[32]
2. Figure/objects in proportion: evidence of possible conflict in specific areas.[32]

3. Drawing fairly centered on paper: general stability with relationship to environment.[32]
4. No transparencies evident: inclusion of transparencies indicates incidence of possible thought disorder.[32,33]

The preceding section has delineated functional component areas and task specific observations utilized in the TOA. This assessment focuses on an individual client's interaction with objects in the environment, and does not evaluate a subject's ability to interact with, or relate to, people in the environment. The following subsection will discuss the design of the Social Interaction Scale (SIS) and its importance in assessing overall functioning.

Social Interaction Scale (SIS)

The SIS is a rating scale that assesses the behavior of an individual in a social situation. The individual's behavior is evaluated across seven different components, or parameters, of social interactions. These parameters reflect normal interactional patterns that are developed in the process of socialization, in which a person interacts with others in the environment. Scores on the SIS are used in addition to scores on the TOA, in which the subject relates to objects within the environment, in assessing overall functioning. The SIS was developed because a review of what was available for assessing social interaction did not meet our needs. There is a multitude of literature, especially in the fields of sociology and social psychology, dealing with the topic of social interaction. However, we were unable to identify a tool by which interaction could be measured quickly and by rehabilitation personnel with little expertise in sociological measurement. An instrument that was specifically applicable to rehabilitation settings was also needed. Therefore, the SIS was developed, utilizing the design of many commonly used psychiatric rating scales which rate global symptomatology.[21,34]

The design of the SIS is that of a behavioral *rating scale,* as opposed to a *behavioral checklist.* It is important to distinguish the difference between these two concepts of behavioral evaluation. A characteristic of a behavioral checklist is that it reports only the presence or absence of certain observable aspects of behavior, whereas a rating scale is characterized by the following:[34]

1. *A defined continuum of dimensions* along which judgments are placed: a graduated sequence of adjectives, phrases, statements, or categories with numbers attached that correspond to an increasing or decreasing amount, severity, or characteristic of what is being observed. For instance, on the instructions for filling out the SIS, examiners are asked to rate the client's behavior along a continuum from dysfunction to function (1-5). Although there are descriptive phrases for each level of the continuum, examiners are asked to rate the behavior along the continuum using the descriptive phrase as a guide, but also to exercise their clinical judgment in rating.

2. *A standard of comparison.* In psychiatric practice, this standard of comparison is a class of persons or reference groups. The task of the rater is to make a comparison between the individual being observed with respect to the appropriate reference group. This reference group for the SIS is the normal, non-client population with respect to their regular interactional activity as well as the expectation of the normal level of interaction within a therapeutic community. (The norms for the SIS and the relationship to the normative data

Judith Bloomer and Susan Williams

collected on a non-client population will be discussed later in this chapter.)

3. *Establishment of equal intervals.* In situations other than psychiatry, scales are expected to establish equal intervals along a graduated continuum, locating an origin, or zero point. In his book, *Psychiatric Rating Scales,* Lyerly states that "equal intervals and the establishment of a zero point cannot be properly performed with typical psychometric data."[34] This reference, which was published by the National Institute of Mental Health (NIMH) speaks to the difficulty of establishing absolute or fixed values in trying to measure a parameter (such as behavior) that is so variable. We have attempted, in the continuum of dysfuntion to function for each parameter of social interaction on the SIS, to help identify the five different intervals through the aid of the descriptive phrases. The phrases are merely behavioral guidelines, to be supplemented by clinical judgment.

We chose the rating scale format for assessing social interaction because it was felt it would be the most useful in meeting the objectives. Typically, rating scales are used for the following purposes: 1) to use as an evaluation procedure that might be more comprehensive than an informal interview; 2) for communication—to provide a consistent frame of reference or baseline of communication from one clinician to another; 3) to record treatment progress, or change in clinical status; and 4) to provide a format where research data or information can be classified and collected quantitatively.[34]

Prior to discussing the development of the SIS, a review and definition of terms are offered:

> *Socialization* is the "process by which a person acquires sensitivity to social stimuli, especially the pressures and obligations of group life. The person then uses this sensitivity to get along with and to behave like others in his/her group or culture."[2] There is a sort of "perceptual give and take" or adaptation, between the person and the environment.

This definition of adaptation or aculturation to a group is important in assessing the social interaction of clients within institutional settings. Institutional environments can influence social behavior and interaction.[35,36] However, in most short-term treatment settings today, the environmental influence is felt to be beneficial to the social development of the client.[36,37,38] In long-term institutionalization, the client often assumes the effects of apathy, or loss of interest and initiation, submissiveness, lack of individuality, and apparent inability to make plans for the future.[35] These characteristics are caused by the extended loss of contact with the outside world, the loss of responsibility, the loss of personal contacts, possessions, and the atmosphere of a long-term facility. These characteristics apply to a chronic, "institutional neurosis," as researched by Barton,[35] and is usually caused by a length of stay greater than two years. Since the data collected in standardizing the BaFPE was done in a relatively short-term treatment setting, negative factors affecting social interaction in an institutional environment are not considered in the design of the SIS.

> *Social Interaction* is defined as "the mutual stimulation of one person by another and the responses that result.[2]
> *Social Behavior* is defined as "behavior controlled by an organized society," whereas;
> *Society* is the network of social groups in which a person lives; it is a social order in contrast to the individual.[2]

The BaFPE

Socially Appropriate Behavior is social behavior that is appropriate to the situation or environment. Appropriate indicates "specifically suitable, fit or proper; belonging to" a particular social code.[1]

To a major part, it is actually social conditions that are the determinants of psychiatric illness.[37] For instance, a person is not usually identified as being psychiatrically ill unless someone else labels this behavior. Although the person can subjectively identify symptoms and feelings associated with psychiatric illness, the point is that the person must express verbal or behavioral manifestations of these symptoms to be considered ill by our society. A society's reaction to mental illness may be culturally determined: for example, some cultures tend to protect a psychiatrically ill individual, whereas others will expel them from the cultural subgroup. A person is not seen as being mentally ill in a vacuum: someone in the environment (family, neighbors, co-workers, friends, etc) usually reacts to unusual behavior or affect exhibited by the individual in question. Therefore, treatment settings need to provide an alternative social condition or environment to provide a structure to facilitate the loss of functional performance experienced in the larger society. Most treatment settings emphasize a therapeutic community or environment (in the areas of practice of psychiatric or physical disability) that fosters optimal functioning.[37]

Behavior within institutions or small groups is still social behavior.[39,40] The main difference is that there may be a different set of norms or expectations of behavior. For instance, at Langley Porter, our clients are expected to participate in program activities—the norm (or relative level of achievement represented with a given population) is therefore considered to be active, functional participation— similar to the social interaction that a normal or non-disabled population would exhibit.

Given the objective of assessing social interaction within rehabilitation settings or programs, the next decision is to determine which aspects of social interaction to measure. We needed an assessment that would look at the normal components of social interaction since one objective of treatment is that the clients would assume normal social interaction. Therefore, we define *normality* as health, or the absence of disease or dysfunction.[41]

Functional Parameters and Behaviors Assessed on the SIS

Seven basic categories of social interaction were chosen, because we felt that each was important in assessing a person's social interaction within an occupational therapy or rehabilitation program. The seven parameters of social interaction and their respective definitions are:

Response to Authority Figures. This parameter assesses the client's interaction with people assuming the role of authority in different situations. Authority is defined as having the "power to influence the outward behavior of others, [and the] status that carries with it the right to command and give final decisions."[2] When evaluating responses to authority figures, the issue of conformity is important to assess. Homans states that response to authority often has to do with the degree of social conformity in a group or individual.[38] There are basically two types of responses to a group or to individual behavior. In Type A, most members tend to behave in a certain natural way, without being told to do so and without the fear of being punished if they do not. Type B is the set of norms or group behavior where people may behave naturally, but contrary to what has been asked of them.

Judith Bloomer and Susan Williams

In assessing the parameter of "response to authority figures" on the SIS, we do not wish to take a moral stand about conformity. However, in the definition of function, optimal functioning is viewed as the conformance to the social values of American society as a whole. It is significant to note that in American culture, the larger middle class work ethic stresses that people are expected to take direction from others, such as supervisors, teachers, parents, military officers, etc. Therefore, direction from authority figures is considered a reality to be dealt with, and response to such direction should be appropriate, non-hostile, and functionally accommodating, relative to the situation at hand.

Verbal Communication. Verbal communication with people in one's environment is considered a "critical mode of social development."[42,43] Doll, author of the *Vineland Social Maturity Scale,* says that social competence is directly related to facility in *means* of communication. The person who cannot speak the language of his environment is definitely impaired in the social expression of his capabilities. (Even, for instance, in the non-verbal deaf person who is competent in utilizing sign language or lip reading there is still the linguistic handicap.) This principle of impairment in verbal communication becomes extended when related to foreign language or to regional differences in languages. When assessing social interaction, the social environment is taken into account. However, in an attempt to take in cultural factors in a multi-ethnic society, the client's primary language is noted. This information can be used for clinical purposes and for interpretation, although if the person being assessed is unable to communicate verbally in the present environment, the client is scored at level 1 on the SIS.

Psychomotor Behavior. This is defined as "pertaining to the motor effects of psychological processes and is used to have dualistic implications."[2] An example of this would be in psycho-motor retardation, where the person's motoric responses and affect are slowed or delayed. If the subject being assessed is taking medication (such as a major tranquilizer) that might contribute to psycho-motor slowness, this is noted, but still scored, as with the parameter of verbal communication. Again, this information might be used for clinical purposes and interpretation of results, but the parameter is scored since the person's functional performance is currently impaired.

Independence/Dependence. Independence is defined as self-reliance and/or self-direction.[2,42] Dependence or dependency is the lack of self-reliance, or the requirement of the support of others in securing minimal requirements for food, shelter, and clothing. Dependency also implies the tendency to seek the help of others in making decisions, carrying out tasks, or for seeking comfort, guidance, or reassurance. Doll's concept of social competence also places heavy emphasis on personal independence and the exercise of individual responsibility and self-sufficiency.

Independence is seen by different indicators of competence along an age/stage continuum. For instance, in early childhood, development of independence is seen as self-help (ie, in eating, dressing, hygiene, locomotion, or toileting). In adolescence, it is seen as the desire for social freedom in personal conduct and the beginnings of desire for separation from parents. In early adulthood, it is seen as the assumption of responsibility and eventual authority for others (eg, as in family life). Self-directed activities are a definite reflection of the successful management of one's own affairs. This management is seen as essential to all acceptable definitions of social adequacy.[42]

Socially Appropriate Behavior. As mentioned earler in this section, socially appropriate behavior is that type of behavior that is specifically "suitable, fit, or proper—belonging to a specific social code."[2] It is important to assess behavior relative to the situation at hand. For example, socially appropriate behavior would include the absence of the type of symptomatology which would be obviously peculiar within an acceptable code of behavior for the situation. Emotional maturity and dynamics are also critical aspects of a person's social behavior and overall social presentation.[42]

Ability to Work with Peers. This ability is considered an integral aspect of socialization—social competence naturally involves social relationships with a peer group. "This social competence of the individual is indicated by the extent to which he is accepted among his fellows as an equal, inferior, or superior relative to age and cultural-economic level."[42] Social performance which involves group relationships is most clearly evident in play activity and cooperative group interests. Normal human living requires collaborative relationships with others.[40,42-44]

Participation in Group/Program Activities. Participation implies taking part in, or the sharing of, some experience. This parameter on the SIS assesses the person's ability to take part in or share experiences in activities that reflect social interaction. As mentioned earlier in establishing norms, our expectation for social interaction is that the person being observed participates in some type of group activity. In the nonpatient community, it could be participating in clubs, committees, competitive team sports, community groups, performing for others, sharing community responsibilities, or any kind of collaborative interactive group.

In the subject population, group activities would include some of the above mentioned groups, normal interactive play activities, table games, and any kind of activity group in the ward's occupational therapy program. Therapeutic activity programs in rehabilitation settings are areas for assessment of participatory group behavior. Participatory behavior of individuals in groups can be categorized in the following major areas:[39]

1. *Interpersonal behavior* such as cooperative problem solving, as in task-oriented groups.
2. *Individual performance* of the person within the group.
3. *The format of interaction,* ie, the type of communication network or channels of communication between members, and the interaction rate, or frequency.

The field of sociology assesses these components of participatory behavior very specifically and very thoroughly.[39,40,44-47] The objective in looking at social interaction is to look at participatory behavior much more generally, as indicated in the continuum of behaviors on the SIS assessing the subject's ability to participate in group or program activities.

In summary, the design of the SIS utilizes a behavioral rating scale format. The SIS measures seven different parameters of social interaction. Each of these components of interaction is relevant and assessable in normal interactional activity within the community, as well as within the social environment of a rehabilitation program. The procedure for administering, or rating, the SIS is detailed in the BaFPE administration manual.

The three components (Pre-Assessment Interview, TOA, and SIS) of the BaFPE can be administered within the same time frame, or can be split up within a 24 hour period. It is important to collect information on the SIS within this 24 hour period to validly reflect functional performance in a social setting, as compared to the more structured setting of the TOA.

The Pre-Assessment Interview should be conducted in a quiet room that offers confidentiality and is free from distractions. The TOA should also be administered in such an environment. The structure of the TOA requires a work space such as a table or desk where the subjects can complete tasks, all of which can be done sitting at the table.

Persons being tested are told the general purpose of the evaluation and are informed that they may ask specific questions about their performance at the end of the testing session. At that time, the examiner gives general feedback regarding performance in any of the functional component areas, and answers specific questions regarding the tasks, if there are any. General testing protocol is maintained throughout the testing session: verbalizations are kept at a minimum, time limits are observed, and standardized administration instructions are followed. Administration of the BaFPE presents no special problems, although it should be remembered that the TOA cannot be administered in a group situation. Although problems with language, vision, limited range of motion, and coordination may interfere with successful completion of the TOA, for example, it is felt that these conditions do, in fact, reflect real limitations in functional performance that need to be considered in an overall assessment of functional ability. The TOA is scored according to the behavioral guidelines specified for each of the 10 functional components. These guidelines were developed to represent a function to dysfunction continuum of behavior. Each of the five tasks are rated across all 10 functional areas and the scores are tallied to a subscore obtained from rating the presence or absence of task specific observations and general behavior indications of perceptual-motor and cognitive functioning. The tallied scores from the TOA are subtotaled and added to the score obtained from the SIS to give a composite profile of functional performance.

The SIS is administered by observing subjects in socially interactive environments and rating their behavior in seven different areas of interaction previously defined. The face value for each of the seven parameters of social interaction is tallied, weighted, and added to the TOA subtotal to give a composite BaFPE score. It is essential that the composite score is always used in interpreting a subject's test scores, as neither the TOA nor the SIS give a comprehensive assessment of functional performance when considered independently.

Research Design of the Standardization Process

As discussed in the previous sections, the intent in developing an evaluation to assess functional performance included the desire for objectivity as well as the need for an assessment that was specific to goals within the field of rehabilitation. We wanted an evaluation that was more objective than the ratings used by many therapists in clinical settings; we wanted one that could be objectively given, scored, and could provide information that was relative to those elements assessed. With these goals in mind, it became clear that the evaluation tool needed to be standardized.

The BaFPE is designed to be used by occupational therapy clinicians; however, many of the clinicians trained at the basic baccalaureate level have not had much background in statistics or research terminology. Therefore, some of the basic terminology related to standardization will be discussed. A description of how these concepts were actually applied in the research project and a discussion of the significance of the data that was collected in standardizing the BaFPE will be offered.

What is a standardized test? A standardized test is one that is substantially uniform and well-established; it is always the same—in content, administration protocol, and scoring procedure. A test becomes standardized through long development and use; the wider the use, the more meaningful the results.

Why standardize? We wanted not only to be able to evaluate behavior, but to do it in a consistent, measurable, and quantitative way that could be used for research purposes. There have been so many adaptations of behavioral checklists, projective batteries (like the Azima, Fidler, and Goodman Batteries), and adaptations of test interpretations that we wanted to develop a tool that could be consistent over time and with different raters. Since there was nothing available, it was decided to standardize the BaFPE.

There are probably many reasons that clinicians have adapted evaluation instruments within the field of occupational therapy. In many cases, an evaluation has been developed exclusively for a specific clinical population and is not easily, or appropriately, used with another population or in another setting. Clinicians, recognizing some of the valuable elements of an evaluation, elect to keep part of the evaluation, but not all of it. The problem here is that the test is no longer consistent, and valid interpretation of the results of the test can no longer be made in the manner that the original test developer intended.

The research edition of the manual was published as a standardized test, although at this writing, a second edition is anticipated some time in the future. The second edition will incorporate improvements and changes that we have systematically reviewed and decided upon through a formal evaluation process which is currently being coordinated through a field testing project at LPPI, University of California, San Francisco. With such evaluative input from test users, a second edition of the BaFPE can be developed that has improved with age and with use.

What is involved in standardizing a test? There are three main elements that must be addressed:

First, test norms must be defined. The term *norm* is derived from the Latin *norma,* which generally means a rule or accepted standard. More specifically, it usually refers to a standard determined by assessing certain characteristics and measures of central tendency among various groups of individuals.[48] Norms refer to the population(s) with whom one is working. It is important to clearly describe this population for reference so that the scores of one individual or population can be compared to the scores of another individual or population. For example, one set of norms may describe an adult inpatient psychiatric population. Another set may describe an adolescent developmentally disabled population. Still another may be the normal population, matched to one of the first two populations in terms of age, sociocultural status, etc.

The norms for the BaFPE included two different populations. The research data was collected on an adult psychiatric inpatient population at LPPI, this being one set of norms used in the manual. Comparative data was collected attempting to match normal, or non-psychiatric control subjects to the ward population in terms of age, sex, and educational/occupational status. It is important to note here that the comparative normal group does not reflect national norms or people-in-general norms, because we were limited to collecting data from the sample of people that were available in the community. Thus, the available norms reflect a small sample of 20 adults residing in a cosmopolitan, metropolitan city (San Francisco). Undoubtedly, normal samples of other areas in the United States, such as the rural midwest, would provide a different set of data.[49] How variable this data would be is undetermined, and can only be assessed through formal data collection. Adding to the comparative data is one of the things we would like to see addressed by contributing research-oriented therapists. (Please see Future Research, pp 302-304).

The comparative normal group ranged in age from 17 to 59 years of age, with an educational level ranging from 11 to 18 years. Racial distribution was 100% caucasian. Occupational status for this group was: 20% housewives, 33% students, 14% clerical/sales and 33% professional, semi-professional, or managerial. Because the premise behind the BaFPE is the assessment of functional performance, we included only those individuals in the comparative normal group who were assuming productive, functional roles within the environment. Thus, there are no representatives in this sample under the classification of "temporarily unemployed." Other characteristics of our comparative normal group, such as the range of scores on the BaFPE, will be discussed in the section on normative and comparative group data.

The clinical research data using adult psychiatric patients came from two inpatient wards at LPPI. There were some differences in ward characteristics, but none so great that we felt unjustified in combining the data for research purposes reflecting a general adult, inpatient population. At the time of the study, the two wards were called the Inpatient Treatment and Research Service (ITRS) and the Crisis Intervention Unit (CIU). ITRS is the major adult research and teaching oriented unit at LPPI. Many patients are referred to this ward for specialized diagnostic workups, and many patients are accepted onto the ward according to the research needs of the service at that time (eg, medication research studies for particular diagnostic groups). ITRS usually maintains a wide variety of diagnostic categories of patients because of teaching needs of the ward. The average length of stay of ITRS is longer than CIU—two months (62.6 days) during the time the data was collected.

The CIU accepts all patients from a certain catchment area in San Francisco. Many of the patients, although acutely ill on admission, have chronic diagnoses. The average length of stay was about two weeks (12.3 days) during the time the data was collected. Previous hospitalization for CIU patients averaged 3.3 times (as opposed to ITRS, in which the average previous hospitalization was 0.5).

The second aspect involved in standardizing a test is to develop a *consistent* protocol and *administration procedure,* as well as a consistent method for rating or scoring what is being evaluated. The standardized protocol for administering and scoring the BaFPE is presented in full in the administration manual.

Finally, in standardizing a test, the instrument's *reliability* and *validity* must be established. The concepts of reliability and validity are crucial elements in assessing the value of any test. It is important to know if: a) what is being measured is being measured in a predictable way; and b) what is being evaluated is really being measured. These terms will be defined in greater detail in Chapter 17. What follows is a discussion of how each is addressed in the development of the BaFPE.

Reliability

In reference to reliability, we consider two types: *intra-rater* reliability and *inter-rater* reliability.

Intra-rater reliability refers to reliability within a rater or test. This is assessed by using the same rater over time, and is referred to as the test-retest method. However, the test—retest method cannot be sufficiently determined when there is a changing subject or trait. For instance, it is not possible for one rater to assess the functional performance of a client who changes in functional status due to clinical improvement and get the same score as the first testing session. Also, a patient who is given the test again shortly after the first administration might do better simply because of a practice effect. Relative to intra-rater reliability, we suggest allowing at least three weeks between administrations of the TOA in an effort to control a practice effect. Also, in developing the TOA, tasks were chosen that did not utilize materials the client might have had extended exposure to within the context of an activity program (such as working with clay when clients often have ceramics as part of their scheduled activities).

Inter-rater reliability is the type of reliability that we have mainly been concerned with in the BaFPE. This type of reliability refers to measurement error between different raters. We have attempted to assess different rater   reliability in two ways: across subjects (two or more raters assessing multiple subjects); and across different raters (multiple raters rating the same subject).

Inter-rater reliability was assessed across subjects in the following manner: we rated 42 subjects concurrently. One of us administered and rated the TOA as the principal examiner and the other rated the TOA during the same administration session as an observer. The scores from these two ratings were compared using a statistical method to obtain the correlation coefficient, or numerical indication of comparative relationship, between the two ratings. Also, we, along with the ward staff, concurrently rated the subjects using the SIS. There were six different raters involved in rating the SIS, although only two at any one time for any one subject. The correlations for the BaFPE were assessed at two different times. One assessment of correlation was completed after administering the TOA and SIS to the first 12 subjects; we then did a second assessment after the next 30 subjects, assessing inter-rater reliability for 42 subjects in total (Table 15.1).

The results show that inter-rater reliability across subjects using two different raters (ourselves) was extremely high; most correlation coefficients were in .80s and .90s (1.0 = perfect correlation between ratings). The lowest correlation was .76 on decision-making. In comparing the results between the first 12 subjects and subsequent 30 subjects, it is apparent that ratings did not differ significantly across time. One thing that this data *might* indicate is that extensive experience in administering the BaFPE is not necessary. In other words, reliability of ratings does not improve that much between the 12th and 40th administration. One note of caution—the inter-rater reliability was assessed using our ratings. Most likely, those that develop a test are more familiar with it and more likely to have higher inter-rater reliability than a less familiar test user. For instance, the correlations of ratings by raters using the SIS were somewhat lower: .81 to .83 (though still high, as far as reliability). These coefficients reflected the ratings of six different raters, including ourselves. Since our inter-rater reliability may be unusually high because of author familiarity, we would like to suggest that potential test users practice administering the BaFPE at least 10 times prior to actually giving it in a clinical situation. This will help the users to become more familiar with it and help to decrease measurement error.

An attempt was made to assess inter-rater reliability for the TOA across raters using the same subject. The method used was to make a color videotape of an actual TOA administration and show this videotape to multiple raters. Twelve therapists in the Rehabilitation Therapy Department at LPPI were utilized. The therapist

Judith Bloomer and Susan Williams

TABLE 15.1

INTER-RATER RELIABILITY
CORRELATION ACROSS SUBJECTS (N=42)

	First 12 Subjects	Subsequent 30 Subjects*
BaFPE (Total)	.97	.99
SIS (6 different raters)....................................	.81	.83
TOA (Total)	.98	.99
TOA Tasks:		
Sorting Shells...	.95	.90
Depost Slip	.96	.99
House Floor Plan..	.98	.97
Block Design	.96	.97
Draw-A-Person	.95	.98
TOA Functions:		
Paraphrase	.95	.96
Decision Making	.76	.87
Motivation	.93	.90
Organization	.95	.95
Mastery	.90	.91
Frustration	.95	.94
Attention Span	.87	.95
Abstraction...	.85	.88
Disorder	.93	.95
Completion	.96	.99

*At .001 level of significance; all others are at .01 level.

composition included occupational therapists (seven, including ourselves) and five other rehabilitation therapists, including music, dance, and recreation therapists. An analysis of variance between four groups (ourselves, all others, occupational therapists, and non-occupational therapists) was used to see if ratings differed significantly between the groups. The results are presented in Table 15.2.

The results of this statistical test showed no significant difference in means, or average scores, between raters in the four groups. The total points possible in the scoring of the TOA is 240 and the raters by group, ranged in their total of TOA scores from 190.0 to 202.5 points—only a 12 point difference. However, it is important to note the range of individual ratings. Although there is no significant difference in the means, or averages, of the four groups of raters, the range of scores are markedly different between groups. Note that in establishing the average ratings for each group, scores at extreme ends of the scoring range—continuum of function to dysfunction: 1-4, should be cancelled out to approximate the mean. As indicated in Table 15.2, the range of scores between groups is widely divergent. We rated the TOA most closely, with only a 1-point difference in the total TOA score. Since we were more familiar with the TOA than any other group, this range is to be expected.

The BaFPE 279

TABLE 15.2

INTER-RATER RELIABILITY (TOA-VIDEO)

Across Raters (N = 12) Analysis of Variance
Between Four Groups

Group	Mean Score	Standard Deviation	Range
I Authors (2)	202.5	00.7	1
II Others (10)	192.5	16.9	64
III OTs (7)	197.0	8.2	23
IV Non-OTs (5)	190.0	23.4	64*
No significant difference in means at .05 level.			

Range is widely divergent.

Occupational therapists, as a group, were closer than non-OTs in rating the total TOA. Their range of ratings is 23 points as opposed to 64 points by other rehabilitation therapists. This might imply that occupational therapists assess task oriented behavior more consistently than other rehabilitation therapists.

Although there is a definite implication that occupational therapists are more skilled at assessing task behavior, it is necessary to note that this study was based on a sample size of only 12 therapists. With such a small sample size, the study most certainly needs replication with a larger group of therapists from each discipline. Until such future studies are completed, however, we suggest that administration of the BaFPE be restricted to occupational therapists. Occupational therapists are specifically trained in their academic and practical experiences to analyze activities, break down these activities or tasks into component areas, and assess task-oriented functioning.

In summary, reliability is concerned with measurement error—both within the evaluation instrument and within and among raters. Reliability can be assessed over time, between raters, and across subjects. Results of the analysis of reliability using the TOA and SIS indicate that the BaFPE is a reliable tool for evaluating performance when used in the suggested manner (adhering to the standardized protocol) by occupational therapists trained at the basic professional level.

Validity

The other important aspect of standardizing a test is to establish the test's validity. The main question in addressing the issue of validity is: *Does the test measure what you think it does?* In other words, how valid is the test as an indicator of functional performance? To carry this line of questioning further:

1. What can be inferred about what is being measured within the test (specific functions on the TOA or social parameters on the SIS)?
2. What can then be inferred about other behavior; for example, general functioning?

In reference to the BaFPE, the following question was proposed: How useful is the assessment of specific functions and total scores on the TOA and the SIS as predictors of functional behavior outside the assessment session?

There are four main types of validity: 1) face validity; 2) content validity; 3) criterion-related validity; and 4) construct validity. Each of these types will be defined in greater detail in Chapter 17. What follows is a discussion of how these relate to standardizing the BaFPE.

Face validity refers to the general appearance and impression of the test. Does the instrument, taken at face value, appear to measure what it is intended to? Does its appearance reinforce general acceptance by potential test users?

We have positive indications that the face validity of the BaFPE is not only acceptable, but good. The BaFPE utilizes terminology common to all OTs—terms used in looking at clients' functional performance in activity sessions and task oriented behavior. It compiles information on behavior that OTs routinely assess in clinical practice, much of the terminology being used in activity check lists.

In addition to potential test users, the BaFPE seems valid for face validity in reference to the reaction of the subject group. Many clients initially questioned the use of the TOA materials. However, after they were administered the test, they seemed to accept the tasks as having some value in assessing the level of their functional performance.

Content validity is concerned with how well the items within the test sample the parameters about which the conclusions are to be drawn. Does the content of the TOA (10 functional component areas across five separate tasks) adequately reflect task oriented behavior? The premises of functioning and the specific functional components and parameters of social interaction were previously defined. They are statistically demonstrated in Table 15.3. We conclude that behaviors exhibited in the TOA session and behaviors exhibited in a social or group setting are representative of task-oriented behavior and social interaction in general.

Criterion-related validity is concerned with how well the test under construction compares to other criteria, or external, independent variables that are already considered to be direct or valid measures of the characteristic or behavior being evaluated.

There are two main types of criterion-related validity: *concurrent* and *predictive* (concurrent and criterion-related are often used interchangeably, but there is a difference). These will be discussed further in Chapter 17.

Concurrent validity is determined when it is assessed how well a score on one test relates to another (external) criterion being measured concurrently, or at the same time. We determined concurrent validity for the BaFPE by comparing scores on the BaFPE to scores on two other evaluation tools. These two evaluation tools were administered to the same clients by the nursing staff on the wards during the same time period the BaFPE was administered to each client. These two other criteria were the *Functional Life Scale* and the *Global Assessment Scale*.

The Functional Life Scale (FLS)[22,23] consists of nine different components, such as Cognition, Activities of Daily Living (ADL), Home and Outside Activities, etc. The FLS was developed for use with physically disabled clients on a physical medicine and rehabilitation unit by the psychiatrist Sarno, and has since been adapted for use with psychiatric patients.

The Global Assessment Scale (GAS)[21] is a rating scale assessing level of functioning and degree of symptomatology along a 10-interval scale divided into percentile rankings.

Both these scales are described more completely in the references under the

TABLE 15.3

CORRELATION MATRIX FOR CONCURRENT VALIDITY.
COMPARISON OF BaFPE COMPONENTS WITH THE GLOBAL ASSESSMENT SCALE (GAS) AND COMPONENTS OF THE FUNCTIONAL LIFE SCALE (FLS) N=62

BaFPE Components: TOA	GAS	FUNCTIONAL LIFE SCALE COMPONENTS									
		Cognition	ADL	Home (unit)	Outside	Social-ization	Total Score	Initi-ation	Frequency	Speed	Efficiency
Tasks:											
Sorting Shells	.25a	.30b	.12	.28a	.12	.20	.27a	.18	.24a	.24a	.31b
Deposit Slip	.48c	.53c	.34b	.36b	.31b	.33b	.46c	.37c	.43c	.43c	.53c
House Floor Plan	.44c	.49c	.29a	.35b	.21a	.25a	.35b	.27a	.35b	.36b	.45c
Block Design	.29b	.39c	.17	.20	.14	.25a	.30b	.24a	.11	.24a	.34b
Draw-A-Person	.43c	.43c	.25a	.36b	.31b	.30b	.42c	.37b	.37c	.37b	.44c
Functions:											
Paraphrasing	.45c	.55c	.34b	.44c	.32b	.34b	.49c	.44c	.30b	.42c	.54c
Decision Making	.42c	.53c	.30b	.37b	.32b	.36b	.48c	.46c	.40c	.43c	.49c
Motivation	.31b	.39c	.13	.29a	.16	.18	.32b	.32b	.18	.29a	.35b
Organization	.46c	.45c	.25a	.29a	.23a	.28a	.39c	.33b	.30b	.33b	.45c
Mastery	.15	.33b	.05	.24a	.15	.09	.23a	.18	.14	.25a	.30b
Frustration	.37b	.38c	.15	.27a	.17	.17	.31b	.28a	.23a	.29b	.38c
Attention Span	.42c	.45c	.26a	.34b	.29a	.26a	.40c	.37c	.32b	.38c	.44c
Abstraction	.47c	.48c	.44c	.30b	.22a	.35b	.45c	.39c	.26a	.37b	.48c
Evidence of Mood or Thought Disorder	.50c	.56c	.36b	.42c	.36b	.38c	.50c	.43c	.37b	.45c	.55c
Completion	.39c	.40c	.21	.25a	.14	.28a	.35b	.30b	.23a	.26a	.36b
TOTAL SCORE TOA Total	.45c	.50c	.27a	.34b	.24a	.31b	.43c	.38c	.31b	.37c	.47c
SIS Total	.53c	.51c	.42c	.37b	.21	.42c	.46c	.42c	.32b	.35b	.49c
BaFPE Composite Score (TOA & SIS)	.57c	.58c	.41c	.43c	.27a	.44c	.52c	.47c	.37b	.42c	.55c

a = $p \leq .05$ b = $p \leq .01$ c = $p \leq .001$

Judith Bloomer and Susan Williams

respective author's name. The scales have been standardized and are used routinely in clinical settings, mostly by nursing staff and physicians. The FLS and the GAS are referred to on Table 15.3.

Concurrent validity reflects only the ratable behavior at a particular time—in this study, within four days of admission and the day before discharge (Table 15.3). The statistical results show that the BaFPE and its components, the TOA and SIS, correlate well with the FLS and GAS. The *total* scores (not all tasks and functions of TOA) correlate well. There is a substantial positive correlation in the following areas:

1. The BaFPE correlates at .52 with the total score of FLS, significant at the .001 level.
2. The SIS correlates at .42 with socialization component of FLS, significant at the .001 level.
3. The BaFPE correlates at .57 with the GAS, significant at the .001 level.

These are all substantially positive correlations. Validity correlations are usually not as high as reliability correlations. There is a good reason for this. A perfect, 1.0 correlation or near perfect correlation (ie, .95) is not preferable. If a correlation this high is gotten, it indicates that the two tests being compared measure essentially the same thing. For instance, although we wanted the SIS to assess social interaction, which the socialization component of the FLS also does, the social interaction is viewed in a somewhat different way specific to OT programming. If the scores on the SIS correlate very highly (.90s) with the socialization component on the FLS, there would be no need to develop a new scale; the FLS would be used instead. The objective is to get some differentiation, such as a positive correlation like .42.

One item of interest on the correlation tables is that the TOA component of mastery did not correlate with the GAS and many of the FLS components. Of the tasks in the TOA, sorting shells and the block design did not correlate as highly with the GAS as the other three tasks. The tasks of the deposit slip and house floor plan have a high level of correlation with the FLS component of cognition (.53 and .49, respectively), a relationship that is not surprising as both tasks emphasize cognitive functioning (addition, subtraction, measurement, etc).

The *composite* score of the BaFPE correlates substantially with the FLS at .52 and the GAS at .57. The components of the BaFPE (TOA and SIS) also correlate with the FLS and GAS (TOA with the FLS at .43, and with the GAS at .45 and the SIS with the FLS at .46, and with the GAS at .53), but it is important to note that neither the SIS nor the TOA, taken alone, correlate as highly with the FLS and GAS as the composite functional score reflected by the BaFPE total.

In summary, then, for criterion-related validity, the BaFPE has been shown to be a valid instrument in concurrently measuring functioning when compared to the two externally standardized scales (FLS and GAS) used to assess functioning in the sample population.

Construct validity is the fourth and final type of validity to be considered in standardizing the BaFPE. Construct refers to a dimension; the construct that has been chosen for assessment is *functional performance*. A psychological construct is a theoretical concept used to explain and organize some aspects of existing knowledge. Construct validity is established when a test is evaluated in light of the specified construct. To obtain information "needed to establish construct validity, the investigator begins by formulating a hypothesis about the characteristic of those who score high on the test in comparison to those who score low."[50] In our study, the hypothesis was that individuals who score high on the BaFPE show better functional ability in most general situations than people who score low. The research results supported the hypothesis in two ways: 1) The more psychotic a person is, the worse he scores on the BaFPE. There is a significant negative correlation—or inverse relationship: The higher the degree of psychotic behavior, the lower the scores on the BaFPE, indicating greater functional impairment; and 2) The research results supported the hypothesis that the functional status of the clients tested are lower on admission than the functional status on discharge. The BaFPE also reflects this change in status, with discharge scores being significantly higher than admission scores. The functional status of the clients is reflected as being higher on discharge on the two external indexes of criterion-related validity that were used in the study, as well as on the scores from the BaFPE. The overall change in clinical status is reflected in Table 15.4 which shows the relative values of the tests.

Construct validity is also considered when reviewing the internal structure of the test. Test users and developers would want to know to what extent certain concepts account for performance on a test. For instance, given our definition of the functional component of paraphrasing, it would be expected that a person who scores high on the house floor plan would also score high on paraphrasing, as correct task completion on the house floor plan requires the understanding and processing of multiple verbal instructions. (See Table 15.5 to review the internal relationships of functions and components on the TOA.)

Table 15.5 shows that high correlations between tasks and functions include:

1. The relationship between the bank deposit slip and organization (.85, at .001 level of significance: $p < .001$).
2. The correlation between task completion and organization (.89, $p < .001$).
3. The relationship between the House Floor Plan task and organization (.80, $p < .001$).
4. The relationship between the Draw-A-Person task and evidence of thought or mood disorder (.81, $p < .001$).
5. Decision-Making and Organization (.89, $p < .001$).
6. Decision-Making and Task Completion (.87, $p < .001$).

TABLE 15.4

CHANGE IN FUNCTIONAL STATUS AS
REFLECTED IN ADMISSION/DISCHARGE GROUP SCORES

	Admission Group			Discharge Group		
	N	X	S.D.	N	X	S.D.
BaFPE Total	44	355.73	69.941	16	390.50	43.945
SIS Scale Total	44	174.36	41.090	16	189.88	27.035
TOA Total	45	182.36	39.716	17	200.94	23.069
FLS Total	45	55.29	22.991	17	77.18	16.191
GAS	45	38.04	17.209	17	45.53	14.786

Judith Bloomer and Susan Williams

TABLE 15.5

CORRELATION MATRIX SHOWING INTERNAL RELATIONSHIPS OF THE TASK ORIENTED ASSESSMENT
(CORRELATING FUNCTIONS AND TASKS)

	SS	DS	HFP	BD	DAP	Para	Dec	Mot	Org	Mast	Frust	Atten	Abst	Disor	Comp
Sorting Shells (SS)															
Deposit Slip (DS)	.68														
House Floor Plan (HFP)	.57	.72													
Block Design (BD)	.69	.67	.74												
Draw-A-Person (DAP)	.67	.71	.67	.68											
Paraphrasing (Para)	.67	.77	.73	.75	.76										
Decision Making (Dec)	.78	.83	.76	.77	.80	.78									
Motivation (Mot)	.67	.73	.79	.76	.70	.67	.72								
Organization (Org)	.79	.85	.80	.81	.78	.78	.89	.75							
Sense of Mastery (Mast)	.62	.65	.63	.58	.66	.49	.64	.74	.64						
Frustration Tolerance (Frust)	.76	.83	.85	.79	.78	.71	.82	.89	.86	.80					
Attention Span (Atten)	.69	.78	.81	.74	.77	.71	.74	.78	.77	.72	.86				
Abstraction (Abst)	.53	.69	.68	.72	.62	.74	.66	.52	.69	.30*	.59	.55			
Evidence of Thought or Mood Disorder (Disor)	.71	.76	.78	.75	.81	.76	.79	.70	.79	.60	.79	.85	.69		
Task Completion (Comp)	.78	.81	.82	.84	.78	.76	.87	.71	.89	.58	.84	.77	.74	.76	

N = 62

All items significant at the .001 level except item marked * (.01 level)

It is interesting to note that a number of these examples are cognitively oriented tasks or functions. It is possible that the performance scores of components such as organization, decision-making, bank deposit slip, house floor plan, etc, would cluster if a factor analysis were done on the internal components of the TOA. A factor analysis is a statistical technique that is used for analyzing patterns or relationships of intercorrelation among many variables in a test.[51] It is often used to simplify a test by eliminating some of the items that may provide repetitive or nondiscriminating data. A factor analysis on the BaFPE needs to be done at some point in the future.

Other items included in Table 15.5 that might warrant discussion are the correlation between abstraction and sorting shells (.53, p < .001) and the lack of significant correlation between abstraction and mastery. Sorting shells is a very concrete task which might explain the slightly lower correlation between this task and abstraction in comparison to other tasks in the TOA. We can offer no reason for mastery to correlate with abstraction, whereas mastery would be expected to correlate higher with the successful completion of the various tasks on the TOA.

Other Statistical Information of Interest

As with any research project, we ended up with more data and more questions than can be integrated at this point in time! However, we did collect and would like to share some additional information that might be of interest to some potential test users.

Task Difficulty. Among the clinical group of norms for psychiatric clients, the Draw-A-Person task was completed most successfully (the average score, or mean among our 62 subjects, was 37.2 out of 44 points possible for the task). The tasks, in order of increasing difficulty for our client population were:

Draw-A-Person, mean = 37.2 (out of 44 points possible)
Sorting Shells, mean = 36.35
Block Design, mean = 34.5
House Floor Plan, mean = 32.6
Bank Deposit Slip, mean = 32.2

Our normative group of non-client subjects scored as follows:

Sorting Shells, mean = 43.0 (out of 44 points possible)
House Floor Plan, mean = 42.8
Bank Deposit Slip, mean = 42.5
Draw-A-Person, mean = 42.4
Block Design, mean = 41.7

Profile of mean scores of TOA components, SIS and BaFPE. For the TOA functional components, the client and non-client groups had the following profiles of mean scores, shown in Table 15.6.

A Task Questionnaire was used to compare client's subjective ratings of personal motivation and frustration during the TOA with the independent ratings of these during the TOA session. The questionnaire asks the test subjects to rate their own levels of frustration and motivation along a continuum of four graduations of subjective feelings for each of the five tasks in the TOA. For instance, the subjects were asked to indicate how interested they were in completing the task to designate their motivation. The graded continuum is varied

TABLE 15.6

NORMATIVE/COMPARATIVE MEAN SCORES ON FUNCTIONAL PARAMETERS

Functional Component	Psychiatric Patients (N = 62)	Normative, Non-patient Group (N = 20)
Paraphrasing	15.6 (out of 20)	19.3 (out of 20)
Decision Making	14.2 (out of 20)*	18.8 (out of 20)
Motivation	16.7 (out of 20)	19.6 (out of 20)
Organization	16.1 (out of 20)	20.0 (out of 20)**
Mastery	15.7 (out of 20)	17.6 (out of 20)*
Frustration Tolerance	16.6 (out of 20)	19.5 (out of 20)
Attention Span	17.5 (out of 20)**	20.0 (out of 20)**
Abstraction	14.4 (out of 20)	19.2 (out of 20)
Evidence of Thought or Mood Disorder	15.3 (out of 20)	20.0 (out of 20)
Task Completion	29.7 (out of 44)	42.4 (out of 44)
TOTAL TOA	187.5 (out of 240)	230.8 (out of 240)
TOTAL SIS Weighted X 7	178.5 (out of 245)	231.7 (out of 245)
TOTAL BaFPE	365.0 (out of 485)	462.8 (out of 485)

*Lowest
**Highest

or alternated in position on the questionnaire in an attempt to control response set bias on the part of the person filling out the questionnaire. The client's subjective ratings were correlated with the ratings of motivation and frustration on the TOA and it was found that the result reflected the literature; ie, that a subjective measurement of motivation and frustration is necessary because these functional components cannot be assessed validly by independent observers.

The specifics of this comparison showed that there were low correlations ranging from .07 (not significant) to .39 on motivation and low correlations ranging from a negative .08 to .48 on frustration. A higher correlation on the deposit slip with frustration may be due to the fact that the deposit slip is cognitively oriented and may be very frustrating for clients who do not have skills in addition and subtraction. A negative correlation (-.08) was found between the scores on the Draw-A-Person task completion item and scores on frustration for the same task. A possible explanation for this relationship might be that higher scoring clients completing the task might have been more frustrated, even though they did well, because instructions for the DAP task are simple, relatively unstructured, and do not offer much in the way of guidelines. High achieving clients may have been more concerned with imperfection, especially when there is no clear-cut sense of accomplishment on the DAP.

When we gave the subjects the bank deposit slip task, the subjects were asked if they had ever had any experience with a bank account. We found that experience in having a checking account did *not* correlate significantly with the deposit slip task completion item. In other words, whether or not they correctly completed the deposit slip task did not seem to have a significant relationship to prior experience with bank accounts. It was hoped that the written instructions (Forms A or B) would clarify the directions without having had prior experience. Prior banking experience does not seem to be an issue here, which was a concern in terms of possible cultural or socio-economic bias.

Range of scores on the BaFPE. For the client group, the range was 65 points (low) to 236 points (high) out of 240 total points possible on the TOA.

For the normative group, the range was 223 points (low) to 237 points (high) out of 240 total points possible for the TOA.

On the SIS, the range of scores for the client group was from 15 to 35 (out of 35 points, unweighted). For the normative group, most normal subjects were rated 4s and 5s on the SIS, ranging from 29 to 35 total points, unweighted. (A rating of 5 is the highest possible score for each of the parameters.) The mean unweighted scores for normative subjects (N = 20) on the seven parameters of social interaction are:

I. Response to Authority Figures, mean = 4.6
II. Verbal Communication, mean = 5.0
III. Psychomotor Behavior, mean = 4.6.
IV. Independence/Dependence, mean = 4.7
V. Socially Appropriate Behavior, mean = 4.9
VI. Ability to Work with Peers, mean = 4.5
VII. Participation in Group Activities, mean = 4.6.

For the composite BaFPE score (TOA plus 7x SIS), the client group scored (out of 485 points possible):

mean = 365.0 (355.7 on admission, 390.5 on discharge—see Table 15.4)
range = 171 to 469

The normative group scored:

mean = 462.8
range = 440 to 478

The range of scores and distribution of the two norm groups will be discussed in more detail later.

Normative and Comparative Group Data

Prior to the clinical interpretation of scores on the BaFPE, it is important to have an understanding of some characteristics of the subject population in comparison with the normal group. This facilitates an assessment of clinical relevance; that is, do the scores of the BaFPE appear to reflect the kinds of interactions with both people and objects in the environment that the subject population might tend to have in the real world? Some of this information might be gathered by comparing demographic data from both the subject group and the normal population. As has been mentioned previously, a Demographic Data Sheet was filled out for each subject that participated in the study.

Demographic data was also compiled for the comparative normal group. We found that the sample from the normal population reflects demographic characteristics similar to the subject group. For example, such things as age, education, and occupational status are important characteristics which are needed as points of comparison between the two groups. People similar in these three characteristics may be expected to have somewhat comparable positions in the world regarding responsibilities, obligations, and contact with the outside environment. Clients may therefore be expected to perform functional activities of similar complexity and to be involved in somewhat similar social, familial, or work-oriented interactional situations in their day-to-day contacts. Given these similarities, then, any significant variance in performance by these two groups on an evaluation such as the BaFPE should reflect a real difference in range of functioning.

In the comparative normal group, the mean age was 33.2 years. This is very close to the mean age in the subject group which was 33.95 years. Similarly, the average number of years of education for the comparative normal group was 13.3 years, closely approximating the average number of years of education for the subject group, which was 12.97 years. Certainly occupational status is an important variable in determination of an individual's responsibilities in relation to the environment. We found that the comparative normal group was similar, although not identical, to the subject group in occupational status. Because of the attempt to produce an evaluation that would have relevance to a broad spectrum of people, we approximated the range of occupational status of the subject group, although did not attempt to exactly duplicate it. In the comparative normal group, the following occupational roles were represented:

Clerical/Sales: 14%
Professional/Semi-professional: 20%
Service/Domestic: 20%
Managerial/Proprietary: 13%
Student: 33%

This means that in the comparative normal group, there is a higher percentage of students, managerial and proprietary persons, and professional and semi-professional persons than in the subject group. However, the percentage of persons involved in service and domestic work was about the same in the two groups. There was a smaller percentage of persons involved in clerical and sales oriented occupations in the comparative normal group than in the subject group. These differences did not appear to be diverse enough to significantly separate the comparative normal group from the subject group and, in fact, indicated that 85% of the subject population was involved in occupational situations represented in the comparative normal group.

The fact that these two groups have important similarities implies that one might assume that differences in scores between the two groups on a functional performance evaluation like the BaFPE would be due to actual differences in functioning. The assumption was made that people residing and functioning in the community should be performing at a higher functional level than people who are hospitalized, in relation to both objects and people in the environment. It is important to see if the range of scores on the BaFPE for the two groups reflect this difference in functional performance.

The BaFPE   *289*

There are considerable differences between the comparative normal group and the subject group in scores on both the TOA and the SIS, even though there were many similarities between the two groups according to the demographic data gathered. As stated earlier, we believe that these differences in scores are due to actual differences in level of functioning between a comparative normal group living in the community and a hospitalized patient group. On both the TOA and the SIS, the range of scores for the comparative normal group is much more clustered than for the subject group. We believe that this is reflective of the fact that people who are identified as patients and hospitalized may tend to be more deficient in specific components of functional behavior (ie, may show more difficulty in task oriented behavior than in social interactional behavior, or vice versa). Some clients score either high *or* low on both TOA and SIS, but most clients score higher on one than on the other. Cases like this, where clients score quite high on one subtest and low on the other, would have an overall tendency to increase the range of scores on both the TOA and the SIS.

We are also interested in the TOA and SIS scores for the subjects in the admission and discharge groups. Although the TOA scores of both groups tend to the high end of the range, the admission group scores are much more variable and the mean is lower, at 182.4, compared to the discharge group mean of 200.9. A t-test of the difference between these two means is significant beyond the .05 level. This indicates that the probability is very small that the difference between the means of the two groups is a chance occurrence. Further validation of the measure of differences in functional performance on the TOA is provided by the results of the other measures of functional level used in this study, the GAS and the FLS. The results of the analysis of these data support the hypothesis that differences in functional performance are measurable in an objective way and that the TOA can be used as such a measure.

The findings on the SIS are similar to those for the TOA. The scores for the admission group were lower than those for the discharge group, implying that people being discharged are better able to relate socially to others in the immediate environment than are people admitted. The mean for the SIS for the admission group was 174.4 and the mean for the discharge group was 189.8.

We want to emphasize the importance of utilizing both the TOA and the SIS in making determinations of overall functional performance. Even though the TOA and the SIS reflect scores indicating higher functional performance on discharge than on admission, this does not mean that therefore one subtest can be validly used independently of the other. It is important to remember that the admission scores for both the TOA and the SIS are more widely distributed than the discharge scores. Therefore, the subject who performed poorly on one subtest and did well on another may have come out with a total BaFPE score looking similar to a subject who had performed in exactly the opposite way. If either of the subtests for these subjects had been considered independently in determining functional performance, the scores would have been highly misleading. The composite BaFPE score must be looked at and scores of both subtests should be available to adequately assess overall functional performance.

It can be implied that scores on the BaFPE may be interpreted to be indicative of overall functioning. This has been shown to be true both in relation to the comparative normal group and also within the subject groups in accordance with general expectations for changes in functioning during a hospitalization. The previous discussion has utilized mostly the comparisons of data from different research groups to support interpretations of scores on the BaFPE. This approach has been related to the research effort, but we are aware that most people wanting to utilize the evaluation will be interested in the clinical application and interpretation of the scores. The next portion of this chapter will consider clinical data gathered from the BaFPE and ways in which this may be interpreted in clinical settings.

Case Studies

In the following text, a clinical case will be briefly summarized and results of the subject's performance on both the TOA and the SIS will be reported. The clinical application of information derived from these scores will be reviewed. In addition, other examples of case material that illustrate client responses to the various tasks on the TOA and their interpretation will be discussed. These examples have been taken from actual clinical examples that were gathered during the research portion of this study.

Case Example: Frank

Identifying Information. Frank T. was a 20 year old, single black male high school graduate who had been living with his parents prior to his hospitalization at LPPI. His high school diploma was from a vocationally oriented school and he attended one year at a community college in general social sciences.

Past History. Frank was the last-born child of a family of nine siblings. Developmental milestones were reported to have been normal. Medical history was unremarkable, with no history of allergies, accidents, or operations. Frank was born and raised in San Francisco and was described as being shy and isolated throughout his school years. His mother, to whom he was very close, stated that it was difficult to engage him in family activities in the home, as he would always prefer to remain alone in his bedroom. His father was described as being nice, but distant, and very disciplinarian. Frank described his mother as "one of my best friends," although she was also seen as demanding and aggressive. Frank stated that his early childhood was "happy" and "normal," and reported that his difficulties began in junior high school with increasing feelings of self-consciousness and sensitivity. He was able, however, at age 17, to get a job as a dishwasher, which enabled him to get his own apartment. He then worked as a clerk for an insurance company, a job that lasted for approximately seven months. He was laid off from his job in 1977, at which time he moved back into his parents' house. After moving back home, Frank was able to get another job as a city landscape worker which lasted from February to April of 1978. He reported this period as one of his best in recent times, although this ended when he met a woman who "did her thing on me," and generated feelings of self-doubt and depression in Frank.

Frank had no psychiatric contact until 1977 when he was hospitalized twice within two months with complaints of depression and feelings of self-doubt. On the second admission, the ward staff also reported violent, agitated, belligerent, and somewhat paranoid behavior, and he was diagnosed as having an acute schizophrenic episode. Frank was discharged after a short hospitalization with the recommendation that he continue to take antipsychotic medication, which he did not do. After his discharge from the second hospitalization, Frank had periods of relatively good intermittent functioning, but his "depression" would always return; his social relationships would become stressful, and he would be unable to hold down his job. This pattern continued (with two short hospitalizations early in

1978) until Frank was referred to LPPI later in 1978 for treatment.

Present Illness. Symptoms on admission included pacing, complaints of depression, difficulty sleeping, loss of appetite, ruminations, and difficulty with concentration. The mental status examination revealed a casually dressed and disheveled young man who appeared anxious and somewhat agitated. Affect was reported to be more distraught than sad, and he was quoted as saying, "I'm at the end of my rope." Thought content was coherent and rational, although verbalizations were slow, methodical, and tedious. There was some loosening of associations, but there were no reported delusions or hallucinations. He was oriented to time, place, and situation. Both recent and remote memory appeared to be intact. Frank presented a diagnostic dilemma to the staff, because he demonstrated some, but not all, of the symptomatology that might be expected in a schizophrenic patient. Although there remained the question of a major affective disorder, Frank was given the diagnosis of schizophrenia, chronic undifferentiated type.

Research information relevant to the BaFPE. Frank was placed in the admission group and was therefore administered the BaFPE on the fourth day after admission. The demographic data sheet was filled out on Frank prior to the administration of the BaFPE during a separate interview in which he was told about the purposes of the assessment. During the interview, he reported that he had held five jobs, the most recent being three months prior to this admission. He stated that the longest job he had held was approximately 10 months. This information was important because it was clear from his history that one of Frank's problems, when he got ill, was that his illness interfered with his functioning on the job. It is also important to remember that Frank was reported to have been shy as a child, and having few friends. This historical data would suggest clinical observations that the therapist would want to be sure to make in attempting to provide relevant information through administration of the BaFPE. For example, was he still isolative? If so, how much might this interfere with overall functioning?

Frank's scores on the TOA and the SIS will be reported and then discussed in relation to clinical application. The following data summarizes Frank's scores on the TOA.

Scores on Functional Components:
(range from 5 to 20)

    Paraphrasing—18
    Decision-Making—15
    Motivation—18
    Organization—18
    Mastery and Self-Esteem—15
    Evidence of Frustration—17
    Attention Span—13
    Ability to Abstract—20
    Evidence of Thought/Mood Disorder—14
    Correct Task Completion—33
      (range = 5 to 40)

Overall Task Scores:
(range from 10 to 40)

Sorting Shells—31
Bank Deposit Slip—29
House Floor Plan—24
Block Design—31
Draw-A-Person—33

General Comments and Task Specific Observations. Frank received a total score of 14 for this section (range from 0 to 20). He received a "NO" on the following observations and thus did not receive credit for them in the total score.

Movements steady/directional (SS)
Personal information OK? Date $\underline{X}$ (DS)
Divide rooms with logical placement (HFP)
Label each room drawn (HFP)
Justify room placement (HFP)
Duplicate design from memory (BD)

Total TOA Score: 195

On the Task Questionnaire given to him after the TOA, Frank gave the following responses to questions about his interest and possible feelings of frustration on each of the tasks.

Sorting Shells: Interested most of the time
    Didn't feel frustrated at all
Bank Deposit Slip: Interested part of the time
    Didn't feel frustrated at all
House Floor Plan: Not interested but tried it anyway
    Didn't feel frustrated at all
Block Design: Interested most of the time
    Felt somewhat frustrated
Draw-A-Person: Not interested but tried it anyway
    Didn't feel frustrated at all

Frank's SIS scores are listed below: (range of individual SIS scores is from 1 to 5)

1. Response to Authority Figures—5
   (5 = almost always appropriate interaction with, or response to, authority figures).
2. Verbal Communication—3
   (3 = verbal interactions appropriate only when directly questioned).
3. Psychomotor Behavior—2
   (2 = agitated behavior or pressured speech).
4. Independence/Dependence—2
   (2 = markedly dependent, does not carry through with general tasks of daily living alone and does not seek assistance).
5. Socially Appropriate Behavior—2
   (2 = markedly inappropriate).
6. Ability to work with Peers—1
   (1 = not able to assess due to degree of dysfunction).

The BaFPE

7. Participation in Group or Program Activities—1
  (1 = not able to assess due to degree of dysfunction).

Total SIS score: 16 (x 7 = 112). Frank's total BaFPE score (TOA plus SIS) is: 195 + 112 = 307.

Frank's overall BaFPE score is lower than the means of either of the research groups, and lower by more than 150 points than the normative group. This indicates that Frank was definitely performing at a level below that of his peers in the hospital environment and far below that of functioning people in the community. In attempting to break this rather global judgment down into more specific areas that may have clinical significance, his TOA versus his SIS scores should be studied.

Frank's total score on the TOA is 195. The mean score for the admission group (of which Frank was a part) is 182.3, so it can be surmised that Frank was functioning approximately at the same level as other people in his research group. However, the mean for the normative group is 230.8, reminding us that Frank was still performing at a level a good deal lower than functional members of the community. It should be remembered that Frank's scores could be compared to those of other subjects in the research project. This may not be possible in many clinical settings in which this evaluation will be administered because the comparative populations may be quite different. However, what is actually being done is looking at the range of scores and seeing where along that continuum the scores of a particular subject lie. Frank's task oriented behavior on the whole was relatively intact. Moreover, when looking at the specific components of the TOA, those areas in which he appears to have the most difficulty can be focused on and the therapist may want to incorporate them into a treatment plan for Frank.

In looking at the scores for the functional components of the TOA, it could be seen that Frank had difficulty in some of the areas that are characteristically difficult for a person who is schizophrenic: thought/mood disorder, attention span, decision making, etc. However, Frank had a high score on ability to abstract, with which many schizophrenics have difficulty. Although these findings appeared discrepant, they accurately reflected the dilemma about Frank's diagnosis that was previously mentioned in the case history: findings were inconsistent in some areas. Additionally, from the functional component scores of motivation and frustration, the rater felt that Frank was fairly well motivated during the tasks (18 out of 20), and somewhat frustrated, although not overly so (17 out of 20). The motivation scores tended to agree with Frank's on his Task Questionnaire. However, his own rating of frustration and the raters tended to differ: Frank denied feeling frustrated on most of the tasks, while the ratings showed at least some evidence of frustration. Research indicates that a person's subjective assessment of frustration must be taken into account. However, the fact that Frank denied feeling frustrated on the House Floor Plan, which was the task on which he received the lowest score, could lead the therapist to consider the possibility that Frank utilized denial in some situations that may have been difficult for him. Frank's score on mastery and self-esteem was also somewhat low (15 out of 20), which may tend to support the possibility of denial. (People who feel a lack of confidence about their ability in general, may tend to mask this through the use of denial or other mechanisms.)

Regarding the task completion scores, it could be seen that Frank did best on the least structured task, the Draw-A-Person, (Fig. 15.1), although even that score is only 33 out of 44. However, remember that this task is scored according to task

Judith Bloomer and Susan Williams

oriented, rather than projective, guidelines. The therapist should look at the drawing to gather other clinical information that may be of value in a projective sense.

Frank did not do well on the Bank Deposit or the House Floor Plan. These are the two most complex tasks as far as the level of instruction goes. Each task involves several steps, and looking at Frank's scores on attention span, this difficulty was reflected on these two tasks, both of which require concentration. The House Floor Plan also involves the necessity of making decisions and utilizing judgment about what rooms to put where. As was indicated in the TOA functional component, Frank had difficulty with decision-making, and it could be expected that this was evidenced clearly in the House Floor Plan (Figure 15.2).

On the task specific observations, Frank received a "NO" on six of the categories. Although this score would not be cause for alarm, the fact that he had difficulty with steady movements, did not know the date, and was unable to duplicate the design from memory should be noted. He also appeared to have poor spatial organization, and although this may be a manifestation of his basic psychiatric disorder and possibly connected to his difficulty with attention span, the therapist should be aware of it. Whether or not there may be some pre-existing perceptual difficulties, Frank was still somewhat impaired in these particular areas at the time of testing, regardless of the etiology of the dysfunction. More would have to be known about the specific responses that Frank made on the House Floor Plan to determine how impaired he was in relation to spatial organization.

In summary, it seems that the following statements are among those that may be made regarding Frank's task oriented functioning as evidenced by his performance on the TOA:

1. Frank has difficulty concentrating. He was observed, during the TOA administration, to be easily distracted by external stimuli and his score on the

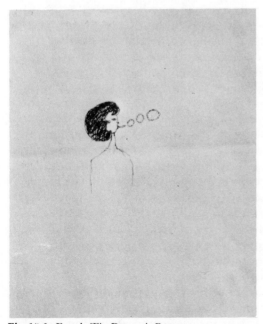

Fig 15.1: Frank T's Draw-A-Person.

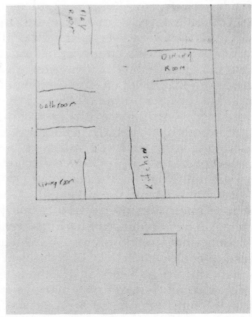

Fig 15.2: Frank T's House Floor Plan.

functional component of Attention Span reflected this. At times during the assessment, he appeared to be responding to internal stimuli (possible hallucinations), although he did not show evidence of a thought disorder in his ability to make abstract associations (as demonstrated in the Abstraction item).

2. He appeared to have overall low self-esteem, which may have influenced his task behavior and facilitated the use of denial.

3. He appeared to do best on tasks that did not involve complicated sets of instructions, although overall task performance would have to have been characterized as impaired.

4. Motivational factors are difficult to assess at this point. While he did not indicate a lack of motivation during the assessment and acknowledged his interest in most of the tasks, he completed the tasks hurriedly, with little attention to detail. It is not clear if motivational factors contributed to his poor overall task performance. It may be that his acknowledgment of interest is a part of his system of denial. Although he said that he felt motivated *during* the assessment, his motivation to participate in the evaluating process seemed questionable *prior* to beginning. Also, he had been noted to show little initiation or motivation within the general rehabiliation program.

5. Some observations made during the assessment indicated poor eye-hand coordination in fine motor tasks, poor spatial organization, and poor visual memory. The degree to which medications and/or motivation may be affecting this area needs to be assessed.

6. There was overall evidence of psychomotor retardation; Frank was very slow in verbal responses and in general task performance.

Frank's overall score of 122 on the SIS is below the mean for either of the research groups (174.4 for the admission group, and 189.1 for the discharge group), and well below the mean for the normative group (231). It begins to become clear that Frank's performance in a task oriented setting may have provided him with structure in which he was able to function quite highly. It seems that he was not able to translate his few task-oriented skills in relating to objects, to skills in relating to people. It can be seen that Frank was so severely impaired in his ability to work with peers that his skill in this area was not even able to be assessed. Looking at these scores on Independence/Dependence and Response to Authority Figures, there emerges the picture of a young man who is overly dependent, and, judging from his other SIS scores, has great difficulty communicating at all in a socially appropriate way. It appears that the task oriented situation may have facilitated this person's best functioning. The examiner served as a strong authority and the TOA session provided a clear structure in which he could work on a task that did not require his interaction with other people. The etiology of his dysfunction in social interaction was not known, but it is known that he was severely impaired in his ability to relate to the people in his environment. This impairment was also reflected through the fact that for Frank, his history of losing jobs was due to his difficulty in relating to superiors or co-workers, and this loss usually precipitated hospitalization.

Looking then, at Frank's overall performance on the BaFPE, it might be said that this young man was impaired in general functional performance. His impairment was in both specific areas of task-oriented behavior, and in overall social interactional behavior, but it appeared that his social interactional behavior was far more impaired than his task-oriented behavior. There are some areas in task behavior that should be watched and further evaluated, such as poor spatial organization, and poor eye-hand coordination that may or may not be situational in terms of perceptual dysfunction. General rehabilitation goals for Frank may include the following:

1. Structured settings in which he can accomplish tasks and begin to build self-esteem.
2. Graded exposure to interactional situations, initially arranged around task behavior, if possible.
3. Further assessment of motivational areas and extent to which they may have influenced dysfunction.
4. Further assessment of perceptual-motor difficulty.
5. Possible referral to vocational rehabilitation for aptitude testing and/or training programs.

Additional Clinical Implications

We have also found that in addition to computing the actual scores on the BaFPE and interpreting data in this framework, the therapist may be able to derive from the TOA additional clinical observations that are not always taken into account in the actual scoring of the TOA. Tasks on the TOA range in content from very structured to unstructured and quite projective. *Projective* refers to tasks that facilitate projection of the internal (or intrapsychic) states of the subjects onto graphic material. Certainly, all the tasks involve verbal projections to some extent. All tasks require that the subject abstract from the specific task to the general goal of the task, and all tasks take into account the subject's thought process and feelings of mastery and self-esteem, both of which may reflect projection of the subject's internal state. We are referring to the graphic evidence of a projective process in the subjects. Two of the tasks on the TOA appear to be most susceptible to this sort of dynamic: The House Floor Plan and the Draw-A-Person tasks. The Sorting Shells, Bank Deposit Slip, and Block Design are all relatively structured with clear instructions that imply a right and wrong way to complete the task. In order to assist the therapist in looking at these tasks (HFP/DAP) from the point of view of content which may be useful in clinical settings, but not always calculated in the scores on the TOA, two examples of the House Floor Plan and the Draw-A-Person were selected from different subjects and will be discussed briefly. The purpose of this discussion is not to introduce any ideas regarding interpretation, but rather to familiarize the therapist with some of the ways in which the tasks may be viewed for assessment of potentially important clinical issues that are not reflected in the functional scores on the BaFPE.

Case Examples: "Floor Plan" and "Draw-A-Person"

The following pictures were selected because they revealed information which is not necessarily reflected in the scores on the TOA. The following House Floor Plan (Figure 15.3) was done by a 24 year old man who had a total TOA score of 200, which is above the mean for the subject group. Although this subject was generally seen as having a thought disorder, the structure of the TOA apparently assisted him in organizing his thoughts, and he was generally able to contain his verbalizations to coherent, logical patterns. However, in the House Floor Plan, when he had the opportunity to project some of his ideas onto the Floor Plan, the difficulty he had

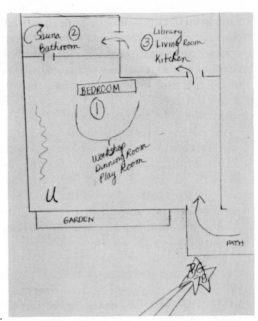

Fig. 15.3: BG's House Floor Plan.

with judgment, decision-making, and logical organization of space, can be seen.

"Room 1" was a bedroom, but was turned into a haphazard combination of three other rooms. The living room and kitchen are one, and although "Room 3" clearly leads into the Sauna/Bathroom (Room 2), there is an arrow leading nowhere in the left side of this room. The subject was greatly concerned because he had forgotten the utility room, even though the instructions informed him that he need not include all the rooms. Therefore, he added the "U" in the left hand corner of the floor plan to symbolize the Utility Room. In addition, he added his initials with a star below the floor plan, which is unusual in itself and not frequently seen in this task. People occasionally sign the Draw-A-Person picture, but seldom would one sign a floor plan, especially in this manner. When this subject was asked why he chose to arrange the rooms as he did, his response (pointing to Room 3, the Living room, Library, Kitchen) was that, "Man needs books to live, to guide him on his way." This response was felt to be an example of a loose associative process, in which he associated the library and the living room in his justification of room placement. It can be seen that just within this one task, there are several content items that warrant clinical comment and/or further investigation.

A second example of the House Floor Plan reveals an entirely different set of clinical information, some of which would be reflected in the TOA scores, but some of which would not. The following House Floor Plan (Fig. 15.4) was completed by a 62 year old woman with a diagnosis of involutional paranoia. Unlike the previous example, her overall TOA score fell in the low to fair functional range, and some of the difficulties revealed in the House Floor Plan are picked up in other tasks as well. However, it is in the House Floor Plan where the most blatant example of her disorganization can be seen.

It is clear from her drawing that she understood some aspects of what she was trying to do, but was not able to organize graphic space in any way that made sense. During the task, she constantly verbalized about what she was putting where, and

Judith Bloomer and Susan Williams

mentioned the "person" in the third "room" from the right on top who was painting the house. From this drawing alone, one would suspect that her visual-spatial and organizational skills were far lower than she demonstrated on the rest of the TOA (she refused to do the Draw-A-Person). There had been ongoing suspicion of an organic process contributing to this client's dysfunction, and this drawing, along with other clinical observations, led to the final diagnosis of organic brain syndrome. It is noteworthy that this woman had refused to cooperate with psychological testing, and it was felt that she was aware of her deficit and had been able to compensate for it to some extent up to that point. It is believed that she was willing to participate in all but the last task of the TOA because of the rapport and trust that she had developed with the occupational therapist during the time she was on the unit. Clearly, this task was an important one in assisting the staff to understand her psychiatric illness and to prescribe appropriate treatment.

The Draw-A-Person has been written about by many clinicians since it was first developed as a projective test. It has been interpreted in many different ways and the purpose here is not to review these. We do wish to point out some of the features of this task that therapists may want to notice when they are utilizing the TOA. The client is asked to draw a picture of a person doing something. The purpose for this is to get some idea of how the subject may project himself in relation to objects or people in the environment. This may be termed a "kinetic" Draw-A-Person task in the sense that movement or activity is implied. The following two examples illustrate two very different responses to this task.

The first Draw-A-Person was done by a 24 year old man who had some previous experience with art and had enjoyed drawing in the past. He drew without hesitation with clear, decisive strokes (Fig. 15.5).

The subject explained that the picture was of a "good crew member who was tending to his garden." He explained that he picked the theme for his picture

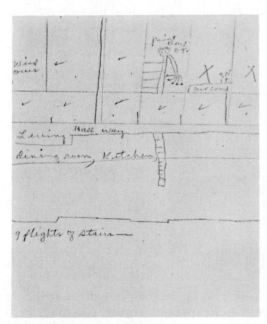

Fig 15.4: RS's House Floor Plan.

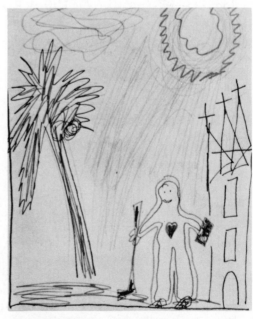

Fig 15.5: BG's Draw-A-Person.

because of "erosion control." When asked if he had any reason for choosing that particular activity, he said, "Because that is the particular activity that is closest to my heart."

It becomes clear that this subject's verbalizations around his picture revealed a good deal of clinical information about his thought process. Although some of this process is reflected in the scores on the TOA (under Task Specific Observations), there was much about his picture that qualified it as a correct completion of this particular task. This picture, although it is not contained within a defined space on the middle of the page, is clearly well spaced and organized. Although there is evidence of transparencies, and themes of religiosity (gardener holding Bible), the graphic organization does not reflect his disorganized psychic processes. These were, however, clearly revealed by his verbalizations about his picture. Graphic organization, in general, should not be automatically taken to reflect psychic organization. In some clients, especially those with paranoid characteristics, tight or very structured graphic organization is commonly seen. In summary, this drawing, coupled with the verbalizations about it, may be more clinically useful than the raw task oriented scores on the TOA would indicate initially.

A second example of the Draw-A-Person task shows a drawing that indicates *graphically* that certain concepts regarding self-concept and body image may be deficient. This is a drawing by a 24 year old woman who described her picture as a "woman singing" (Fig. 15.6).

Several aspects of this drawing that are unusual were picked up on the Task Specific Observations. However, the overall fragmentation and the paucity of detail revealed more than was generally indicated in the TOA score for this task. Interestingly, this woman was admitted to the hospital in a wheelchair complaining of paralysis in her legs, a condition which was thought by staff, and later proved to be, of a hysterical nature. In her drawing, the legs are completely severed from the body. The characteristics of her drawing would obviously not reveal the etiology of her "paralysis," but it would indicate to the therapist that the separation of specific body parts from the rest of the body and accompanying lack of differentiation of body parts may be indicative of conflict around body image. The lack of sexual differentiation in this picture, and the accompanying verbalization that this picture is of a "woman singing," may indicate confusion and/or conflict around psychosexual areas. It was later learned that this client did have severe problems with sexual identity. Overall, this picture, in the gestalt sense, gives an impression of shallowness, fragmentation, distortion, lack of detail, and lack of differentiation of body parts. These observations may be clinically very important but are not reflected with such poignancy if only the task scores for the Draw-A-Person task are looked at.

In summary, this section on case studies from the BaFPE has considered both the translation of statistically derived data to clinically useful information regarding functioning, as well as the presentation of some examples which it is hoped will be useful in a purely clinical application of the BaFPE. Although it is difficult to discuss the exact implications of the data, one *can* say that the BaFPE appears to be able to measure components of functioning that seem to be consistent with other measures of functioning (eg, GAS, FLS). One can also say that the BaFPE does seem to reflect levels of functioning along a continuum from dysfunction to function.

Current Status of the BaFPE Research Project

The initial goals in undertaking this project were simply to develop a reliable and valid tool that could be used to assess the outcome of occupational therapy intervention. This objective mandated a project that is neither simple nor one that we feel can be completed without collaborative national effort.

What we have accomplished is the development of an evaluation tool, the BaFPE, that has been standardized with a small population of psychiatric clients in the San Francisco area. Although the method of test design has resulted in a tool that has been shown to be reliable and valid, we are acutely aware of the BaFPE's limitations. There is a need for widespread field testing in different geographic regions of the United States to further validate the instrument. The sample size of the normative population needs to be increased, and the content of the TOA revised to be more sensitive to lower functional levels.

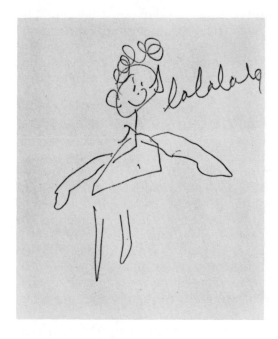

Fig. 15.6: JC's Draw-A-Person

The culmination of the first three years of work on the BaFPE research project resulted in the publication of the 1979 Research Edition of the BaFPE Administration Manual (see References). This edition basically documented the research project, giving readers of the manual specific instructions and test forms so that a potential test user could administer the test. The dissemination of the research edition has allowed for widespread field testing which will result in the collection of additional data using the test. We hope that test users will contribute data to add to the size of the sample used in standardizing the BaFPE, and thus, further validate it.

The BaFPE research project, at the time of this writing, is being continued through the Rehabilitation Therapy Department at Langley Porter Institute. The primary focus of this phase of the project is to coordinate, collect, and analyze data supplied from contributing test users nationwide. Ideas regarding the data collection project, research questions generated from what has already been done, and projection for further study will be addressed next.

Future Research

The BaFPE test developers have a number of ideas for continuation of the BaFPE Project and for potential projects that others interested in research in the area of functional performance might pursue. We would like to invite others to participate in data collection, share data and feedback regarding the test and, finally, to expand upon the work that has been done to date.

Invitation for Participation. One of the main concerns a test developer has is the continued development, validation, and improvement of any instrument that has been introduced. Coming from an occupational therapy background, we are especially interested in "facilitating the growth and development" of the research effort.[5] Consequently, we would like to suggest some areas that invite further study, and to share some objectives established by the *Test Service Bulletin.*[49] The foremost objective is that in order to develop improved tests, test data must be shared by practicing clinicians, test developers, and researchers. Of interest are the norms or distributions for well-defined groups, completed reports, or raw data contributing to validation studies. Other data such as studies of reliability, the effect of training and retesting, and the relation of test scores to variables such as age and education are important, and will be discussed later in the book.

The sharing of research data requires the structure of a feedback system, and constitutes the framework for a data collection project. We would like users and reviewers of the BaFPE to share their impressions and experiences through the mechanism of a "BaFPE Feedback Questionnaire" supplied with each administration manual, or through open-ended correspondence. We would like to encourage psychiatric special interest groups of the AOTA Mental Health Speciality Section to participate in a collaborative effort among therapists working in this area of practice. Furthermore, we would also be interested in hearing from members of other specialty sections and would like to assess the feasibility of using the BaFPE with other (non-psychiatric) patient populations. Finally, we would especially like to encourage student participation. Many students could obtain experience in research methodology simply by replicating and expanding the data base of what has already been done, or better yet, by addressing any of the research questions posed in the following pages.

The next section will list many of the questions that have developed through the work on the development and standardization of the BaFPE. For ease of reference these ideas are classified into 12 categories. For each of the questions listed, the most relevant classification(s) will be indicated by the Roman numeral corresponding to the following categories:

    I. Applicability to Different Client Populations
    II. Establishment of Normative Data
    III. Reliability
    IV. Validity
    V. Cultural Implications
    VI. Geographic Considerations
    VII. Content-Task Oriented Assessment
    VIII. Content-Social Interaction Scale
    IX. Use of Demographic Data
    X. Administration/Training

XI. Scoring/Interpretation

XII. Implications for Occupational Therapy Practice and/or Education

Research Questions

1. What would be the range of scores and applicability of the BaFPE for the following groups: Outpatient adult psychiatric clients; adolescent clients within an adolescent treatment program; adolescents or adults who are developmentally disabled or have the diagnosis of mental retardation; clients with head injuries due to traumatic brain damage; and those who have suffered cerebral vascular accidents? (I)

2. Would subjects from different geographic areas of the United States score differently on the BaFPE? Would there be significant differences between rural vs. urban vs. suburban groups? (VI)

3. Would subjects from different cultural backgrounds within the United States score significantly different on the BaFPE? If so, what would be the characteristics of the differences? (V)

4. Can professionals from other disciplines reliably administer and interpret the BaFPE? If so, which disciplines? If not, what restrictions should be made, if any, concerning the availability of the BaFPE? (III, IV, X, XI, XII)

5. How many practice administrations of the TOA are needed for basic competency in administration? Are training sessions necessary, or is reading the administration manual sufficient for background information and administration procedures? (X, VII)

6. What is the extent of clinical contact needed (ie, three hours, two days, one day) for reliable and valid assessment, using the Social Interaction Scale? (III, IV, VIII, X, XI)

7. Are any of the tasks biased for different cultural groups within the United States? If so, what are the limitations of the use of the TOA? (V, VII, XI, XII)

8. What differences in socio-economic class, educational level, or job history affect performance on the BaFPE? Would these differences be reflected among the normative group? (II, IX, XI)

9. How can the time element (the time it takes a subject to complete the TOA) be taken into consideration in the scoring procedure? (VII, XI)

10. If any of the tasks were to be deleted in future revisions of the TOA, which task(s) would be excluded? (VII, IV)

11. If a factor analysis were done on the TOA once additional data is collected, what factors provide the same, or different information among the tasks and functional components? (VII)

12. If a factor analysis were done on the seven components of the SIS, which components would prove to be most valuable in assessing functional performance in relating to others in the environment?(VIII)

13. Is the BaFPE applicable to populations in other countries, from other cultures? (I, II, V, VI, IX, XI)

14. What new tasks might supplement the information obtained in the TOA? (VII)

15. How can the TOA be made to more accurately reflect lower levels of functioning? (VII)

16. What interview format or other evaluation instrument would provide information that is supplemental and harmonious to information obtained on the BaFPE? Is supplemental information needed? (VII, VIII, XII)

17. How can the Task Questionnaire be numerically incorporated into the TOA scoring process? What is the best way to consider the subjective and objective ratings of motivation and frustration? (VII, XI)

18. Would the block design task be improved if multicolor blocks were available to provide more of an opportunity for color discrimination? (VII)

19. What is the effect, if any, upon a subject's performance by having an observer, or second rater, present during a TOA administration? (X, XI, XII)

20. What can be learned from studying the content of the Draw-A-Person task? What are the research implications involving differences in portrayal of kinetic person drawings, body image, etc? (XII)

21. How much time should be allowed between administrations of the TOA to control for possible "practice effect?" (X, IV, XI)

22. Is the BaFPE useful as a tool for assessing functional status given the objective of measuring the effectiveness of occupational therapy intervention? (IV, XI, XII)

23. Can the BaFPE be used to substantiate occupational therapy practice by measuring the clinical status of clients pre- and post- OT intervention? (XII)

24. Can the BaFPE be used to predict functional performance in the community? Or, are scores on the BaFPE valid for predictive validity? (XI, IV)

25. Will the BaFPE project prove to be useful in stimulating occupational therapy research in the area of functional performance? (XII)

26. How can occupational therapy clinicians be stimulated to participate in a data collection project in order to standardize an evaluation instrument on a nationwide basis that is specific to the discipline of occupational therapy?

Conclusion

The fact that something about the components of functioning can be measured, should mean that a treatment plan based on consistent, reliable information can be developed. The effectiveness of the treatment plan could then be evaluated through re-administration of the evaluation tool, the BaFPE. Far-reaching implications for the development of the BaFPE are that occupational therapists may be able to substantiate and validate their treatment goals and modalities more clearly than they have been able to in the past, particularly in the specialty area of psychiatry. It is clear that the development of the BaFPE is just the first step toward clarifying for clinicians our role as therapists in mental health. It is, however, an important first step which we hope will provide a useful tool for assessment of overall functional performance.

References

1. Webster's New International Dictionary. Springfield, MA; G & C Merriam Co, 1961, pp 920-921, 106, 146.
2. English HV, English AC: A Comprehensive Dictionary of Psychological and Psychoanalytic Terms. New York, Longmans, Green & Co, 1958, pp 218, 103, 139, 365, 217, 104, 3, 507-510, 427.

The BaFPE Administration Manual (2nd printing) is available from Consulting Psychologists Press, Inc., 577 College Avenue, Palo Alto, California, 94306.

3. Goldenson R: The Encyclopedia of Human Behavior, Psychology, Psychiatry, and Mental Health. New York, Doubleday & Co, Inc, 1970, pp 48, 16.
4. Herrnstein R, Boring E: A Source Book in the History of Psychology. Cambridge, MA, Harvard Univ Press, 1965, p 507.
5. Llorens LA: Facilitating growth and development: The promise of occupational therapy—1969 Eleanor Clarke Slagle lecture. A J Occu Ther 24:93, 1970.
6. Llorens LA: Application of a Developmental Theory for Health and Rehabilitation. Rockville, MD, The American Occupational Therapy Association, 1977.
7. Mosey AC: Three Frames of Reference for Mental Health. Thorofare, NJ, Charles B. Slack, 1970, pp 10, 17.
8. Meyer A: The philosophy of occupational therapy. A J Occu Ther 1:1-5, 11, 1922.
9. Matsutsuyu J: Occupational behavior—a perspective on work and play. A J Occu Ther 25:291-294, 291, 1971.
10. Shapiro D, Shanahan P: Methodology for teaching theory in occupational therapy basic professional education. A J Occu Ther 30:217-224, 1976.
11. Reilly M: The educational process. A J Occu Ther 23:299-307, 1969.
12. Reilly M: A psychiatric occupational therapy program as a teaching model. A J Occu Ther 20:61-67, 1966.
13. Black M: The occupational career. A J Occu Ther 30:225-228, 1976.
14. Moorhead L: The occupational history. A J Occu Ther 23:329-334, 1969.
15. Heard C: Occupational role acquisition: A perspective on the chronically disabled. A J Occu Ther 31:243-247, 1977.
16. Burke J: A clinical perspective on motivation: Pawn vs. origin. A J Occu Ther 31:254-258, 1977.
17. Reilly M: Play as Exploratory Learning: Studies in Curiosity Behavior. Beverly Hills, CA, Sage Publishing Co, 1974.
18. King LJ: Occupational therapy research in psychiatry: A perspective. A J Occu Ther 32:15-18, 433, 1978.
19. Spencer EA: Functional restoration. In Hopkins, Smith (eds): Willard and Spackman's Occupational Therapy, Fifth Edition. Philadelphia, JB Lippincott Co, 1978, pp 336, 347, 354.
20. Diasio K: Psychiatric occupational therapy: Search for a conceptual framework in light of psychoanalytic ego psychology and learning theory. A J Occu Ther 22:400-406, 1968.
21. Endicott J, Spitzer RL, Fleiss JL, Cohen J: The global assessment scale. Arch Gen Psychiat 33:766-771, 1976.
22. Sarno JE, Sarno MT, Levita E: The functional life scale. Arch Phys Med Rehabil 54:214-220, 1973.
23. Underwood P: Nursing Care as a Determinant in the Development of Self-Care Behavior by Hospitalized Adult Schizophrenics. Dissertation, University of California, San Francisco, 1978.
24. Allen C: Performance Status Examination. Evaluation instrument presented at the Annual Conference of the American Occupational Therapy Association, San Francisco, November, 1976.
25. Morris W (Ed): The American Heritage Dictionary of the English Language. New York, Houghton Mifflin Co., 1969, pp 951, 6.
26. Cofer CN, Appley MH: Motivation: Theory and Research. New York, John Wiley & Sons, Inc, 1964, pp 8, 782.
27. Fiske DW: Measuring the Concepts of Personality. Chicago, Aldine Publishing Co, 1971.
28. Hunt JM: Personality and the Behavior Disorders. New York, The Ronald Press, 1964, p 380.
29. Eysenck JA, Arnold W, Meili R (eds): Encyclopedia of Psychology. New York, Herder & Herder, 1972, pp 377, 291.
30. Ayers AJ: Sensory Integration and Learning Disorders. Los Angeles, Western Psychological Service, 1973, pp 111, 248.
31. Taber CW: Taber's Cyclopedia-Medical Dictionary. Philadelphia, FA Davis, 1970, pp 82, D-54, A-10.
32. Hammer EF: The Clinical Application of Projective Drawings. Springfield, IL, Charles C Thomas, 1958, pp 63, 105, 106, 69-71, 182.
33. Buck JN, Hammer EF: Advances in the House-Tree-Person Technique: Variations and Applications. Los Angeles, Western Psychological Services, 1969, p 174.
34. Lyerly SB: Handbook of Psychiatric Rating Scales. Rockville, MD, NIMH, DHEW Document 73-9061, 1973, pp 1, 2.
35. Barton R: Institutional Neurosis. Bristol, England, John Wright & Sons, Ltd, 1966, p 62.
36. Camp WP: Social change in the mental hospital. A J Occu Ther 19:339-343, 1965.
37. Granlnick A (ed): Humanizing the Psychiatric Hospital new York, Jason Aronson, Inc, 1975, p 13.

The BaFPE

38. Lander J, Shulman R: Impact of the therapeutic milieu on the disturbed personality. Social Casework 41:227-234, 1960.
39. Hare AP: Handbook of Small Group Research. New York, The Free Press, 1976, pp 5, 6.
40. Homans GC: Social Behavior, Its Elementary Forms. New York, Harcourt, Brace, Jovanovich, Inc, 1974, pp 356, 98-110.
41. Offer D, Sabshim M: Normality: Theoretical and Clinical Concepts of Mental Health. New York, Basic Books, 1966.
42. Doll EA: The Measurement of Social Competence: A Manual for the Vineland Social Maturity Scale. USA, Education Test Bureau, Educational Publishers, Inc, 1953, pp 185, 231, 232.
43. Argyle M: Social Interaction. New York, Atherton Press, 1969.
44. Bales RF: Personality and Interpersonal Behavior. New York, Holt, Rinehart & Winston, Inc, 1970.
45. Borgatta EF, Crowther B: A Workbook for the Study of Social Interaction Processes: Direct Observation Procedures in the Study of Individual and Group. Chicago, Rand McNally & Co, 1965.
46. Roby TB: Small Group Performance. Chicago, Rand McNally & Co. 1968.
47. Triandis HC: Interpersonal Behavior. Belmont, CA, Wadsworth Publishing Co, Inc, 1977.
48. Ricks JH: Local norms—when and why. Test Service Bulletin 58(August):1, p 1, 1971.
49. Seashore HG, Ricks JH: Norms must be relevant. Test Service Bulletin 38(December):11-19, 1950.
50. APA Standards for Educational and Psychological Tests. Washington, DC, American Psychological Association, 1974, p 30.
51. Isaac S, Michael W: Handbook in Research and Evaluation. San Diego, Robert R Knapp, Publisher, 1971, p 116.

Bibliography

Allard I: The influence of occupational therapy on the perceptual inaccuracies of the schizophrenic. A J Occu Ther 23:115-121, 1969.

Allen C: 1976 Mental Health Task Force Report. Report presented to the Delegate Assembly of the American Occupational Therapy Association, October 1976.

Androes L, et al: Diagnostic test battery for occupational therapy. A J Occu Ther 19:53, 1965.

Aumack L: Social adjustment behavior rating scale. J Clin Psychol 4:436-441, 1962.

Azima H, Wittkower ED: A partial field survey of psychiatric occupational therapy. A J Occu Ther 11:1-9, 1957.

Azima H, Azima FJ: Outline of a dynamic theory of occupational therapy. A J Occu Ther 13:215-218, 1959.

Bales R: Interaction Process Analysis. Cambridge, MA, Addison-Wesley Press, 1951.

Berkowitz L, Lurie A: Socialization as a rehabilitative process. Community Ment Health J 2(1):55-60, 1966.

Brayman S, et al: Comprehensive occupational therapy evaluation. A J Occu Ther 30:94-100, 1976.

Buck RE, Provancher MA: Magazine collage as an evaluation technique. A J Occu Ther 26:36-39, 1972.

Casanova JS, Ferber JA: Comprehensive evaluation of basic living skills. A J Occu Ther 30:101-105, 1976.

Chernewski E: The social determinant of mental illness and psychosomatic disease. A J Occu Ther 25:193-195, 1961.

Clark JR, et al: A factor analytically derived scale for rating psychiatric patients in occupational therapy: Part I, Development. A J Occu Ther 19:14-21, 1965.

Dinis JS: Occupational therapy: Historical introduction. A J Occu Ther 30:1-7, 1976.

Doll EA: Vineland Social Maturity Scale, Condensed Manual of Direction, 3rd ed. Circle Pines, MN, American Guidance Service, Inc, 1965.

Doppelt JE: Watch your weights. Test Service Bulletin 52(December):2-5, 1957.

Ellsworth PD, Coleman AD: A model program: The application of operant conditioning principles to work group experience. A J Occu Ther 23:495-501, 1969.

Etheridge DA: Prevocational assessment of rehabilitation potential of psychiatric patients. A J Occu Ther 22:161-168, 1968.

Etzioni A: Interpersonal and social structure of a psychiatric hospital. Psychiat 23(November): 17-24, 1960.

Fidler GS, Fidler JW: Occupational Therapy: A Communication Process in Psychiatry. New York, MacMillan, 1963.

Flanagan M, Wolf K: Initial Evaluation Battery: Psychosocial Dysfunction. Evaluation instrument presented at the Annual Conference of the American Occupational Therapy Association, October 1975, Milwaukee; and November 1976, San Francisco.

French JR: The social environment and mental health. J Soc Issues 19(4):39-56, 1963.

Harlock S: A Study of the Correlation Between the Activity Interests and Skills of a Selected Group of Subjects and their Interpersonal Interaction During a Series of Activity Group Experiences. Master thesis, San Jose State University, 1972

Hasselkus BR, Safrit MJ: Measurement in occupational therapy. A J Occu Ther 30:429-436, 1976.

Jantzen AC: Definitions of mental health and mental illness. A J Occu Ther 23:249-253, 1969.

Kaye JH, et al: Contingency management in a workshop setting: Innovation in occupational therapy. A J Occu Ther 24:413-417, 1970.

King LJ: A sensory integrative approach to schizophrenia. A J Occu Ther 28:529-536, 1974.

King LJ: Toward a science of adaptive responses—1978 Eleanor Clarke Slagle lecture. A J Occu Ther 32:429-437, 1978.

Laurencelle P: An analysis of the social and sociological implications of rehabilitation. A J Occu Ther 22:329-331, 1968.

Lawn EC, O'Kane CP: Psychosocial symbols as communication media. A J Occu Ther 27:30-33, 1973.

Lewisohn PM, Clark JR: A factor analytically devised scale for rating psychiatric patients in occupational therapy: Part II, Concurrent validity. A J Occu Ther 19:72-81, 1965.

Linn L, et al: Occupational Therapy in Dynamic Psychiatry, Washington, DC, American Psychiatric Association, 1962.

Linnell KE, et al: Resocialization of schizophrenic patients. A J Occu Ther 29:288-290, 1975.

Llorens LA, et al: Work adjustment program. A J Occu Ther 18:15-19, 1964.

Llorens LA, et al: The effects of a cognitive-perceptual-motor training approach on children with behavior maladjustment. A J Occu Ther 23:502-512, 1969.

Meyers C (Ed.): Twenty-Five Year Cumulative Index of the American Journal of Occupational Therapy. Rockville, MD, American Occupational Therapy Association, 1973.

Morimoto F, Greenblatt M: Personal awareness of patients' socializing capacity. A J Psychiatry 110:443-447. 1953.

Mosey AC: Dependency and integrative skills as they relate to affinity for and acceptance by an assigned group. A J Occu Ther 23:348-349, 1969.

Odhner F: Verbal ascendency in process and reactive schizophrenics. A J Occu Ther 25:7-9, 1971.

Odhner F: A study of group tasks as facilitator of verbalization among hospitalized schizophrenic patients. A J Occu Ther 24:7-12, 1970.

Reilly M: Research potentiality of occupational therapy. A J Occu Ther 14:206-208, 1960.

Sanchez V: Relevance of cultural values for occupational therapy programs. A J Occu Ther 18:1-5, 1964.

Shapiro D: Personal communication on behalf of the Mental Health Specialty section of the American Occupational Therapy Association.

Shoemyen CW: A study of procedure and media: Occupational therapy orientation and evaluation. A J Occu Ther 24:276-279, 1970.

Solomon AP: Occupational therapy, a psychiatric treatment. A J Occu Ther 1:1-7, 1947.

Stein F: Three facets of psychiatric occupational therapy: Models for research. A J Occu Ther 23:491-494, 1969.

Weinman B: Treating the social symptomatology of the chronic mental health patient. Pa Psych Q 7(3):2-12, 1967.

West WL: Changing Concepts and Practices in Psychiatric Occupational Therapy, New York: American Occupational Therapy Association, 1959.

Wolff RJ: A behavior rating scale. A J Occu Ther 15:13-16, 1961.

Yerxa EJ: Research seminar. A J Occu Ther 30:509-514, 1976.

Zilborg G, Henry G: History of Medical Psychology. New York, Norton, 1941.

Acknowledgments

We have been encouraged by the support of colleagues in the field of occupational therapy to whom we have presented numerous workshops, and by the financial support of the Santa Clara and Golden Gate Chapters of the California Occupational Therapy Association. This support was used to publish the Research Edition of the administration manual. The BaFPE Project was also supported through a BioMedical Research Grant awarded through the University of California in San Francisco which provided funds to produce a color videotape depicting an administration session of the Task Oriented Assessment. This tape was made to be used for training purposes and is available through: Educational Television Department, University of California, San Francisco, 1855 Folsom Street, Room 646A, San Francisco, California 94103.

Judith Bloomer and Susan Williams

16
The Creative Clay Test And an Exploration of Task Structure

E. Nelson Clark, O.T.R.
Michael S. Cross, Ph.D.

Literature Review

The Concept of Structure

The concept of structure and the act of structuring time and tasks have been readily accepted in the history of occupational therapy. The need to organize time, balance work and play, and structure the tasks of living is emphasized by Adolf Meyer in the now classic reference on the philosophy of occupational therapy.[1] The profession developed using Dr. Meyer's concept of providing multi-leveled tasks, leisure activities, and play to aid in promoting a balance in the lives of clients considered dysfunctional. In the following years, literature in occupational therapy generally describes the analysis of activities in the area of analytical theory, behavioral development, physical restorative properties, and neuro-behavior.[2] In virtually all of these areas, structure is mentioned as a component to be evaluated without a thorough-going analysis or definition of the concept. Proponents of assessment devices[3] and therapeutic strategies[4] allude to structure as an important variable in client performance in the absence of precise definitions or supporting research. In brief, while the general concept of structure has long been a part of the vocabulary of occupational therapists, the existing occupational therapy literature reveals a lack of precise and consistent usage, and a dearth of substantive research about this concept.

Despite the lack of a precise working definition, some clues to the relationship between task structure and performance have emerged from various disciplines. Kuhn describes job ambiguity as an important factor contibuting to job stress, which in turn, results in detrimental physical and mental changes in employees.[5] In related studies, Cobb[6] and French[7] reach similar conclusions utilizing variations in the structure of work as a means of assessing job stress. Rubin[8] reports that the element of structure in community meetings affects client participation on psychiatric wards in that more structured meetings (ie, greater proportionate staff participation) promote greater client participation. Rubin interprets these findings in terms of executive ego deficits in mental health clients for which the external structure of the milieu provides compensation. Rapaport[9] indicates that an

Editor's Note: *The opinions and assertions contained herein are those of the writers, and are not to be construed as official or reflecting views of the Department of the Navy.*

individual will structure his environment according to the defenses available to him in unstructured situations. Thus, in projective (unstructured) testing situations (eg, Rorschach, TAT), the mentally ill client shows poor performance relative to normals. In a similar vein, many authors argue that lack of structure or organization in surroundings produces anxiety, which in turn, inhibits productivity and performance.[10-13] Over the past few years, it has been our observation that clients diagnosed as schizophrenic perform poorly on occupational therapy tasks which might be considered unstructured, but often perform quite satisfactorily on more structured tasks. Thus, information from a variety of sources suggests that the degree of structure present in a situation influences the quality and level of performance of the individual in that situation.

In summary, it appears that occupational therapists and others have attached significance to the influence of structure on performance. This view has developed in the absence of a single, precise definition of the concept, and in the absence of systematic investigation. The observation that the acutely-ill psychiatric client performs poorly in an unstructured setting and thereby, may benefit from the structuring of time and tasks has important implications for occupational therapists, and merits further investigation. There is a need for occupational therapists to have a systematic way of measuring the degree of structure inherent in a particular task, and to understand the extent to which structure affects the client's response to treatment.

The Analysis of Structure

Dr. Mary Reilly, in an address to the military occupational therapists in June, 1979, stated, "We have to take the idiot's position and question those basics that we have always assumed to be defined." The concept of task structure appears to be one of those basics that bears re-examination. *Webster's New World Dictionary* (1970) defines structure as the "manner of building, constructing, or organizing...the arrangement or interrelation of all the parts of a whole." This definition provides only a starting point for application to occupational therapy tasks, and the available literature does not provide much additional elaboration. Therefore, we have developed a concept of structure which is based upon a logical analysis of the fundamental components of tasks.

In this conception, the structure of a task is considered to be determined by three factors: 1) the specificity of the outcome of the task; 2) the specificity of the procedures necessary to accomplish the task; and, 3) the nature of the materials used in the task. For example, a highly structured task would be assembling a set of nuts and bolts in a specified manner and in a specified time period. In this task, the outcome of the activity is clear, the procedure (assembly and time alloted) is specified, and the materials have very little flexibility of usage. On the other hand, a relatively unstructured task has less clearly defined elements. The client must impose some elements of structure onto the task in order to reach a final outcome. For example, occupational therapists frequently ask clients to create objects from a ball of clay. In this task the outcome is determined by the subject. The procedure is specified only to a limited degree (ie, time limits). The material is totally pliable and suggests no particular outcome or means.

Rationale

Utilizing this concept of structure, a determination of the degree of structure inherent in any task must involve an analysis of each of the three dimensions mentioned above. Each of these dimensions may be thought of as varying along a continuum from clearly defined or specified at one end to undefined or unspecified at the other. Clearly, there are an infinite number of points on each continuum, and a wide variety of combinations of points for all three dimensions taken together. However, for purposes of practical application, each dimension may be viewed as having major divisions—for example, three categories such as: highly specified, unspecified, and an intermediate category. Structure can then be assessed by rating a task on each of the three dimensions and examining the overall result. In this way, tasks can be compared as to the degree of structure they present to the client. At present, this approach provides only a rough estimate of structure since many tasks may have a mixed structure (ie, specified on one dimension but unspecified on others). The implications of such combinations are unclear, and require further investigation.

How can this concept of structure be of use to the occupational therapist? We are presently pursuing applications in three areas: task analysis; therapist self-assessment; and research. A brief disussion of each follows.

Task analysis. By using the general means described above for analyzing task structure, the occupational therapist can inventory the tasks available in the clinic, and order these with respect to the degree of structure. In the same way, assessment tools can be rated. The resultant inventory can aid in prescribing tasks for clients. The occupational therapist can match performance on assessment tasks to the therapeutic tasks which the client is then most likely to successfully complete at a particular point in treatment. In keeping with the observation that as the psychiatric client improves and can gradually tolerate less structured tasks, the therapist can utilize the task inventory in moving the client through a gradual series of therapeutic experiences.

Therapists often enjoy creating, or need to create, new tasks for clients. Use of the dimensions of structure provides a means for systematic variations of old tasks and a basis for the creation of new tasks. If the therapist creates new tasks, the three dimensions permit assessing these tasks for degree of structure before administration.

Therapist self-assessment. When coming to an occupational therapy clinic, the client senses the expectations of his behavior in that clinic whether or not these are made explicit. The client's perception of that role may vary tremendously, depending upon tasks assigned to him and the manner in which he is treated. Thus, the clinical approach and personality of the therapist will affect the client and his performance, as well as the general milieu in the clinic. While this may seem patently obvious, it is mentioned here because we see the dimensions of structure as a means of self-assessment for the therapist to better understand the impression that is made on the client. The occupational therapist can ask himself: "Do I generally make clear the behavioral goals and expectations for clients in the clinic? Do I make clear the means by which clients may attain these goals or am I ambiguous about these? In general, do I tend to favor certain types of materials in therapy tasks?" In brief, the therapist can address the question: "Am I a structuring clinician, or one who imposes less structure on my clients?" Through self-inventory and feedback from others, the therapist may be able to gain helpful personal insights, learn to alter his professional approach, and obtain information relative to therapeutic failures and successes.

Research. Finally, we want to mention the application of the tridimensional concept of structure to research. The discussion up to this point emphasizes the need for a more definitive, scientifically-based concept of structure for use in occupational therapy settings. However, the definition, based largely on clinical experience and logic, provides only an initial step in that direction. Both precise measurement of client task performance in structured and unstructured situations, and research regarding issues of client response to such tasks are needed to further our knowledge.

Valid and reliable measurements of task performance are prerequisite for research. Several assessment tools are now being used in occupational therapy clinics, primarily in the evaluation of physical disabilities, which could serve to measure structured task performance. For example, normative data are available on such tasks as the Purdue Pegboard,[14] the Minnesota Rate of Manipulation,[15] the Nine Hole Peg Test,[16] and the Bennett Tool Test.[17] While these evaluations were originally intended to measure motor coordination, they readily meet the criteria for highly structured tasks. However, norms and means of measuring performance on unstructured tasks are not readily available. This led to the development of the Creative Clay Test which quantifies performance on an unstructured task.

The Creative Clay Test: Administration

The Creative Clay Test was developed in order to objectively measure and quantify performance on an unstructured task. Administration of the clay test involves presenting the subject with a ball of clay and instructing him to create as many different objects as he can in a specified time period. During testing, the administrator records and scores the subject's performance in accordance with specific criteria.

Materials.
A ball of clay (gray modeling) 10 inches in circumference
A plexiglass or smooth board 15 *x* 17 inches
A timer clock (at least five minutes duration)
No other tools permitted

Procedure. The therapist says, "The object of this task is to make as many different objects or things as you can in five minutes. You may use all or part of the clay to make the objects. You may re-use the clay to make objects. Please name each object as you complete it so that I (we) may make note of it. Remember, the object of this task is to make as many different things or objects as you can in five minutes. Questions?"

The examiner may repeat any part of the initial instructions during the test. If the client inquires as to time remaining, the examiner may reply.

Scoring.

(Example)	OBJECTS	IDENTIFIABLE PARTS	SHAPE-ETCH
	car	5 (4 wheels, body)	
	face	4 (nose, head, 2 ears)	x x
	golf club	1	(nose pulled "shaped", mouth and eye etched in
Total	3	10	with fingernail)

E. *Nelson Clark and Michael S. Cross*

Objects.
1. Object names may be brief. Clients tend to assign long names to some of their creations.
2. One object name per creation. A client may not make an object (ie, ball) and assign multiple names to the object (ie, ball—grape, orange, baseball).
3. Each object must be created from scratch. Parts may be used to reform new objects.
4. Objects expanded or improved on are considered the same object with additional parts (ie, a man with 6 parts has been created. The client adds 2 parts, breasts, and calls it a woman. The object is recorded as human figure with 8 parts. If the client destroys the man and re-creates the woman, then the client is credited with the 2 objects and the parts they contain.

Parts.
1. Parts must be identifiable. Autistic shaping/responses (example: a mass with gashes and holes, with spikes over it, and described as the universe with mountains and valleys, etc) are counted as 1 object and 1 part.
2. Pictures or outlines are considered one part unless separate parts are constructed (example: House—windows and doors added; Car—wheels added).
3. Parts may be formed separately, or they may be pulled or shaped from the central body of the object. The examiner must pay particular attention to pulling and shaping techniques as these parts are harder to identify at times.
4. Objects usually considered as one are recorded as one part (example: spoon, golf club, knife).
5. Attention to detail may be counted as parts in some instances. Objects having separately fashioned parts, such as knife with a handle and blade, are credited with 2 parts. A football with lacing was credited with 4 parts: the ball itself and three separate, individual pieces of clay for the lacing.
6. Letters of the alphabet and numbers are considered 1 part. They are considered an object of unity.
7. Objects having a large number of identical parts (example: a bunch of grapes, log cabin, etc) are recorded as such with number of parts. This is sometimes diagnostic in itself as with 1 object with 25 parts. (eg, passive aggressive, grandiosity, persevering).
8. Bits, parts, or pieces of clay fashioned or shaped as a whole are recorded as one part (example: bits formed together as a cup, ship hull, box, etc.) However, if the bits are definitely identifiable, such as rose petals, individual leaves, etc, that are individually placed to form a whole, they are counted as separate parts.

Shaping/Etching.
1. An X is placed in the shape-etch column to denote this particular task behavior.
2. Shaping is defined as forming the clay by pulling the parts from the central body, or forming the clay by pushing in the fingers to shape cups, hulls of boats, pinching out the parts such as handles, wings on a plane, the nose of a face, etc. Research has pointed out that schizophrenics tend to pinch and push on clay not for constructive purposes, but to achieve sensory awareness.[21]
3. Etching is usually done with the fingernail, as no other tools are allowed in the clay test. When etching is done, this is not counted as a part. It is noted with an X in the etch column.
4. Only 1 shape and 1 etch notation may be given per object.

The Creative Clay Test   *313*

Comments.

The directions given for the Creative Clay Test are believed to cover most constructive behaviors as observed in pilot projects spanning 3 years. Certainly there are exceptions to the rule when dealing with a projective media. In those instances, the use of the therapist's own intuition and discretion is encouraged.

Previously, it was mentioned that schizophrenic clients have been observed to perform poorly on unstructured tasks in occupational therapy. In addition, general performance deficits in clients diagnosed as depressed have been observed. Initial observation suggests that patterns of performance on structured and unstructured tasks may correlate highly with major psychiatric diagnostic categories. Performance on the clay test appears to reflect the psychological status of the psychiatric client as described in the following case studies.

Case Studies

Case Example 1. A 26 year old male with a diagnosis of paranoid schizophrenia was referred to occupational therapy within one week of his initial hospital admission. He was administered a routine occupational therapy assessment battery to evaluate work, play, self care, cognitive, and interpersonal skills. Among the tests administered was the Creative Clay Test on which the client constructed 1 object having four parts. During his hospitalization, he attended occupational therapy regularly for a total of 41 clinic visits. He participated in a variety of tasks designed to aid him in problem areas. He was retested seven weeks following admission and just prior to discharge from the hospital. At this time the client constructed eight objects having a total of eleven parts on the clay test.

Case Example 2. A 22 year old male diagnosed as acute psychotic episode was referred to occupational therapy within the first week of his admission to the hospital. The client was evaluated with a standard assessment battery and administered the clay test. Results as demonstrated were:

Objects	Parts	Shape-Etch
Face	5	X
Soccerball	1	X

The client attended occupational therapy regularly for approximately two months and participated in a variety of tasks according to a treatment program. At time of discharge, the results of the clay test were:

Objects	Parts	Shape-Etch
Snowman	3	
Cigarette	1	
Bottle	2	
Pipe	2	X
Donut	1	
Dinosaur	7	

E. Nelson Clark and Michael S. Cross

Case Example 3. A 21 year old male diagnosed as possible drug ingestion (possibly PCP) was referred to occupational therapy within two weeks of hospital admission. Earlier referral was not possible, due to his psychotic and violent behavior. Upon initial occupational therapy evaluation he responded well and appropriately to the structured tasks (eg, tool test, pegboard, formboard). However, during the course of the clay test he began to associate loosely and manipulate the clay vigorously. He produced the following:

Objects	Parts	Shape-Etch	
Smokey Mountain	1	X	X
Mountain	1	X	X

This client attended occupational therapy sporadically and pursued a highly variable hospital course. A clay test following four weeks of treatment revealed an ability to produce seven objects with a total of 12 parts. Two months later, the client was tested again and attempted to construct a log cabin having 32 logs. One month later at time of discharge the client constructed four objects having 13 parts.

Case Example 4. A 20 year old male evaluated as having a thought disorder was given a provisional diagnosis of organic brain syndrome secondary to chronic drug abuse. The client was referred to occupational therapy within one week of his initial admission. The clay test was administered, with the client producing 10 objects with a total of 15 parts and four shape-etch notations. The client participated sporadically in an occupational therapy treatment program. During 16 weeks of hospitalization, he pursued a fluctuating course and was generally considered unimproved by the staff. Upon transfer of the client to another facility for further psychiatric care, his clay test performance had declined to nine objects with a total of 10 parts.

Case Example 5. A 23 year old male with a physical disability of right elbow fracture was referred to occupational therapy for evaluation and treatment. In addition to work related assessments, the Creative Clay Test was administered to evaluate upper extremity manipulation of unstructured media. This client produced 17 objects having 42 parts in the standard five minute time limit.

As these case studies illustrate, the psychiatric client's initial status and general course of progress in treatment was reflected in performance (quantified scoring) on the clay test. Although we are still in the process of developing normative data for the Creative Clay Test, it seems clear from these cases that the more acutely ill clients create very few objects and parts, whereas the less impaired and improved clients, as well as non-psychiatric clients, produce a greater number of objects and parts. In addition, it appears that excessive manipulation of the clay (ie, shaping and etching) occurs in higher proportion in the objects created by the more regressed clients.

Performance data such as those presented above have been used to aid in both diagnosis and treatment planning with clients referred to occupational therapy. With regard to occupational therapy treatment itself, the clay test has provided important information regarding the client's need for structure. A poor clay test performance suggests the need for a more structured environment.

Suggested Research

Many research questions are forthcoming. We may ask about the full nature and range of task performance deficits in acutely ill clients. Changes in task performance with treatment need to be documented. A major question arises as to the relative importance of the different dimensions of task structure in affecting client performance. The effects of various combinations of materials, procedures, and outcomes have great practical relevance to occupational therapy. In brief, there is abundant opportunity for occupational therapists to participate in the investigation of task structure.

Conclusion

The long-standing use of the concept of structure in occupational therapy attests to its face validity as an important variable affecting client task performance. Information from other disciplines supports this view. In this chapter, we have offered a new structured treatment in an effort to: 1) stimulate awareness regarding usage of the term; 2) provide a working definition; and 3) encourage application and research. We believe that more precise use of this term, and application of the suggestions developed in this chapter would benefit both clients and therapists in occupational therapy. In addition, the Creative Clay Test offers occupational therapists an objectively scored, unstructured task for use in the evaluation of psychiatric clients. Addition of the clay test to the occupational therapist's assessment tools provides a greater range of tasks on the structured-unstructured continuum.

In the effort to focus on the issue of task structure, we have necessarily de-emphasized other potentially important factors in task performance, such as client motivation, nature of the task, task complexity,[18,19] and the creative aspect of tasks.[20] Relationships among such factors require thorough investigation.

We believe that the degree of structure inherent in activities is a significant variable affecting human behavior, with special implications for occupational therapy, and that there is a clear need for further refinement and investigation.

References

1. Meyer A: The Philosophy of Occupational Therapy. A J Occu Ther 31:639-642, Nov-Dec, 1977.
2. Hopkins H, Smith H: Willard & Spackman's Occupational Therapy. Philadelphia, JB Lippincott Co, 1978.
3. Evaskus MG: Goodman Evaluation Battery. See Chapter 7.
4. Goldstein AP, Gershaw JN, Sprafkin RP: Structured learning therapy: Development and education. A J Occu Ther 33:635-639, October, 1979.
5. Kuhn RK: Conflict, ambiguity, and overload: Three elements in job stress. Occupational Mental Health 3:2-9, Spring, 1973.
6. Cobb S: Role responsibility: The differentiation of a concept. Occupational Mental Health 3:10-14, Spring, 1973.
7. French JR: Person role fit. Occupational Mental Health 3:15-20, Spring, 1973.
8. Rubin RS: The community meeting: A comparative study. A J Psychiat 136:708-715, May, 1979.
9. Rapaport D: The theoretical implications of diagnostic testing. Congr Int Psychiat 2:241-271, 1950.
10. Kubie LS: Neurotic distortion of the creative process. Lawrence, KS, Univ Kansas Press, 1958.
11. Leeb S: Empirical application of a cognitive framework to rigidity, aspects of creativity, anxiety, and adjustment. Psychological Reports 37: 651, 1975.
12. Fried E, et al: Artistic productivity and mental health, Springfield, IL, Charles C Thomas Publisher, 1964.
13. Myden W: An interpretation and evaluation of certain personality characteristics involved in creative production. Perceptual Motor Skills 9:139, 1959.

14. Purdue Pegboard: Lafayette Instruments Co, Box 1279, Lafayette, IN.
15. Minnesota Rate of Manipulation: Univer Minnesota Press, Minneapolis, MN.
16. Nine Hole Peg Test: Technical Manual: Hand strength and dexterity tests, Sister Kenny Institute Publication No 721, Sister Kenny Institute, Minneapolis, MN, 1971.
17. Bennett Hand Tool Dexterity Test: The Psychological Corporation, 304 E 45th Street, New York, NY, 10017.
18. Huff FW: Learning and psychopathology. Psychological Bull 61:459-468, 1964.
19. Buss AH, Lang PJ: Psychological deficit in schizophrenia: Affect, reinforcement, and concept attainment. J Abnormal Psych 70 2-24, 1965.
20. Weisberg P, Springer K: Environmental factors in creative function. Arch Gen Psychiat 5:554-564, 1961.
21. Schachtel EG: Metamorphosis. New York, Basic Books, 1959.

PART 5
RESEARCH
METHODOLOGY IN DEVELOPING
AN ASSESSMENT TOOL

17
The Principles of Developing Assessment Tools

Mary Garfield, Ph.D., O.T.R.

Whether an individual is developing or utilizing an assessment tool, the statistical components of validity, reliability, and standardization must be thoroughly understood. The therapist needs to be assured that the results of an assessment tool represent accurate information, and that the information is valid for the use for which it is intended. When dealing with variables concerning psychological abnormalities, the task of developing or correctly utilizing a tool becomes even more difficult because of the extreme variances in human behavior.

This chapter contains an overview of the types of reliability and validity as well as the process of standardization. The individual desiring to develop an assessment tool would be advised to review a few of the books from the recommended list at the conclusion of this chapter.

Reliability

Reliability is a technical matter and is not as difficult to obtain as validity. In reliability the measuring part of the instrument is examined. Synonymous with reliability are terms such as accuracy, stability, dependability, and predictability. The researcher seeks the answer to the question: If this test is administered over and over again to the same or comparable subjects, will the same or similiar results be obtained? In other words, how dependable is the test? The researcher also wants to be assured that the measures being obtained are accurate measures of the property measured, and not created measures of error in the instrument.

Errors of measurement relate to the study of the variance of the test. There are two components of variance—a true component and an error component. The degree of error component is the degree of unreliability of the instrument, and depicts the inaccuracy of the instruments. The higher the true component of variance, the higher the reliability of the instrument.

To obtain a high degree of reliability the researcher must write the items of the instrument so that they can be interpreted in only one way. If many people read the item, they should all interpret it the same way. There should be no double meanings. The instrument should be given a pilot test to eliminate unclear or unrelated items. In the BH Battery, for example, items not obtaining a 60% agreement were removed from the battery.

Reliability is increased by having a large number of items in the test. A few items increase the possibility of error variance because the random principle cannot operate. An increased number permits a balancing out of error variance and increases reliability.

A common type of reliability used to establish consistency of measures is intra-rater reliability. The method is referred to as test-retest, and consists of an individual repeating the test. Given that all else is equal, the individual should score the same the second time. If time intervenes between testing, other factors such as learning, or improving health status due to experiences in the lapsed time could account for changed scores. Correlation between the two scores is an indicator of reliability.

Inter-rater reliability takes more effort to establish. There, the researcher examines the correlation between scores of two or more raters evaluating the same subject. When the evaluation contains subjective decisions by the raters, reliability is apt to be lower. Training of evaluators is frequently done to improve reliability.

Directions for the administration of the test should be written clearly and presented in a standardized manner. There should be no variance in the administration of the instrument or error variance, which decreases reliability, could be obtained.

Validity

Validity is best defined by the question: Does this test measure what it is supposed to? The emphasis should be on what is being measured and not on the measurement process itself. If the researcher desires to assess an individual's understanding of the necessity for social interaction skills and administers an instrument which measures the level of interaction skills the individual has obtained, that test is invalid for the purpose. It does not measure understanding, but rather, achievement of skills.

The most common classification of types of validity is put forth by the American Psychological Association.[1] Three types of validity are presented: content, criterion-related, and construct. Although these will be discussed separately, it is important to know that most instruments employ more than one type of validity and there is often overlap between types.

Content Validity. Assessment tools should be a reflection of the behavior being examined. The items of the tool should represent skills or behaviors which could be observed in the universe. This representativeness of content is content validity. Usually a measure of content validity is obtained through the judging process. The items should be examined closely to determine the relevance to the variable being explored. Other professionals experienced with the content should be asked to judge the items and their relevance. In the development of items for assessment of adolescent role behavior, for example, the researcher could ask sociologists or psychologists who specialize in this area to evaluate the items for accuracy. Because it is difficult to know if a satisfactory content validity has been obtained, the user of an assessment tool must judge content validity for his use. If the instrument appears to be representative of the behaviors the user is desirous of assessing and the user is aware of the constraints of content validity, the tool can be beneficial.

Criterion-related validity. In criterion-related validity, the emphasis is on the criterion and its prediction rather than on what the test measures. Concern is with how well the tool compares to other criteria or external variables known to measure the attributes under study. An example of criterion-related validity is described in Chapter 4. Weaknesses identified through the Adolescent Role Assessment were also suggested in assessments on Rowenberg's Self-Esteem Scale, Bills' Indexes of Adjustment and Values, etc. If a person can achieve a good rating or score on the assessment tool, does that mean a better state of wellness exists? Criterion-related validity may not be obtained initially, because of a lack of accumulated predictors in the field of Occupational Therapy. Follow-up studies relating scores on assessment tools to behaviors at a later date are needed and will provide the information necessary to obtain criterion-related validity. Presently, there is difficulty obtaining a universally accepted criteria for wellness. What is "good" mental health?

For the most part, assessment tools are used in occupational therapy to ascertain the level of functioning of an individual on a scale of wellness. When the level has been obtained, a treatment program is begun which will provide opportunities for the client to gain skills and/or understanding necessary to change behavior toward a state of mental health. With this in mind, it seems that criterion-related validity is a concept which occupational therapists must work towards achieving in all assessment tools.

Construct validity. In construct validity the researcher is not just validating the test or tool, but is validating the theory behind the tool. The researcher wants to find the meaning of the test. How and why do the constructs relate to each other?

There are three parts to construct validity: 1) description of the constructs which account for test performance; 2) composition of hypotheses proposing the relationship of the constructs; and 3) empirically testing the hypotheses. Construct validity is theory building in that a hypothesis is put forth, it is tested, and revised, according to new evidence. The Bay Area Functional Performance Evaluation (BaFPE) and the Adolescent Role Assessment have begun the process toward construct validity. Both instruments were founded on theory with implicit hypotheses. Hypotheses have to be stated and tested. Revision of theory then begins, as the revised hypothesis is presented, tested, etc. As a profession, occupational therapy is in need of tested theories for a basis on which to build practice.

Another type of validity which is referred to by the authors of the BaFPE, is face validity. Does the instrument appear to measure what it is intended to? If the tool is to measure intrinsic motivation, do the questions or observations appear to seek that information? There is no measurement of face validity, but rather a subjective feeling toward the instrument. Professionals use their judgment in accepting the tool.

In summary, it appears that content and criterion-related validity are most important to occupational therapy as a profession at this time. Useful criteria must first be obtained through careful, precise, and accurate observation. Occupational therapists are beginning to gather data which can be pooled to use as criteria (content validity). Researchers in occupational therapy are beginning to examine this criteria and make predictions. Some clinicians are making predictions, but not always from carefully scrutinized criteria. There are a few instruments in use which put forth hypotheses to be tested in an effort to develop theories (construct validity). Occupational therapists need to use these instruments and pool their findings in order to help validate them.

Standardization

Standardization has two components: standardizing the administrative procedure in utilizing the test, and collecting normative data for predictive use of the results. It goes without saying that the process of standardizing the administration or collecting norms is not started until there is reasonable assurance that the test is reliable and valid for use. There are no magical numbers or formulas to indicate the correct range of validity and reliability. Initially, an instrument might have low ratings because of poor items or untrained raters, but with increased use and refinement, the test can become quite efficient in validity and reliability.

Standardization of Procedures

Standardizing procedures means that the test can be administered in exactly the same way at different times and places. The test should be printed so that there are no additions or omissions. Instructions for taking the test should be written clearly, and read to the client.

Objective tests (eg, true, false or multiple choice) are comparatively easy to standardize because a scoring guide can be used, and no personal judgment is involved. Subjective tests (eg, observing and scoring behaviors), such as the BaFPE, the BH Battery, and the Adult Psychiatric Sensory Integration Evaluation, are more difficult to standardize. Raters or observers must be trained by a standard procedure. This training can be by film, video tape, instructional manual, or in person. Each method has advantages and disadvantages and takes hours of work; but unless raters are trained to observe and score behavior in the same way the test will be of no value. If a therapist is to examine a finger painting and place numerical values on aspects of it, such as color or strokes, the raters must be trained to recognize colors, shades, and strokes according to the test standards. A statistical test, inter-rater reliability, can be performed to obtain a degree of standardization of procedure.

Normative Data

Interpretation of the results from tests, instruments, and assessment tools are in relationship to the population on which it was normed. In order for the results to be used appropriately, the sample for the norms must be similiar to the individual being tested. Norms for adults 35-40 years of age could not be generalized to a 17 year old. Conversely, it is not appropriate to compare scores obtained by an adult on a test normed for children.

Normative data includes such things as: a description of the community or the institution; the type (ie, public school, institution for the mentally retarded); the sample population description (ie, professionals, blue collar workers); age groupings; sex; racial mixture, economic level; geographic area (ie, urban, rural, west, east); and religious or cultural learnings. Anything which is unique about the population sample which could make a difference in predictability for the assessment should be categorized and reported. The user can then determine appropriate use of the tool.

The process of standardization is long, arduous, and most often costly, both in time and money. Unless a test is standardized, its usefulness is questionable at best.

Conclusion

Occupational therapists might move ahead faster in developing good assessment instruments if therapists would use a few of the more finely developed instruments and work toward standardizing them. Norms could be collected from around the country in a short period of time. The author of such an instrument could seek funding for the expenses related to this process. Perhaps graduate students could study and observe some of the basic criteria and add to the validity of an instrument already in development.

References

1. Standards for educational and psychological teasts and manuals. Washington, DC, American Psychological Assoc, 1974.

Bibliography

Blood DF, Budd WC: Educational Measurement and Evaluation. New York, Harper and Row. 1972.

Cronbach LJ: Essentials of Psychological Teasting. New York, Harper & Row, 1970, Chapters 5 and 6.

Ellingstad V, Heimstra NW: Methods in the Study of Human Behavior. California, Brook/Cole, 1974, pp 37-43.

Forcese DP, Richer S: Social Research Methods. New Jersey, Prentice-Hall, 1973.

Goldman L: Using Tests in Counseling. New York, Appleton-Century-Crofts, Inc. 1961.

Hendrick C, Jones RA: The Nature of Theory and Research in Social Psychology. New York, Academic Press, 1972. Chapter 1-5.

Kerlinger FN: Foundations of Behavioral Research. New York, Holt, Rinehart & Winston, Inc, 1973, Chapters 26 and 27.

Labovitz S, Hagedorn R: Introduction to Social Research. New York, McGraw-Hill, Inc. 1971, Chapters 2, 3, and 5.

Magnusson D: Test Theory. Stockholm, Addison-Wesley, 1966.

PART 6
APPENDIX

Appendix A

Name _____   Date _____

Work Experience
   Type: Pay/Volunteer: Length:

Frequency/length of unemployment:

   Work Skills:

   Like most about working:

   Like least:

   Jobs done well at:

   Jobs done poorly at:

      Reasons:

   Parent's attitudes about your work:

   Parent's expectations for you:

   Most satisfying aspects:

Primary occupation at this time:

   Least satisfying aspects:

   Have most difficulty with:

Vocational Plans and Interests
   Please list:

Education
   Grade level completed: Average grade:
   Favorite subjects:

   Least favorite subjects: Average grade:

   Interests in further education/learning:

      Reasons:

   Reading, writing, speaking skill levels:

   Family attitudes about education/learning:

Activity Patterns
   Favorite games frequently played as a child:

   As an adolescent:

   School activities:

   Present hobbies, leisure time interests:

   How frequently done:

   Like to learn/improve skill in:

   Father's hobbies/interests: frequency:

Mother's hobbies/interests: frequency:

Siblings' hobbies/interests: frequency:

Parent's/siblings' principle job(s):

Parent's/siblings' education:

Housekeeping/home maintenance responsibilities:
  who did/does which tasks:

Personal activity configuration: Summary of a typical week's activity:

Your special abilities, assets, strengths, skills:

Appendix B

I. *Childhood-Play*

   1. Activities

      Kids spend a lot of time playing. When you were a child, what was your favorite age and why? What kinds of things did you like to do? Alone or with friends?

      + — Identifies favorite age and names activities

      0 — Hesitant or vague response

      - — Unable to identify favorite age, pessimistic

   2. Rules

      What games or physical sports did you do as a child? Did you play team games or other games with rules?

      + — Identifies games with rules

      0 — Vague or only games without rules

      - — No games or sports

   3. Interactions

      As a child did you play with kids your own age, other than brothers and sisters?

      + — Able to interact with same age peers

      0 — Vague or marginal interaction

      - — No interaction or inability to interact without fights

   4. Fantasy

      When you were a kid did you daydream or have make-believe friends or make-believe games?

      + — Identifies fantasy

      0 — Vague, not sure

      - — Can identify no fantasy

   5. Role Models

      When you were a kid how did you learn to do things such as ride a bike, tell time, etc?

      + — Identifies role models

      0 — Vague or difficulty remembering

      - — Unable to do skills or unable to identify role models

   6. Interests

      Sometimes, as people grow their interests change. What kinds of interests did you have as a kid? How do those interests compare with current interests?

      + — Identifies childhood interests, able to discriminate from current interests

      0 — Few interests, basically same as now

      - — Lack of childhood interests

II. *Adolescence-Socialization*

   A. Family

      7. Interactions

         Teenagers often hassle with their families. How would you describe your relationship with your family? Do you do anything to agitate your family? What are the positive qualities about your family? Negative qualities?

         + — Relatively positive relationship, recognizes strengths and weaknesses

         0 — Moderate relationship with vague recognition of strengths and weaknesses

         - — Negative relationship with no recognition of positive qualities

      8. Responsibilities

         What kinds of responsibilities do you have at home? Are these responsibilities reasonable? Do you usually do them on time?

         + — Age-appropriate responsibilities, usually completed on time

         0 — Lack of clarity of responsibilities usually completed on time

         - — No responsibilities, inappropriate responsibilities, or refusal to do responsibilities on time

---

Assessment originally published in Am J Occup Ther 30:73, 1976. *Permission to reprint the assessment granted by American Occupational Therapy Association.*

9. Economics

How do you obtain spending money? Are you satisfied with the amount and arrangement for obtaining it? Who decides how you will spend it?

+ — Manages own money

0 — Vague plan for obtaining money with few personal decisions on where spent

- — No plan for obtaining money or no personal decisions on how it is spent

B. School

10. Consistent Behavior

What grade are you in? What kinds of marks do you achieve? Throughout your life as a student have your marks been consistent?

+ — Consistent marks of average to high range

0 — Average to low range of marks, some drop in consistency

- — All low marks or significant drop in consistency

11. Responsibilities

Are you usually prepared for class with assignments completed on time? Do you attend your classes? Are you often late? Do you study regularly or only for tests?

+ — Class attendance regular, usually prepared, regular study habits

0 — Occasionally late for class, occasionally unprepared, studies mainly for tests

- — Often unprepared, often misses classes, few study habits

12. Feedback

Are you satisfied with your school performance? What could you do to improve your school experience? Do you ever follow your teachers' suggestions on improvement?

+ — Identifies ways to improve, uses feedback

0 — Recognizes improvement potential, but has difficulty using feedback or recognizing ways to improve

- — Denies improvement potential or does not use feedback

13. Effect of Role Models

Are you treated fairly by teachers? Are you ever removed from class for your conduct? Do you have any favorite teachers? If so, what qualities make them your favorites?

+ — Usually fair treatment, conforms to norms, identifies positive qualities in a teacher

0 — Questionable treatment, occasionally removed from class

- — Unfair treatment, often removed from class, or no positive qualities in teachers

14. Activities

What activities are you involved in at school? What activities do you do with friends (include clubs)? What activities do you do alone?

+ — Several activities, age appropriate

0 — Hesitant with few activities or some inappropriate activities (eg, stealing)

- — No activities or many inappropriate activities

C. Peers

15. Activities

After school are you usually alone? With one friend? With a group? Are your friends older? Same age? Younger? What do you like about your social situation? What do you dislike?

+ — Positive relationships

0 — Mixed feelings about relationships or most friends older or younger

- — Poor relationships, few friends

16. Time

How many hours a week do you spend in the following activities? How do you decide upon your time schedule? Do you usually complete activities? Is scheduling a problem?

School work (outside of school)

Reading for pleasure

Watching television

Doing nothing

Daydreaming

Working

Making yourself or your clothes look good

Dating

Hanging around talking with friends
Playing tennis, swimming, etc.
Other
+ — Balanced, completed activities with no scheduling problems
0 — Concentrated time spent in a few activities, some incompleted activities, or some scheduling difficulties
- — No activities or multiple disjointed activities without completion, serious scheduling difficulties

17. Community
What do you know about your neighborhood? Where is the nearest food store, park, library? If public transportation is available, do you know how to use it?
+ — Knowledge of community
0 — Vague
- — No knowledge of community

III. *Adolescent-Occupational Choice*
18. Work Attitudes
Have you ever worked? What kinds of work have you done? What did you like about working? What did you dislike? From your experience, what are your attitudes toward work in general (eg, necessary evil, valuable, etc.)?
+ — Positive attitudes
0 — Mixed attitudes
- — Negative attitudes

19. Stage of Choice
What occupation would you *like* to enter? How did you make this selection? What are your plans for further education or training? Do you know anyone in this occupation? What occupation do you think you will *actually* be in ten years from now?
+ — Selection based on interests, capacities, or values, with plans for implementation
0 — Selection based on fantasy or interests with few implementation plans. May be role model and recognition that actual occupation is more realistic than idealized
- — No selection or selection based on fantasy with no role model or no plans for implementation

IV. *Adulthood-Work*
20. Goals
When you think about your future, what things do you think will be important to you (eg, money, free time, career, family, etc.)? How can you prepare yourself for these goals?
+ — Some ideas on goals with preparation ideas
0 — Vague ideas on goals
- — Not future-oriented, no goals or no preparation ideas

21. Fantasy
If your future could be whatever you wanted, what would you want? If you could change anything in the world, what would you change? When you daydream, what do you dream about?
+ — Able to fantasize about the future
0 — Some fantasizing, but minimal
- — Unable to fantasize, very concrete

Appendix C

ADOLESCENT ROLE ASSESSMENT — SCORING SHEET

	+	0	–

I. *Childhood-Play*

    1. Activities

    2. Rules

    3. Interactions

    4. Fantasy

    5. Role Models

    6. Interests

II. *Adolescent-Socialization*
  A. Family

    7. Interactions

    8. Responsibilities

    9. Economics

  B. School

    10. Consistency

    11. Responsibilities

    12. Feedback

    13. Role Models

    14. Activities

  C. Peers

    15. Activities

    16. Time

    17. Community

III. *Adolescent-Occupational Choice*

    18. Work

    19. Choice Stage

IV. *Adulthood—Work*

    20. Goals

    21. Fantasy

Appendix D

AZIMA DIAGNOSTIC RATING SCALE

DIAGNOSTIC INDEXES

D-Drawing

F-Finger Paint

C-Clay

P-Plasticene

I. *ORGANIZATION OF MOOD*
   A. ELATION-DEPRESSION
   1. Use and Handling of Color (F, C, P)
      a) Degree of control—from *very controlled* to *no control.*
      b) Intensity of color—from *very intense* to *no intensity.*
      c) Extensity of color—from *mixed* to *small.*
      d) Range and purity of color—from *mixed* to *no color.*
      e) Texture of color—from *very thick* to *none.*
   2. The Use and Handling of Form (D, F, P, C)
      a) Control of form—from *controlled* to *symbolic.*
      b) Form-movement—from *very mobile* to *immobile.*
      c) Extensity of form—from *whole* to *part.*
      d) Purity of form—from *mixed* to *impure.*
   3. Speed of Response—from *very fast* to *slow.*
   4. Tone of Content—from *very happy* to *very sad.*
      — from *animate* to *inanimate.*
      — from *human* to *non-human.*
      — from *symbolic* to *comprehensible.*
   5. Number of Responses (objects made in each media)
      — from *many* to *unique.*
   B. ANXIETY
   1. Use and Handling of Color
      a) Color shock—from *marked* to *none.*
      b) Clarity—from *very clear* to *chaotic.*
   2. Use and Handling of Form
      — Distinct-shading-indistinct.
      — Continuity-discontinuity.
      — Controlled-uncontrolled.
      — Smooth-shaky.
   3. Movement
      — Blocking-rapid movement.
      — Smooth flow-choppy.
   4. Tone of Content
      — Overt anxiety.
      — Covert anxiety.
   5. Texture
      — Degree of shading.
      — Degree of smoothness.
      — Degree of fuzziness.

II. *ORGANIZATION OF DRIVES*
   A. THE NATURE OF DRIVES
   1. Libidinal drives
      a) Content: overt libidinal content; covert libidinal content (symbolic).
      b) Degree of form control.
      c) Degree of intensity of color, texture, movement.
      d) Mode of object handling (stroking, rubbing, messing, soiling, smearing, licking).
      e) The behavior toward the therapist and objects.

Appendix

2. Aggressive drives
   a) Content: overt aggressive content, covert aggressive content.
   b) Degree of form control.
   c) Degree of intensity of movement (energy output).
   d) Mode of object handling (scratching, nailing, twisting, pressing, cutting, breaking, smashing, etc).
   e) Behavior toward therapist and objects.
B. CONTENT OF DRIVES
   1. Oral (libidinal-aggressive)
      — active to passive responses
      — overt to covert and symbolic responses.
   2. Anal (libidinal-aggressive)
      — active to passive responses.
      — overt to covert and symbolic responses.
   3. Phallic (libidinal-aggressive)
      — active to passive responses.
      — overt to covert and symbolic responses.

III. *ORGANIZATION OF EGO*
   A. SYNTHETIC FUNCTIONS
      1. Degree of organization of form, color, and movement
      2. Degree or organization from one medium to another.
      3. Use of the battery.
      4. Total approach to the battery.
      5. Completeness-incompleteness.
      6. Comprehensibility-incomprehensibility
         (the degree of preponderance of secondary and primary processes).
   B. DEFENSIVE FUNCTIONS (inferred from creations and associations).
      1. Repression
      2. Reaction formation
      3. Isolation
      4. Undoing
      5. Projection
      6. Splitting
      7. Introjection
      8. Withdrawal
      9. Denial
     10. Regression

IV. *ORGANIZATION OF OBJECT RELATIONS*
   A. RELATION TO THE THERAPIST
      1. Libidinal-aggressive
      2. Indifferent
      3. Inhibited
      4. Problematic
      5. Realistic
   B. RELATION TO THE OBJECT
      1. Libidinal-aggressive
      2. Indifferent
      3. Inhibited
      4. Problematic
      5. Realistic
   C. CONTENT OF THE OBJECT
      1. Human (mobile-immobile)
      2. Animal (mobile-immobile)
      3. Vegetable
      4. Inanimate
      5. Void
      6. Bizarre

D. STRUCTURE OF THE OBJECT
  1. Recognizability
  2. Culture-sytonicity
  3. Relation of parts
  4. Completeness-incompleteness
  5. Realistic-symbolic

Adapted from Azima: Diseases of the Nervous System, Monograph Supplement, 22, 1961.

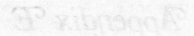

Appendix E

Name _____ Hospital # _____

Address _____

Diagnosis _____ Age _____ Sex _____

Chief Complaint _____ Date of Admission _____

Physician _____ Occupational Therapist _____

Education _____

Occupation(s) _____

Special Interests or Aptitudes _____

Family Structure:
  Mother: Spouse:

  Father: Children:

  Siblings:

_____

Precautions and/or Limitations _____

Development History:

History of Present Illness:

Appendix F

SHOEMYEN BATTERY

OCCUPATIONAL THERAPY DEPARTMENT
SHANDS TEACHING HOSPITAL
UNIVERSITY OF FLORIDA
PSYCHIATRY SERVICE

Patient Name _____
Hospital # _____
Date Completed _____

OCCUPATIONAL THERAPY EVALUATION SUMMARY

1. Patient's reaction to:

   Orientation and evaluation experience _____

   _____

   Follow-up discussion _____

   _____

   Therapist _____

   Others present _____

2. Response to tasks and instructions _____

   _____

3. Response to media _____

   _____

4. Organization _____

   _____

5. Range of attention and persistence _____

   _____

6. Suggestibility _____

7. Creativity _____

8. Dexterity _____

9. Level of independence _____

   _____

COMMENTS
Tile:

Clay figure:

Finger painting:

Sculpture:

Appendix

345

1. MOSAIC TILE

*Complexity of Design scale

Color—warm/cool scale

Color—contrast scale

Representational Design scale

Symmetry of Design scale

Order attempted   Time spent

2. HUMAN FIGURE

Brief description

Apparent physical identity

Identification by patient

Detail

Positioning

Methods & treatment

Order attempted   Time spent

3. FINGER PAINTING

Brief description

Content

Colors used

Overall impression

Technique

Spacing

Order attempted   Time spent

4. SCULPTURE

Brief description

Use of block

Content

Treatment

Use of tools

Order attempted   Time spent

**Bendroth, Sally and Southam, Marti: "Objective Evaluation of Projective Material", AJOT, Vol. 27, #2, March 1973, pp. 78-80.*

In this study it was found that the scale which most significantly predicted diagnoses was complexity.

Appendix G

SHOEMYEN BATTERY*

KEY AND GUIDELINES
to Information Summary and
Occupational Therapy Evaluation

OCCUPATIONAL THERAPY DEPARTMENT
SHANDS TEACHING HOSPITAL
UNIVERSITY OF FLORIDA

The first page is designed for completion during or soon after the client's admission conference. Information relating to headings should be entered as concisely and completely as possible.

The second page is completed if routine Univ. of Florida procedure has been used. It requires short statements or phrases concerning the whole procedure and inconsistencies or differences considered pertinent.

The third page records specifics of each activity. Space is provided for suggested observations.

Suggested Observations and Reactions

Information derived from Univ. of Florida Routine Evaluation Procedure.

1. Client's reaction to:

   Orientation & evaluation experience
       Enthusiastic, perceives it as a challenge
       Participates from sense of duty or to please therapist
       Reluctant, encouragement needed
       Negative attitude
       Perceives as irrelevant to self
       Threatened by evaluation potential
       Withdraws
       Appears to see some value in process

   Follow-up discussion
       Hesitant to become involved
       Expresses pleasure and/or surprise at own achievement
       Remains threatened and withdrawn
       On basis of this experience, approaching OT positively
       Volunteers no information and/or only superficial answers
       Evasive
       Communicates easily

   Therapist
       Is very compliant and submissive
       Accepts and cooperates
       Questions authority, seems to resent supervision
       Flippant and testing
       Attempts to impress and/or downgrade
       Openly defiant and/or hostile
       Appears to find personally threatening

   Others Present
       Apparently oblivious
       Interested in their activity
       Competitive towards. . .
       Seeks ideas from. . .
       Enlists support
       Increased anxiety
       Perceives as supportive

2. Response to tasks and instructions
       Apparently threatened by need to perform

Appendix   *347*

        Considers childish or degrading
        Concerned with completion
        Concerned with process
        Attempts hardest first
        Attempts hardest last

3. Response to media
        Equally accepting
        Comfortable with structure, distaste for messy and expressive activities
        Enjoyed expressive, disliked structured activities
        Particularly distressed by destructive activity
        Regressive response
        Positively challenged by most activities
        Enjoyed showing off
        Preferred structured activities
        Preferred expressive activities
        Minimal response

4. Organization
        Plans ahead and follows through
        Works well from intuition without plan
        Encounters difficulty from inadequate planning
        Appears unable to preplan

5. Range of attention and persistence
        Responds appropriately to task and surroundings
        Easily distracted by fringe activity
        Unable to handle tasks adequately because of distractibility
        Persists in spite of distraction
        Short attention span

6. Suggestibility
        Not apparent
        Obviously influenced by environment
        Extremely suggestible

7. Creativity
        Creative, with talent or technique
        Creative, resourceful approach
        Can implement own ideas
        None observed

8. Dexterity
        Easily performs fine motor skills
        Average in motor skill performance
        Poor manual dexterity
        Has difficulty with most manual skills

9. Level of independence
        Relies heavily on therapist or others
        Performs independently
        Demonstrates specific concern over dependence-independence, ie, figure or other activities
           or tasks
        Denies influence of others

SPECIFICS

1. Mosaic Tile

        Color—Warm/Cool scale
        all warm colors (no neutrals)
        predominantly warm
        equal warm/cool or predominantly neutrals
        predominantly cool
        all cool colors (no neutrals)

Color—Contrast scale
very strong contrast (black/white)
strong contrast (black/yellow, red/white)
moderate contrast (brown/yellow, blue/orange, colors used randomly, all or nearly all colors used, red/black)
slight contrast (green/yellow, orange/brown, red/blue, blue/yellow)
very slight contrast—same hue (blue/green, beige/yellow)

Representational Design scale
pictorial (building, figure)
symbolic (initials, religious, numbers)
symmetrical abstract (single border with symmetrical interior design)
asymmetrical abstract
concentric borders
single border around edge (without interior design evident)
solid stripes of colors (vertical, horizontal, diagonal stripes comprise design)
checkerboard
attempted pattern
random (no design)

Complexity of Design scale
highly complex pattern (symbol, abstract, pictorial)
complex pattern (concentric borders, single border with interior design)
simple pattern (checkerboard, two-color design, single border without interior design)
failed pattern
no pattern (random)

Symmetry of Design scale
complete (color pattern identical in four directions)
partial (color pattern identical in two directions)
portions or elements of symmetry (not symmetrical in entirety but portions or color patterns symmetrical within individual pattern parts)
not all pattern parts symmetrical within themselves (definite color groupings, artistically balanced color, failed symmetrical attempt)
total asymmetry (random design, no symmetrical parts)

COLORS:	*WARM*	*COOL*	*NEUTRAL*
	Chinese Red, Lemon Yellow, Burnt Orange, Medium Brown, Beige	Aqua, Medium Blue, Lime Green	Black, White

2. Human Figure

Apparent physical identity
male, female, female child, male child, neuter, self

Identification by patient
not identified...but animated
identified: self, relative, friend, other

Detail
clothing added or suggested, all facial, ears, single features emphasized, accessories

Positioning
standing, seated, prone, supine, in motion

Methods and Treatment
sections modeled before joining, modeled from one piece, other
concern for whole, one view only, surfaces rough, surfaces smooth, detail added, detail incised, combination

3. Finger Painting

   Content
     abstract
     representational: human, animal, building, land or sea scape, symbol, other

   Colors used
     red, blue, yellow
     used separately, blended

   Overall impression
     cool, warm, balanced,
     light, dark, symmetrical

   Technique
     experimental, goal directed, one finger, several fingers, whole hand or more

   Spacing
     paper covered, bare background, edge frame

4. Sculpture

   Use of block
     basic shape maintained, altered, one surface only

   Content
     abstract
     representational: human, animal, building, symbol, other

   Treatment
     surface smooth, surface rough, superficial

   Use of tools
     hesitant and/or threatened, with apparent ease, aggressive, skillful

---

Reprinted by permission of the American Occupational Therapy Association, Inc. Copyright 1970, AJOT, Vol 24, No 4.

Appendix H

GOODMAN BATTERY RATING SCALE: ABILITY TO ORGANIZE

TILE	DRAWING S	DRAWING P	CLAY		COMMENTS
				1. Minimal or no attempt at task.	
				2. Initiates task, but proceeds with poor organization (e.g. fragmented placement of tile, drawing not related in form or content, primitive production in clay, ex. ball). Difficulty in conceptualizing whole.	
				3. Works in somewhat organized, though indecisive manner making changes because of poor planning, but completes task adequately.	
				4. Easily organizes situation to accomplish task efficiently.	
				5. Somewhat compulsive in his need to organize his approach to task, but able to proceed satisfactorily without constant rechecking and reworking.	
				6. Very careful and exacting; many time-consuming methods of organization (e.g. overly careful in gluing or spacing of tiles, much comparison with tile model; excessive detail and overworking of drawing and clay). Overly concerned with messiness.	
				7. Extremely compulsive to extent that patient does not complete task.	

KEY:
1 — increasingly dysfunctional state
2 — (more inner directed, passive)
3
4 = most functional response to task
5 — increasingly dysfunctional state
6 — (more outer directed, aggressive)
7

DEVELOPED BY:
MARSHA GOODMAN EVASKUS, O.T.R.
JANE VAN de BOGERT, O.T.R.

REVISION OF 9/75

Appendix 7

GOODMAN BATTERY RATING SCALE: INDEPENDENCE

TILE	DRAWING S	DRAWING P	CLAY		COMMENTS
				1. Does not initiate any productive activity in response to instructions given and non-directive therapist (e.g., more generalized inability, immobilized or lost in process of task).	
				2. Asks many questions regarding work process, seeking directions and decision-making from examiner (e.g., "how do I find the right colors"). Has difficulty completing task.	
				3. Asks several questions after instructions are given, seeking clarification, permission to proceed, etc. Task completed adequately.	
				4. Completes task in self-reliant manner.	
				5. Impatient to begin but waits until instructions are given. Task completed adequately.	
				6. Begins without waiting for instructions to be completed. Has difficulty completing task.	
				7. Ignores instructions and layout of materials, proceeds in his own manner (e.g. may change order of tasks, not copy tile model, etc.) or defiantly refuses to do task.	

KEY:

1
2 — increasingly dysfunctional state (more inner directed, passive)
3

4 = most functional response to task

5
6 — increasingly dysfunctional state
7 (more outer directed, aggressive)

DEVELOPED BY:
MARSHA GOODMAN EVASKUS, O.T.R.
JANE VAN de BOGERT, O.T.R.

REVISION OF 9/75

Appendix

Appendix J

GOODMAN BATTERY RATING SCALE — SELF-ESTEEM: PERFORMANCE

TILE	DRAWING S	DRAWING P	CLAY		COMMENTS
				1. May make minimal attempt to perform tasks. Increased hesitancy, becomes immobilized and does not complete task.	
				2. Hesitant, increased changes, erasures, and rebuilding; productions may be small, hidden from examiner; drawings may be faint, incomplete.	
				3. Some hesitancy, erasures and/or changes; may use light, sketchy lines. Task completed adequately.	
				4. Completes task in self-assured manner within reasonable amount of time.	
				5. Works somewhat quickly and boldly: Task completed adequately.	
				6. Approaches task very quickly and boldly, working in careless manner; makes a few corrections; productions may be large; graphics heavy.	
				7. Discounts, pushes aside, or actually destroys work, placing blame for poor results on external sources (e.g. inferior materials, poor directions, etc.) Does not complete task.	

KEY:

1 ⎫ increasingly dysfunctional state
2 ⎬ (more inner directed, passive)
3 ⎭

4 = most functional response to task

5 ⎫ increasingly dysfunctional state
6 ⎬ (more outer directed, aggressive)
7 ⎭

DEVELOPED BY:
MARSHA GOODMAN EVASKUS, O.T.R.
JANE VAN de BOGERT, O.T.R.

REVISION OF 9/75

Appendix K

GOODMAN BATTERY RATING SCALE — SELF-ESTEEM: VERBAL

TILE	DRAWING		CLAY		COMMENTS
	S	P			

1. Comments indicate hopeless, helpless attitude toward ability; minimal engagement with task. Does not complete task.

2. Comments become increasingly self-depreciatory during work process; may sigh, groan, and/or grimace, etc. Has difficulty completing task.

3. Initially questions ability to do task but proceeds to complete task adequately.

4. Completes task adequately in confident manner.

5. Arrogant in approach; comments indicate superiority to task but proceeds to complete task adequately.

6. Comments become increasingly expansive and arrogant during work process; some externalizing in response to problems encountered. Has difficulty completing task.

7. Unable to tolerate discrepancy between his expansive ideas and actual performance, placing total blame for poor results on external sources. Does not complete task.

KEY:

1 — increasingly dysfunctional state
2 — (more inner directed, passive)
3

4 = most functional response to task

5 — increasingly dysfunctional state
6 — (more outer directed, aggressive)
7

DEVELOPED BY:
MARSHA GOODMAN EVASKUS, O.T.R.
JANE VAN de BOGERT, O.T.R.

REVISION OF 9/75
© Marsha Goodman Evaskus, all rights reserved.

Appendix L

THE BH BATTERY
MOSAIC TILING RATING SCALE

PHASE I: Observations during performance. (process analysis)

II. APPROACH TO THE MEDIUM

    A. *Posture: feet*
    Feet or toes on floor
        0(absent)   1(present)
    Feet or toes around chair
      (legs crossed)
    Standing
        0(absent)   1(present)

    A. *Posture: arms*
    Both arms free to work
        0(absent)   1(present)
    Leans on one arm
        0(absent)   1(present)

    B. *Attitude*

Normal speed	1
Lazily	2
Pause	3
Begins and then refuses	4
Refuses	5

III. USE OF SPACE

    D. *Order*

Sequential	1
Arranges pattern on table	2
Rearranges tile on board	3
Rearranges tile after gluing	4
Places tile chaotically	5

VI. CHARACTERISTIC OF MOSAIC DESIGN

    F. *Direction of movement*
    (multiple response)
    Left to right
        0(absent)   1(present)
    Right to left
        0(absent)   1(present)
    Away from self
        0(absent)   1(present)
    Toward self
        0(absent)   1(present)

V. VERBALIZATION DURING THE ACTIVITY

    A. *Characteristics*

Satisfied	1
Apologetic	2
Dissatisfied	3
Boastful	4
Nonverbal	5

    B. *Verbalization about the tile*

Hotplate (trivet)	1
Plaque	2
Geometric	3
A mosaic	4
No use	5

TIME

Appendix

MOSAIC TILING RATING SCALE

PHASE II: Observations following performance (concept analysis)

I. COLOR: (multiple response)

Black	0(absent)	1(present)
Blue	0(absent)	1(present)
Red	0(absent)	1(present)
Yellow	0(absent)	1(present)
Green	0(absent)	1(present)
White	0(absent)	1(present)

III. USE OF SPACE

A. *Surface coverage*

49 tiles	1
48 - 36 tiles	2
35 - 24 tiles	3
23 - 2 tiles	4
beyond edges	5

B. *Texture*

Sufficient glue	1
Not enough glue	2
No glue used	3
Profuse glue	4
Glue on top of tile	5

E. *Overlapping*
   0 (absent)   1 (present)

IV. FORM

A. *Distribution*

All over board	1
Center	2
Corner	3
Slanting	4
Across center	5

V. CHARACTERISTIC OF MOSAIC DESIGN

A. *Number of design/s*

One	1
Two	2
Three	3
Four	4
Five	5

B. *Use of space*

Compact to edge	1
Equally distributed	2
Compact in center	3
Scattered	4
Beyond	5

C. *Position of design*

No edge vacant	1
1 edge vacant	2
2 edge vacant	3
3 edge vacant	4
4 edge vacant	5

D. *Design (one response)*

Scattered
   0(absent)   1(present)
Plain
   0(absent)   1(present)
Random
   0(absent)   1(present)
Random w boarder
   0(absent)   1(present)
Simple checkerboard
   0(absent)   1(present)
Simple checkerboard
   w obvious center
   0(absent)   1(present)
Complex checkerboard
   w obvious center
   0(absent)   1(present)

E. *Symmetry*
   0(absent)   1(present)

Appendix *M*

THE BH BATTERY

FINGER PAINTING RATING SCALE

PHASE I: Observations during performance (process analysis)

II. APPROACH TO THE MEDIA

A. *Posture: feet*
Feet or toes on floor
0(absent)   1(present)
Feet or toes around chair
(legs crossed)
0(absent)   1(present)
Standing
0(absent)   1(present)

A. *Posture: arms*
Arms free to work
0(absent)   1(present)
Leans on one arm
0(absent)   1(present)

B. *Attitude*
Normal speed   1
Lazily   2
Pauses   3
Begins and then refuses   4
Refuses   5

D. *First daub*
Top:
½ 0(absent)   1(present)
¼ left
0(absent)   1(present)
¼ right
0(absent)   1(present)
Middle:
½ 0(absent)   1(present)
½ left
0(absent)   1(present)
½ right
0(absent)   1(present)
Bottom:
½ 0(absent)   1(present)
¼ left
0(absent)   1(present)
½ right
0(absent)   1(present)

E. *Parts of the hand used*
(multiple response)

Finger nails
0(absent)   1(present)
Finger tips
0(absent)   1(present)
Extended fingers
0(absent)   1(present)
Index finger
0(absent)   1(present)
Thumb
0(absent)   1(present)
Knuckles
0(absent)   1(present)
Heel of hand
0(absent)   1(present)
Wrist
0(absent)   1(present)
Whole hand
0(absent)   1(present)
Side of hand
0(absent)   1(present)
Back of hand
0(absent)   1(present)
Arm
0(absent)   1(present)

III. USE OF SPACE

B. *Motion*
(multiple response)
Smearing
0(absent)   1(present)
Scrubbing
0(absent)   1(present)
Scribbling
0(absent)   1(present)
Pushing
0(absent)   1(present)
Pulling
0(absent)   1(present)
Patting
0(absent)   1(present)
Slapping (striking)
0(absent)   1(present)
Scratching
0(absent)   1(present)
Stubbing
0(absent)   1(present)
Picking (plucking)
0(absent)   1(present)
Tapping
0(absent)   1(present)

D. *Order*

Takes paint from jars	1
Puts paint on table before placed on paper	2
Starts over on same sheet of paper	3
Wants another sheet of paper	4
Places paint in a chaotic manner	5

C. *Type of Story*

Fantasy
    0(absent)   1(present)
Fictional
    0(absent)   1(present)
Factual
    0(absent)   1(present)
Cultural
    0(absent)   1(present)
Mythological
    0(absent)   1(present)

E. *Overlapping*
    0(absent)   1(present)

TIME:

IV. STROKES (if present)

  A. *Direction*
    (multiple response)
    Away from self
      0(absent)   1(present)
    Towards self
      0(absent)   1(present)
    Left or right
      0(absent)   1(present)
    Right to left
      0(absent)   1(present)

VI. VERBALIZATION DURING THE ACTIVITY

  A. *Characteristics*

Satisfied	1
Apologetic	2
Dissatisfied	3
Boastful	4
Nonverbal	5

  B. *Occurrence of Verbalization*
    (multiple response)
    Preparation
      0(absent)   1(present)
    Process
      0(absent)   1(present)
    Clean-up
      0(absent)   1(present)

FINGER PAINTING RATING SCALE

PHASE II: Observations following performance (content analysis)

I. COLOR (multiple response)
Yellow   0(absent)   1(present)
Red   0(absent)   1(present)
Blue   0(absent)   1(present)
Black   0(absent)   1(present)
Mixed   0(absent)   1(present)
Mud   0(absent)   1(present)

Dark line
    0(absent)   1(present)
Medium
    0(absent)   1(present)
Light white line
    0(absent)   1(present)
Tearing
    0(absent)   1(present)

II. APPROACH TO THE MEDIA

C. *Format*
    Paper placed horizontal
        0(absent)   1(present)
    Paper placed vertical
        0(absent)   1(present)

D. *Multiplicity of strokes*

None	1
1 - 2	2
3 - 4	3
5 - 6	4
more than 6	5

III. USE OF SPACE

A. *Surface coverage*

All	1
12 - 15 squares	2
8 - 11 squares	3
0 - 7 squares	4
Beyond edges	5

C. *Texture*

Smooth and wet	1
Smooth and dry	2
Little paint but very wet	3
Lumpy and dry	4
Lumpy and wet	5

F. *Shape and length*
    (multiple response)
Angular (more 6")
    0(absent)   1(present)
Angular (less 6")
    0(absent)   1(present)
Horizontal (more 6")
    0(absent)   1(present)
Horizontal (less 6")
    0(absent)   1(present)
Vertical (more 6")
    0(absent)   1(present)
Vertical (less 6")
    0(absent)   1(present)
Curved
    0(absent)   1(present)
Zigzag
    0(absent)   1(present)
Open
    0(absent)   1(present)
Closed
    0(absent)   1(present)

IV. STROKES (if present)

B. *Width of lines*
    (multiple response)
Thin (finger nails)
    0(absent)   1(present)
Medium (index finger)
    0(absent)   1(present)
Bold (heel of hand)
    0(absent)   1(present)

C. *Pressure* (if present)
    (multiple response)

V. FORM

A. *Detail*

Few but essential	1
None but unessential	2
No details	3
Minutus	4
Unrelated detail	5

B. *Shape of Objects*
(multiple response)
Vague (faint)
0(absent)   1(present)
Clear
0(absent)   1(present)
Sharp
0(absent)   1(present)

Enter time from tile

_____

Enter Total in time block _____

TIME: ENTIRE ACTIVITY

1 - 14 min.	1
16 - 30 min.	2
31 - 45 min.	3
46 - 60 min.	4
Beyond 1 hour	5

C. *Size of objects*

Mixture	1
Larger than 8	2
Between 6 - 8"	3
Smaller than 6"	4
Smaller than 1"	5

D. *Distribution of objects*

Equally distributed	1
Center	2
Corner	3
Slanting	4
Across Center	5

E. *Symmetry*
0(absent)   1(present)

VI. THEME

A. *Content*

Plain	1(present)
Repetition	1(present)
Lettering	1(present)
Handprint	1(present)
Landscape (scenic)	1(present)
Building	1(present)
Abstract	1(present)
Animals	1(present)
People	1(present)
Plants	1(present)
Objects	1(present)
Religion	1(present)
Symbol	1(present)
Geometric	1(present)

Enter time for painting

_____

Appendix N

Formal Variables

1. Color of construction paper selected:
   A) red   B) yellow   C) orange   D) green
   E) blue   F) purple   G) black   H) white
2. Number of pictures or cuttings:
   A) 1   B) 2-5   C) 6-10   D) 11-15
   E) 16 and over
3. Color of most cuttings:
   A) black/white   B) colored   C) mixed
4. Over-all color effect:
   A) vivid   B) subdued   C) mixed
5. Manner in which most cuttings are cut out:
   A) square fashion
   B) cut around in detail
   C) part of an object cut off or out
   D) another object cut out of existing object
   E) printing cut out of picture   F) torn out
6. Degree of neatness:
   A) very good   B) good   C) average   D) poor
7. Pictures glued on upside-down or sideways:
   A) all   B) none   C) some
8. Overlapping of cuttings:
   A) all   B) none   C) some
9. Pictures glued completely over another:
   A) all   B) none   C) some
10. Achievement of an over-all balance:
    A) yes   B) no
11. Fragmentation (little cuttings put in with no relevance to others):
    A) yes   B) no
12. Dimensionalizing (folding, accordioning paper, etc.):
    A) yes   B) no
13. Cutting out and use of words:
    A) yes   B) no
14. Framing (either band of color left or border cuttings put on):
    A) yes   B) no

Content Variables

1. Number of people:
   A) 1   B) 2-5   C) 6-10   D) 11-15   E) 16 and over
2. Age and sex of people:
   A) geriatric (A1—male A2—female)
   B) adult (B1—male B2—female)
   C) adolescent (C1—male C2—female)
   D) child (D1—male D2—female)
   E) infant
   F) caricature
3. Feelings people expressed:
   A) pleasure   B) pain   C) anger   D) sadness   E) conflict
4. Activity state of people:
   A) aggressive   B) passive   C) competitive
   D) inactive (sleeping)   E) sensual
5. Emphasis on body part:
   A) eyes   B) head   C) breasts   D) other
6. People clothed in costumes, uniforms, or unusual attire:
   A) yes   B) no

7) Achievement of a central theme:
    A) yes   B) no
8. Number of animals:
    A) 1   B) 2-5   C) 6-10   D) 11-15   E) 16 and over
9. Emphasis on objects:
    A) yes   B) no
10. Type of objects:
    A) food   B) alcohol   C) apparel   D) floral
    E) home oriented   F) scenic or travel
    G) architectural   H) design   I) other
11. Use of appropriate title:
    A) yes   B) no

Patient-Therapist Variables
1. Seeks repetition of directions:
    A) yes   B) no
2. Seeks reassurances of doing it correctly:
    A) yes   B) no
3. Time taken to complete the college:
    A) 0-15 minutes   B) 16-30 minutes   C) 31 minutes to 1 hour
    D) 1-2 hours   E) over 2 hours

Appendix O

Division

Name _____ Age _____ Marital Status _____

Number of children _____ Ages _____

With whom were you living prior to hospitalization? _____

What type of residence: Home _____ Apartment _____ Other _____ (Specify) _____

Why are you seeking treatment? _____

_____

What would you like to change about yourself? _____

_____

EDUCATION

High school grade completed _____ College years completed _____

Major and Degree _____ Vocational Training/Other Education

_____

Do you have future educational plans? If so, what? _____

_____

WORK HISTORY

What type of work do you do? Full or Part Time _____

How many jobs have you held in the past 10 years? _____

How long has it been since your last employment? _____

If you could work at any type of job, what would it be? _____

RECREATIONAL

Approximately how much free time do you have per day? _____

What do you do in your free time for entertainment and/or relaxation?

(Hobbies, sports, community involvement) _____

What do you consider your outstanding abilities, talents, or strong points?

What do you think you do well? _____

_____

What do you think you will be doing 6 months from now? _____

One year from now? _____

Therapist _____ Date _____

Choose a typical weekday in your life: for example, Monday. Fill in the following schedule which deals with how you spend the day.

Time Period   Schedule

6 am — 8 am

_____

8 am — 10 am

_____

10 am — 12 pm

_____

12 pm — 2 pm

_____

2 pm — 4 pm

_____

4 pm — 6 pm

_____

6 pm — 8 pm

_____

8 pm — 10 pm

_____

10 pm — 12 am

_____

*Adapted from a form developed by Richard Spahn of the Austin-Riggs Foundation. Paper presented at the March, 1965 Meeting of the American Orthopsychiatric Society.

Appendix P

ACTIVITIES OF DAILY LIVING QUESTIONNAIRE

Name _____ Age _____ Date _____ Division _____

Interviewer _____

I. *Personal Hygiene*
   1. Do you take care of your personal hygiene independently? (bathing, care of hair, teeth, nails, shaving) _____

II. *Child Care*
   1. Are there any children living at home with you? _____
   2. Which member/members of the family takes care of the child's:
      a. Hygiene _____
      b. Food requirements _____
      c. School requirements _____

III. *Food Management*
   1. How many meals a day do you eat? _____
   2. Where do you eat most of your meals? (home or out) _____
   3. Who does the grocery shopping? _____
   4. Do you know how to cook? _____
   5. How often do you cook? _____
   6. What is the number of people you are accustomed to cooking for? _____
   7. Who does the majority of the cooking at your residence? _____
   8. Would you be interested in attending a group discussion on nutrition in OT? _____
   9. Would you be interested in planning and cooking a meal in OT with a small group of patients? _____

IV. *Homemaking Tasks*
   A. *Cleaning*
      1. Who does the housekeeping at your residence? _____
      2. Do you see a future need for learning or improving cleaning techniques? _____

   B. *Laundering*
      1. Who does the laundry at your residence? _____
      2. Do you do your own ironing? _____
      3. Do you see a future need for learning or improving ironing and laundering techniques? _____

V. *Sewing*
   1. Who does the basic sewing repairs? (hems, buttons, seams) _____
   2. Can you use a sewing machine? _____
   3. Are there any sewing techniques you would like to learn? _____
   4. If you answered yes, check which ones you would be interested in learning:
      a. how to sew buttons, hems, seams _____
      b. how to read a pattern _____
      c. how to lay out and cut a pattern _____
      d. how to sew a pattern _____

VI. *Home Repairs*
   1. Who does the basic home repairs in your house or apartment (ie, repairing leaking faucets, lamp cords, lamp switches, broken window panes)? _____
   2. Would you like to attend a minor home repairs group? _____

VII. *Money Management*
   1. *Banking*
      a. do you have your own savings account? _____
                          checking account? _____

      b. can you balance your checkbook with the monthly statement? _____

      c. would you like to learn how to get a checking or savings account? _____

  2. *Budgeting*

      a. who handles you or your family's money? _____

      b. at the end of the month do you usually have more bills than money? _____

      c. would you like to increase your skills in budgeting? _____

  3. *Smart shopping*

    Would you like to learn hints for smart shopping? (ie, food, household articles, energy conservation) _____

_____

VIII. *Transportation*

  1. Do you have a driver's license? _____

  2. Would you like to learn how to get a driver's license? _____

  3. Are you familiar with how to use public transportation? (rapid, buses) _____

  4. If not, would you like to learn? _____

Appendix Q

COMPREHENSIVE ASSESSMENT PROCESS:
A GROUP EVALUATION

STANDARDIZED ASSESSMENT PROCEDURE

(Prior to commencement of the interviews, the therapist should introduce himself and explain the purpose and goals of the interviews.)

I. Initial Evaluation Interview

  A. Given to client
    1. 1:1 (therapist/client)
    2. Away from client group (in AT or on the ward)
    3. Questions asked by therapist and recorded as client responds

  B. For Assessment of
    1. Eye contact
    2. 1:1 interaction — ie, cooperation, rambling, loose, guarded, responsive, suspicious, delusional, rapid and/or pressured speech, etc.
    3. Affect
    4. Client's insight into illness
    5. Level of self-esteem
    6. Use of leisure time at home
    7. Educational background
    8. Work history

II. Activities of Daily Living Questionnaire

  A. Given to client
    1. 1:1 (therapist/client)
    2. Away from client group (in AT or on the ward)
      a. Questions asked by therapist and recorded as client responds or
      b. Hand form to client to fill out and review questionnaire with client. If he filled it out, ascertain whether or not the client understands what he has answered and requested.

  B. Evaluating (independence, dependence on others for, client's desire to increase skills in):
    1. Personal Hygiene
    2. Child Care
    3. Food Management
    4. Homemaking
    5. Sewing
    6. Minor Home Repairs
    7. Money Management
    8. Transportation

III. Record Keeping

  A. Place initial evaluation interview in client's occupational therapy file.

  B. Record observations and other pertinent data in the client's occupational therapy file.

  C. Inform the therapist in charge of the activities of daily living group what the client has requested in activities of daily living.

IV. Evaluation Group
Note: All clients should know the purpose of this group prior to beginning (we will be assessing their work and interaction skills). Note what client does during each session (use Progress Note—checklist as a guide).

  A. Day 1 — Procedures
    1. The leader is responsible for making sure the supplies are set up before the group starts.

2. Re-explanation of the group
    a. Assessment of work skills and interaction skills to enable the occupational therapy staff to devise a treatment program specific to each client's needs.
    b. Important to attend all 3 days of group from 11:00 am — 12:00 noon.
    c. Try to reschedule appointments that are during the evaluation group.
3. Name introductions (client and staff).
4. Hand out written directions.
5. Tell clients they have 50 minutes to finish the first day's instructions.
6. Give the clients the time midway through the session, when there are five minutes left to finish the hot plate, and if and when client asks for the time.
7. Five minutes before group ends, stop clients.
8. Special Noting:
    a. Can client read directions?
    b. If the client asks for verbal input with directions, the therapist should first point to the appropriate numbered instruction(s) on the printed direction sheet.
    c. If a client still needs help, give oral instructions.
    d. If a client continues to need help, give demonstrated instructions.
9. Ending the group session:
    a. The client may clean up when he finishes his hot plate or five minutes before the group is to end.
    b. The evaluation leader is responsible for making sure the supplies are adequately stocked at the end of each day for the next assessment group.
    c. The leader is also responsible for making sure that every client who does not finish gluing his tiles must do so by the second day of the evaluation group. The leader must therefore contact the client's occupational therapist from activities therapy to inform the therapist that the client has not finished. It is then the responsibility of that therapist to have the client complete the tile hot plate before the next day's evaluation session.

B. Day 2 — Procedures
    1. The leader is responsible for the grouting supplies being set up before the group starts.
    2. Name re-introductions.
    3. Procedures for grouting
        a. Have clients put down newspaper and get their hot plates.
        b. Hand out written directions.
        c. Tell clients they have 30 minutes to complete the grouting.
        d. Announce remaining time after 15 minutes.
        e. Observe if clients clean up independently or need to be reminded.
    4. Procedures for group decision
        a. Present the 3 choices:
            1) Individual Magazine Collage—"How I want people to see me." You may select one or more pictures from available magazines and glue them onto paper. You will then be asked to discuss the meaning of the pictures at the end of the session.
            2) Group Mural—Utopian Place—a place of ideal perfection. You will be given a large sheet of paper and magic markers and will be asked to draw a Utopian Place as a group. You will then be asked to discuss your drawing and what it means to you.
            3) Hypothetical Problem—as a group you will be handed a problem that has nothing to do with your personal or emotional problem and will not be a mathematical problem. You will be asked as a group to solve the problem. (The leader should not explain what hypothetical means, but a client may).
        b. The leader should state that the group has until the end of the group session (whatever is left of the hour) to decide on a choice. Repeat the three choices. Also state that staff will not participate in the decision-making process.
        c. Note what each client's first choice is.

C. Day 3 — Procedures
    1. The leader is responsible for supplies being set up before the group begins.
    2. Name re-introductions.

3. Ask for a volunteer to restate the group's decision.
4. Completing the 3 choices:
    a. Individual Magazine Picture Collage
        1) Inform the client they have 40 minutes to complete the collage (find pictures and glue) on, "How I want others to see me."
        2) After 30 minutes, announce remaining time.
        3) After 40 minutes the clients are asked to individually share with the group what their pictures mean to them (within 20 minutes).
    b. Group Mural—Utopian Place
        1) Inform the clients that it is up to them as a group to decide how the mural will be done and that they have 40 minutes to complete it.
        2) Remove chairs from around table.
        3) Announce time at midway point.
        4) At end of 40 minutes have the group place mural on the wall and have each client explain what they drew (within 15 minutes).
        5) Upon completion of the explanation, ask the group what they would like to do with the mural, and then how they feel they worked as a group.
    c. Hypothetical Problem
        1) Hand out directions and pencils.
        2) Ask for a client volunteer to read directions.
        3) Give clients 10 minutes to individually rank the items.
        4) Then give group 30 minutes to arrive at a mutual decision on rank order.
        5) Announce time left after 15 minutes and 5 minutes before the end of 30 minute time limit.
        6) At the end of the 30 minutes, ask group how they think they worked as a group.
        7) Read correct NASA answers.
5. Let each client know that his primary occupational therapist will be getting back to each of them with the observation results of the evaluation group and OT treatment recommendations.

Appendix R

COMPREHENSIVE ASSESSMENT PROCESS:
A GROUP EVALUATION
TILE HOT PLATE

1st Day

1. Select the needed materials: board, glue, tiles.

2. Write your name on a piece of masking tape and stick it to the underside (rough side) of your board.

3. Plan a design that will cover the *entire* board (smooth side).

4. Start gluing the tiles by placing a thin line of glue along the edges of the board.

5. Place the tiles on the glue about 1/8 of an inch apart.

6. Continue gluing the tiles to the board, working from the edges toward the center, until the entire board is covered with glued tiles.

7. Let the glue dry for several hours.

2nd Day

1. Collect the necessary materials: paper cup, tongue depressor, white grout powder, tile hot plate.

2. Fill your cup 1/2 full of the grout.

3. Very slowly, add a few drops of water to the grout, stirring until smooth (the mixture should be the consistency of thick mashed potatoes).

4. If you want to color your grout, add coloring (in small jars) 1 teaspoon at a time.

5. Using the tongue depressor, spread the grout mixture all over the hot plate, pressing the mixture down between the tiles and along the edges.

6. Press down the grout with your finger until all the air bubbles are out.

7. Take the tongue depressor and scrape off the excess grout, being careful not to remove grout from between the tiles (grout should be even with top of tiles).

8. Let the hot plate dry 24 hours.

9. After the grout has completely dried:
    a. Scrape off excess grout from tiles with a tongue depressor.
    b. Wipe the hot plate with a *damp* sponge.
    c. Apply silicone sealer according to bottle directions.

371

Appendix

Appendix S

NASA Exercise Individual Worksheet*

INSTRUCTIONS: You are a member of a space crew originally scheduled to renedezvous with a mother ship on the lighted surface of the moon. Due to mechanical difficulties, however, your ship was forced to land at a spot some 200 miles from the rendezvous point. During landing, much of the equipment aboard was damaged, and, since survival depends on reaching the mother ship, the most critical items available must be chosen for the 200-mile trip. Below are listed the 15 items left intact and undamaged after landing. Your task is to rank order them in terms of their importance to your crew in allowing them to reach the rendezvous point. Place the number 1 by the most important item, the number 2 by the second most important and so on, through number 15, the least important. You have 10 minutes to complete this phase of the exercise.

_____	_____	_____	Box of matches
_____	_____	_____	Food concentrate
_____	_____	_____	50 feet of nylon rope
_____	_____	_____	Parachute silk
_____	_____	_____	Portable heating unit
_____	_____	_____	Two .45 calibre pistols
_____	_____	_____	One case dehydrated Pet milk
_____	_____	_____	Two 100-lb. tanks of oxygen
_____	_____	_____	Stellar map (of the moon's constellation)
_____	_____	_____	Life raft
_____	_____	_____	Magnetic compass
_____	_____	_____	5 gallons of water
_____	_____	_____	Signal flares
_____	_____	_____	First-aid kit containing injection needles
_____	_____	_____	Solar-powered FM receiver-transmitter

Appendix T

NASA EXERCISE ANSWER SHEET*

RATIONALE		CORRECT NUMBER
No oxygen—matches will not burn	15	Box of matches
Can live for some time without food	4	Food concentrate
For travel over rough terrain	6	50 feet of nylon rope
Carrying	8	Parachute silk
Lighted side of moon is hot	13	Portable heating unit
Some use for propulsion	11	Two .45 calibre pistols
Needs H_2O to work	12	One case dehydrated Pet milk
No breathable air on moon	1	Two 100-lb. tanks of oxygen
Needed for navigation	3	Stellar map (of moon's constellation)
Some value for shelter or carrying	9	Life raft
Moon's magnetic field is different from earth's	14	Magnetic Compass
You can't live long without this	2	5 gallons of water
No oxygen—flares will not burn	10	Signal flares
First-aid kit might be needed but needles are useless	7	First-aid kit containing injection needles
Communication	5	Solar-powered FM receiver-transmitter

Appendix U

OCCUPATIONAL THERAPY PROGRESS NOTES

Name _____
Hosp. No. _____ Date _____
Sex ____ Age ____ Dr. _____
Service _____
Division _____ Room No. _____

I. *GENERAL APPEARANCE*	Good	Needs Improvement	COMMENTS
A. Grooming			
B. Level of Awareness			
C. Orientation			
D. Affect			
E. Motor Level			
F. Self-Esteem			
II. *WORK SKILLS* A. Attendance			
B. Self-Directed			
C. Task Investment			
D. Independence			
E. Concentration			
F. Follows Instructions			
G. Problem Solving			
H. Decision-Making Ability			
I. Frustration Tolerance			
J. Work Tolerance			
K. Planning/Organization			
L. Workmanship			
M. Relationship to Authority			
III. *INTERACTION SKILLS*			
A. Eye Contact			
B. Effective Use of Verbal/Nonverbal Expression			
C. Casual Interaction			

D. Meaningful Interaction			
E. Self-Assertion			
F. Group Membership			
G. Leadership Skills			

IV. ACTIVITIES OF DAILY LIVING (as indicated by patient)	Independent	Dependent on others	Wants to Learn	
A. Personal Hygiene				
B. Child Care				
C. Food Management				
D. Homemaking Tasks				
E. Sewing				
F. Minor Home Repairs				
G. Money Management				
H. Transportation				

TREATMENT PLAN

Therapist _____ Date _____

Appendix V

ACTIVITY LABORATORY QUESTIONNAIRE

Name _____   Date _____

Unit _____

Please check the answer which best applies to you on each question.

1. *I think I did quite well:*
   ( ) On all the activities
   ( ) On a few
   ( ) On one
   ( ) On none

2. *I did poorly:*
   ( ) On all the activities
   ( ) On a few
   ( ) On one
   ( ) On none

3. *I found:*
   ( ) All the activities difficult
   ( ) A few difficult
   ( ) One difficult
   ( ) None difficult

4. *I feel:*
   ( ) Good about my performance on these activities
   ( ) Satisfied with what I have been able to do
   ( ) I would like to have done better
   ( ) Badly about my performance on these activities

5. *In comparison with others:*
   ( ) I did better than most others
   ( ) I did as well as the others
   ( ) I did more poorly than the others
   ( ) I did the most poorly

6. *Others in the group would judge my performance on these activities as:*
   ( ) Very good
   ( ) Generally good
   ( ) Poor
   ( ) Failing

7. *I think the person directing these activities would rate my performance as:*
   ( ) Very good
   ( ) Generally good
   ( ) Poor
   ( ) Very poor

8. *I think the person directing these activities expected that:*
   ( ) I would do much better than I have done
   ( ) I would do about as well as I have done
   ( ) I would do more poorly than I have done
   ( ) Had no expectations for me

9. *My performance in these activities was most influenced by:*
   ( ) The noise around me
   ( ) Other people observing me
   ( ) Medication
   ( ) Desire to do a good job
   ( ) None of these. My performance was influenced
       by _____

Appendix   **379**

10. *The most pleasant part of these activities was:*
    ( ) Getting to know the other people here
    ( ) One of the things I made
    ( ) Having the chance to be active
    ( ) Seeing what I could do
    ( ) None of these. The most pleasant part was
    _____   _____

11. *The most unpleasant part of these activities was*
    ( ) Being observed by others
    ( ) Having to compete
    ( ) My lack of skill
    ( ) The activities were too simple and easy
    ( ) None of these. The most unpleasant part was
    _____

Please rate each of the activities according to your preferences. Mark the one you liked best (1), the one you liked next best (2), and so on with the one you liked least (5).
    ( ) Cutout and crayon
    ( ) Finger painting
    ( ) Collage picture, design
    ( ) Obstacle course
    ( ) Circle ball tag

Other comments you would like to make about these experiences:

Appendix W

DATE																
I. GENERAL BEHAVIOR	1	2	3	4	5	6	7	8	9	10	11	12	13	14	15	16
A. Appearance																
B. Non-Productive Behavior																
C. Activity Level (a or b)																
D. Expression																
E. Responsibility																
F. Punctuality																
G. Reality Orientation																
Sub-Total																
II. INTERPERSONAL BEHAVIOR	1	2	3	4	5	6	7	8	9	10	11	12	13	14	15	16
A. Independence																
B. Cooperation																
C. Self Assertion (a or b)																
D. Sociability																
E. Attention Getting Behavior																
F. Negative Response From Others																
Sub-Total																
III. TASK BEHAVIOR	1	2	3	4	5	6	7	8	9	10	11	12	13	14	15	16
A. Engagement																
B. Concentration																
C. Coordination																
D. Follow Directions																
E. Activity Neatness or Attention To Detail																
F. Problem Solving																
G. Complexity And Organization Of Task																
H. Initial Learning																
I. Interest In Activity																
J. Interest In Accomplishment																
K. Decision Making																

L. Frustration Tolerance																		
Sub-Total																		
TOTAL																		

Scale   0 — Normal,   1 — Minimal,   2 — Mild,   3 — Moderate,   4 — Severe

Comments

_____

_____

_____

_____

_____

_____

_____

_____

_____

_____

(Therapist's Signature)

Appendix X

COMPREHENSIVE OCCUPATIONAL THERAPY
EVALUATION SCALE
DEFINITIONS

PART I. GENERAL BEHAVIOR

A. APPEARANCE

The following six factors are involved:
1) clean skin, 2) clean hair, 3) hair combed, 4) clean clothes, 5) clothes ironed, and 6) clothes suitable for the occasion.

0 — No problems in any area
1 — Problems in 1 area
2 — Problems in 2 areas
3 — Problems in 3 or 4 areas
4 — Problems in 5 or 6 areas

B. NONPRODUCTIVE BEHAVIOR

(Rocking, playing with hands, repetitive statements, appears to be talking to self, preoccupied with own thoughts, etc.)

0 — No nonproductive behavior during session
1 — Nonproductive behavior occasionally during session
2 — Nonproductive behavior for half of session
3 — Nonproductive behavior for three-fourths of session
4 — Nonproductive behavior for the entire session

C. ACTIVITY LEVEL (a or b)

(a)0 — No hypoactivity
2 — Hypoactivity attracts the attention of other clients and therapists but participates
3 — Hypoactivity level such that can participate but with great difficulty
4 — So hypoactive that client cannot participate in activity

(b)0 — No hyperactivity
1 — Occasional spurts of hyperactivity
2 — Hyperactivity attracts the attention of other clients and therapists but participates
3 — Hyperactivity level such that can participate but with great difficulty
4 — so hyperactive that clients cannot participate in activity

D. EXPRESSION

0 — Expression consistent with situation and setting
1 — Communicates with expression, occasionally inappropriate
2 — Shows inappropriate expression several times during session
3 — Show of expression but inconsistent with situation
4 — Extremes of expression—bizarre, uncontrolled or no expression

E. RESPONSIBILITY

0 — Takes responsibility for own actions
1 — Denies responsibility for 1 or 2 actions
2 — Denies responsibility for several actions
3 — Denies responsibility for most actions
4 — Denial of all responsibility—messes up project and blames therapist or others

F. PUNCTUALITY

0 — On time
1 — 5 to 10 minutes late
2 — 10 to 20 minutes late
3 — 20 to 30 minutes late
4 — 30 minutes or more late

G. REALITY ORIENTATION

0 — Complete awareness of person, place, time, and situation
1 — General awareness but inconsistency in one area
2 — Awareness of 2 areas
3 — Awareness of 1 area
4 — Lack of awareness of person, place, time, and situation (who, where, what, and why)

PART II. INTERPERSONAL

A. INDEPENDENCE

0 — Independent functioning
1 — Only 1 or 2 dependent actions
2 — Half independent and half dependent actions
3 — Only 1 or 2 independent actions
4 — No independent actions

B. COOPERATION

0 — Cooperates with program
1 — Follows most directions, opposes less than one half
2 — Follows half, opposes half
3 — Opposes three-fourths of directions
4 — Opposes all directions and suggestions

C. SELF-ASSERTION (a or b)

(a)0 — Assertive when necessary
   1 — Compliant less than half of the session
   2 — Compliant half of the session
   3 — Compliant three-fourths of the session
   4 — Totally passive and compliant

(b)0 — Assertive when necessary
   1 — Dominant less than half the session
   2 — Dominant half the session
   3 — Dominant three-fourths of the session
   4 — Totally dominates the session

D. SOCIABILITY

0 — Socializes with staff and patients
1 — Socializes with staff and occasionally with other patients or vice versa
2 — Socializes only with staff or with patients
3 — Socializes only if approached
4 — Does not join others in activities, unable to carry on casual conversation even if approached

E. ATTENTION GETTING BEHAVIOR

0 — No unreasonable attention getting behavior
1 — Less than one-half time spent in attention getting behavior
2 — Half-time spent in attention getting behavior
3 — Three-fourths of time spent in attention getting behavior
4 — Verbally or nonverbally demands constant attention

F. NEGATIVE RESPONSE FROM OTHERS

0 — Evokes no negative responses
1 — Evokes 1 negative response
2 — Evokes 2 negative responses
3 — Evokes 3 or more negative responses during session
4 — Evokes numerous negative responses from others and therapist must take some notion

PART III. TASK BEHAVIOR

A. ENGAGEMENT

0 — Needs no encouragement to begin task
1 — Encourage once to begin activity
2 — Encourage 2 or 3 times to engage in activity

Rate either Activity Neatness or Attention to Detail, not both.

3 — Engages in activity only after much encouragement
4 — Does not engage in activity

B. CONCENTRATION

0 — No difficulty concentrating during full session
1 — Off task less than one-fourth time
2 — Off task half the time
3 — Off task three-fourths time
4 — Loses concentration in less than 1 minute

C. COORDINATION

0 — No problems with coordination
1 — Occasionally has trouble with fine detail, manipulating tools or materials
2 — Occasional trouble manipulating tools and materials but has frequent trouble with fine detail
3 — Some difficulty in gross movement-unable to manipulate some tools and materials
4 — Great difficulty in movement (gross motor), virtually unable to manipulate tools and materials (fine motor.)

D. FOLLOW DIRECTIONS

0 — Carries out directions without problems
1 — Occasional trouble with more than 3 step directions
2 — Carries out simple directions—has trouble with 2
3 — Can carry out only very simple one step directions (demonstrated, written, or oral)
4 — Unable to carry out any directions

*E. ACTIVITY NEATNESS

(a)0 — Activity neatly done
   1 — Occasionally ignores fine detail
   2 — Often ignores fine detail and materials are scattered
   3 — Ignores fine detail and work habits disturbing to those around
   4 — Unaware of fine detail, so sloppy that therapist has to interevene

(b) ATTENTION TO DETAIL

0 — Pays attention to detail appropriately
1 — Occasionally too concise
2 — More attention to several details than is required
3 — So concise that project will take twice as long as expected
4 — So concerned that project will never get finished

F. PROBLEM SOLVING

0 — Solves problems without assistance

1 — Solves problems after assistance given once
2 — Can solve only after repeated instructions
3 — Recognizes a problem but cannot solve it
4 — Unable to recognize or solve a problem

G. COMPLEXITY AND ORGANIZATION OF TASK
0 — Organizes and performs all tasks given
1 — Occasonally has trouble with organization of complex activities that should be able to do
2 — Can organize simple but not complex activities
3 — Can do only very simple activities with organization imposed by therapists
4 — Unable to organize or carry out an activity when all tools, materials, and directions are available

H. INITIAL LEARNING
0 — Learns a new activity quickly and without difficulty
1 — Occasionally has difficulty learning a complex activity
2 — Has frequent difficulty learning a complex activity, but can learn a simple activity
3 — Unable to learn complex activities; occasional difficulty in learning simple activities
4 — Unable to learn a new activity

I. INTEREST IN ACTIVITIES
0 — Interested in a variety of activities
1 — Occasionally not interested in new activity
2 — Shows occasional interest in a part of an activity
3 — Engages in activities but shows no interest
4 — Does not participate

J. INTEREST IN ACCOMPLISHMENT
0 — Interested in finishing activities
1 — Occasional lack of interest in a long-term activity
2 — Interest or pleasure in accomplishment of a short-term activity-lack of interest in a long term activity
3 — Only occasional interest in finishing any activity
4 — No interest or pleasure in finishing an activity

K. DECISION MAKING
0 — Makes own decisions
1 — Makes decisions, but occasionally seeks therapist's approval
2 — Makes decisions, but often seeks therapist's approval
3 — Makes decision when given only 2 choices
4 — Cannot make any decisions or refuses to make a decision

L. FRUSTRATION TOLERANCE
0 — Handles all tasks without becoming overly frustrated
1 — Occasionally becomes frustrated with more complex tasks, can handle simple tasks
2 — Often becomes frustrated with more complex tasks but is able to handle simple tasks
3 — Often becomes frustrated with any task but attempts to continue
4 — Becomes so frustrated with simple tasks that client refuses or is unable to function

Appendix Y

COTE RATING SCALE

III. TASK BEHAVIOR

A. ENGAGEMENT
- 0 — Needs no encouragement to begin task
- 1 — Encourage once to begin activity
- 2 — Encourage 2 or 3 times to engage in activity
- 3 — Engages in activity only after much encouragement
- 4 — Does not engage in activity

B. CONCENTRATION
- 0 — No difficulty concentrating during full session
- 1 — Off task less than one-fourth time
- 2 — Off task half the time
- 3 — Off task three-fourths time
- 4 — Loses concentration on task in less than one minute

C. COORDINATION
- 0 — No problems with coordination
- 1 — Occasionally has trouble with fine detail, manipulating tools or materials
- 2 — Occasional trouble manipulating tools and materials but has frequent trouble with fine detail
- 3 — Some difficulty in gross movement—unable to manipulate some tools and materials
- 4 — Great difficulty in movement (gross motor), virtually unable to manipulate tools and materials (fine motor)

D. FOLLOW DIRECTIONS
- 0 — Carries out directions without problems
- 1 — Occasional trouble with more than three step directions
- 2 — Carries out simple directions—has trouble with two
- 3 — Can carry out only very simple one step directions (demonstrated, written, or oral)
- 4 — Unable to carry out any directions

E. ACTIVITY NEATNESS OR ATTENTION TO DETAIL
(a) Attention to Neatness
- 0 — Activity neatly done
- 1 — Occasionally ignores fine detail
- 2 — Often ignores fine detail and materials are scattered
- 3 — Ignores fine detail and work habits disturbing to those around
- 4 — Unaware of fine detail, so sloppy that therapist has to intervene

(b) Attention to Detail
- 0 — Pays attention to detail appropriately
- 1 — Occasionally too concise
- 2 — More attention to several details than is required
- 3 — So concise that project will take twice as long as expected
- 4 — So concerned that project will never get finished

F. PROBLEM SOLVING
- 0 — Solves problems without assistance
- 1 — Solves problems after assistance given once
- 2 — Can solve only after repeated instructions
- 3 — Recognizes a problem but cannot solve it
- 4 — Unable to recognize or solve a problem

G. COMPLEXITY AND ORGANIZATION OF TASK
- 0 — Organizes and performs all tasks given
- 1 — Occasionally has trouble with organization of complex activities that should be able to do
- 2 — Can organize simple but not complex activities
- 3 — Can do only very simple activities with organization imposed by therapists
- 4 — Unable to organize or carry out an activity when all tools, materials, and directions are available

H. INITIAL LEARNING
- 0 — Learns a new activity quickly
- 1 — Occasionally has difficulty learning a complex activity
- 2 — Has frequent difficulty learning a complex activity but can learn a simple activity
- 3 — Unable to learn complex activities; occasional difficulty learning simple activities
- 4 — Unable to learn a new activity

I. INTEREST IN ACTIVITIES
- 0 — Interested in a variety of activities

1 — Occasionally not interested in new activities
2 — Shows occasional interest in a part of an activity
3 — Engages in activities but shows no interest
4 — Does not participate

J. INTEREST IN ACCOMPLISHMENT
0 — Interested in finishing activities
1 — Occasional lack of interest or pleasure in finishing a long term activity
2 — Interest or pleasure in accomplishment of a short term activity; lack of interest in a long term activity
3 — Only occasional interest in finishing any activity
4 — No interest or pleasure in finishing an activity

K. DECISION MAKING
0 — Makes own decisions
1 — Makes decisions but occasionally seeks therapist's approval
2 — Makes decisions but often seeks therapist's approval
3 — Makes decision when given only two choices
4 — Cannot make any decisions or refuses to make a decision

L. FRUSTRATION TOLERANCE
0 — Handles all tasks without becoming overly frustrated
1 — Occasionally becomes frustrated with more complex tasks, can handle simple tasks
2 — Often becomes frustrated with more complex tasks, but is able to handle simple tasks
3 — Often becomes frustrated with any tasks, but attempts to continue
4 — Becomes so frustrated with simple tasks that client refuses or is unable to function

Appendix Z

OCCUPATIONAL THERAPY
FUNCTIONAL EVALUATION RATING SCALE

Date	1	2	3	4	5	6	7	8	9	10	11	12
I. ACTIVITIES OF DAILY LIVING												
A. Bathing (Upper Extremity)												
B. Bathing (Lower Extremity)												
C. Dressing (Upper Extremity)												
D. Dressing (Lower Extremity)												
E. Grooming												
F. Feeding												
G. Kitchen Activities												
Sub-Total												

II. MOTOR SKILLS	1	2	3	4	5	6	7	8	9	10	11	12
A. Gross-Motor Lue												
B. Gross-Motor Rue												
C. Fine-Motor Lue												
D. Fine-Motor Rue												
E. Handwriting												
Sub-Total												

III. SENSORY MOTOR	1	2	3	4	5	6	7	8	9	10	11	12
A. Perception												
Sub-Total												

IV. SENSATION	1	2	3	4	5	6	7	8	9	10	11	12
A. Stereognosis Lue												
B. Stereognosis Rue												
C. Temperature Lue												
D. Temperature Rue												
E. Sharp/Dull Lue												
F. Sharp/Dull Rue												
G. Proprioception Lue												
H. Proprioception Rue												
Sub-Total												

V. Endurance	1	2	3	4	5	6	7	8	9	10	11	12
A. Sitting Balance												
B. Sitting Tolerance												
C. Standing Balance												
D. Standing Tolerance												
E. General Endurance												
Sub-Total												

VI. COGNITION	1	2	3	4	5	6	7	8	9	10	11	12
A. Orientation to Person												
B. Orientation to Place												
C. Orientation to Time												
D. Recall												
E. Handwriting												
F. Ability to Handle Money												
G. Ability to Tell Time												
H. Ability to use Telephone												
I. Follow Directions-Written												
J. Follow Directions-Verbal												
K. Problem Solving												
L. Attention Span												
M. Decision-Making												
Sub-Total												

VII. APPEARANCE	1	2	3	4	5	6	7	8	9	10	11	12
A. Sociability												
B. Cooperation												
C. Affect												
D. Lability												
E. Safety Awareness												
F. Frustration Tolerance												
Sub-Total												

SCALE:

1 — Independent or within normal limits

2 — Mild Dysfunction

3 — Moderate Dysfunction

4 — Severe dysfunction or dependent

5 — Unable to perform

Appendix AA

FUNCTIONAL EVALUATION RATING SCALE

DEFINITIONS

PART I. ACTIVITIES OF DAILY LIVING

A. UPPER EXTREMITY BATHING
  1 — Independent
  2 — Minimal Assistance
  3 — Moderate Assistance
  4 — Maximal Assistance or Dependent

B. LOWER EXTREMITY BATHING
  Same As Above

C. UPPER EXTREMITY DRESSING
  Same As Above

D. LOWER EXTREMITY DRESSING
  Same As Above

E. GROOMING
  1 — Independent In All Areas
  2 — Independent In 2 Or More Areas
  3 — Independent In 1 Area
  4 — Dependent in All Areas

F. FEEDING
  1 — Independent
  2 — Needs Set-Up/Meat Cut
  3 — Able To Hold Utensil Only
  4 — Able To Chew and Swallow
  5 — Unable To Chew and Swallow

G. KITCHEN ACTIVITIES
  1 — Independent
  2 — Minimal Assistance
  3 — Moderate Assistance
  4 — Maximal Assistance

PART II. MOTOR SKILLS

A. GROSS-MOTOR   LUE
  1 — Within Normal Limits
  2 — Minimal Impairment
  3 — Moderate Impairment
  4 — Maximal Impairment

B. GROSS-MOTOR   RUE
  Same As Above

C. FINE-MOTOR   LUE
  1 — Within Normal Limits
  2 — Manipulates Objects Less
     than 1 inch
  3 — Manipulates Objects Less than
     3 inches
  4 — Unable to Manipulate Objects
     Larger than 3 inches

D. FINE-MOTOR   RUE
  Same As Above

E. HANDWRITING
  1 — Within Normal Limits
  2 — Able To Write but Illegibly
  3 — Holds Pen Only
  4 — Unable To Hold Pen or Mark
     Paper

PART III. SENSORY MOTOR

A. PERCEPTION
  1 — Within Normal Limits
  2 — Minimal Impairment
  3 — Moderate Impairment
  4 — Maximal Impairment

PART IV. SENSATION

A. STEREOGNOSIS   LUE
  1 — Within Normal Limits
  2 — Minimal Impairment
  3 — Moderate Impairment
  4 — Maximal Impairment

B. STEREOGNOSIS   RUE
  Same As Above

C. TEMPERATURE   LUE
  Same As Above

D. TEMPERATURE   RUE
  Same As Above

E. SHARP/DULL   LUE
  Same As Above

F. SHARP/DULL   RUE
  Same As Above

G. PROPRIOCEPTION   LUE
  Same As Above

H. PROPRIOCEPTION   RUE
  Same As Above

PART V. ENDURANCE

A. SITTING BALANCE
  1 — Within Normal Limits
  2 — Up To 15 Minutes
  3 — 5 Minutes To 15 Minutes
  4 — Less Than 5 Minutes

B. SITTING TOLERANCE
  Same As Above

C. STANDING BALANCE

1 — Within Normal Limits
2 — Up To 15 Minutes
3 — 5 Minutes To 15 Minutes
4 — Less Than 5 Minutes

D. STANDING TOLERANCE
Same As Above

E. GENERAL ENDURANCE
1 — Within Normal Limits
2 — Up To 30 Minutes
3 — Up To 15 Minutes
4 — Less Than 5 Minutes

PART VI. COGNITION

A. ORIENTATION TO PERSON
1 — Within Normal Limits
2 — Knows Staff Working with Patient
3 — Knows Own Name Only
4 — Does Not Know Name (Unable To Evaluate)

B. ORIENTATION TO PLACE
1 — Within Normal Limits
2 — Knows Residence of Family
3 — Knows Hospital Presently In
4 — Knows Own Residence Only
5 — Does Not Know Residence (Unable to Evaluate)

C. ORIENTATION TO TIME
1 — Within Normal Limits
2 — Knows The Month
3 — Knows The Year
4 — Knows Day of Week Only
5 — Does Not Know Day of Week (Unable to Evaluate)

D. RECALL
1 — Within Normal Limits
2 — Remembers Events of Past Week
3 — Remembers Events of Past 24 Hours
4 — Does not Remember Current Therapy Session (Unable to Evaluate)

E. HANDWRITING
1 — Within Normal Limits
2 — Writes Alphabet Correctly
3 — Writes Numbers 1-10 Correctly
4 — Writes Name Correctly
5 — Unable to Write Name Correctly (Uable to Evaluate)

F. ABILITY TO HANDLE MONEY
1 — Within Normal Limits
2 — Makes Change For One Dollar
3 — Counts Out Specific Amounts
4 — Able To Distinguish Different Coins
5 — Unable To Distinguish Different Coins (Unable to Evaluate)

G. ABILITY TO TELL TIME
1 — Within Normal Limits
2 — Recognizes Half Hours
3 — Recognizes Numbers On Clock
4 — Does Not Recognize Numbers On Clock (Unable to Evaluate)

H. ABILITY TO USE TELEPHONE
1 — Within Normal Limits
2 — Able To Dial Familiar Phone Numbers
3 — Able To Dial Any Number
4 — Able To Pick Up and Hold Receiver
5 — Unable To Pick Up and Hold Receiver (Unable To Evaluate)

I. FOLLOW DIRECTIONS—WRITTEN
1 — Within Normal Limits
2 — Follows One Step Commands
3 — Follows One Step Commands With Extra Cueing
4 — Follows One Step Commands With Manual Demonstration
5 — Unable To Follow One Step Commands With Manual Demonstration (Unable to Evaluate)

J. FOLLOW DIRECTIONS—VERBAL
1 — Within Normal Limits
2 — Follows One Step Direction
3 — Follows One Step Directions With Verbal Cueing
4 — Follows One Step Directions With Manual Demonstration
5 — Unable To Follow One Step Directions with Manual Demonstration (Unable To Evaluate)

K. PROBLEM SOLVING
1 — Within Normal Limits
2 — Solves Problems After Instructions Given Once
3 — Solves Problems After Repeated Instructions
4 — Unable To Solve Problems
5 — Unable To Evaluate

L. ATTENTION SPAN
1 — Within Normal Limits
2 — Up To 15 Minutes
3 — Up To 10 Minutes
4 — Up To 5 Minutes

M. DECISION MAKING
1 — Within Normal Limits
2 — Makes Decisions Only With Approval From Staff
3 — Makes Decisions When Given Only Two Choices
4 — Refuses Or Unable To Make Decisions
5 — Unable To Evaluate

PART VII. APPEARANCE

A. SOCIABILITY
  1 — Within Normal Limits
  2 — Socializes With Staff
  3 — Socializes Only When Approached
  4 — No Socialization Indicated

B. COOPERATION
  1 — Within Normal Limits
  2 — Cooperates 50% of Time
  3 — Cooperates 25% of Time
  4 — Cooperates less than 25% of Time
  5 — Totally Uncooperative (Unable
      to Evaluate)

C. AFFECT
  1 — Within Normal Limits
  2 — Appropriate Affect 50% of Time
  3 — Appropriate Affect 25% of Time
  4 — Appropriate Affect less than 25% of
      Time
  5 — Unable To Evaluate

D. LABILITY
  1 — No Lability
  2 — Labile 25% of Time
  3 — Labile 50% of Time
  4 — Labile More Than 50% of Time
  5 — Unable to Evaluate

E. SAFETY AWARENESS
  1 — No Impulsive Behavior
  2 — Impulsive 25% of Time
  3 — Impulsive 50% of Time
  4 — Impulsive More Than 50% of Time
  5 — Unable to Evaluate

F. FRUSTRATION TOLERANCE
  1 — Within Normal Limits
  2 — Low At Times But Does Not
      Hinder Function
  3 — Low and Hinders Function 50%
      of Time
  4 — Low and Hinders Function More
      than 50% of Time
  5 — Unable to Evaluate

NAME INDEX

A

Alard, I., 212
Allport, G., Vernon, P., 128
Alschuler, R., Hattwick, L., 134
Anastasi, A., Foley, J.P., 89, 105, 106
Androes, L., Dreyfus, E., Bloesch, M., 85
Ayres, A.J., 9, 176, 228, 232, 233
Azima, H., 8, 85, 90, 127
Azima, H., Azima, F., 85, 141

B

Bach-y-Rita, G., Lion, J.R., Climent, C.E., et al., 235
Baldessarini, R.J., 230
Barton, R., 271
Beals, R.G., 211, 212
Bender, L., Woltmann, A., 90
Bendroth, S., Southam, M., 67, 79
Berman, S. and Loffol, J., 178
Black, M., 260
Brick, M., 131
Buck, J.N., 89, 107, 108, 122
Buck, R., Provancher, M., 140, 141

C

Choungourian, A., 131
Clark, J.R., Roch, B.A., Nichols, R.C., 212, 222
Cobb, S., 309
Coggins, D., 64
Cohn, R., 170, 174, 179, 187
Crow, T.J., Johnstone, E.C., 234

D

deQuiros, J.B., Schranger, O.L., 232
Dewey, J., 256
Diamond, B.L., Schmale, H.T., 87
Diasio, K.B., Jones, M.S., 47
Diefendorf, A.R., Dodge, R., 232
Doll, E.A., 272, 273
Dorken, H., 130

E

Edwards, B., 190
Egal, C., Lindgren, H.C., 174
Esser, T.J., 213

F

Fawzi, S.D., 187
Fidler, G.S., 6, 8, 64, 85
Fidler, G.S., Fidler, J., 8, 90, 127, 128, 211, 212
Fingert, H., Kagan, J., Schilder, P., 190
Fiske, D.W., 267
Frank, L., 90, 128
French, J.R., 309
Freud, S., 173

G

Gillette, N., 64, 96
Ginzberg, E., 50
Ginzberg, E., Ginzberg, S.W., Axelrod, S., Herman, J.L., 50
Golomb, C., 91, 92
Goodenough, F., 106, 173, 188
Gurr, R.E., 234

H

Hall, G.S., 49
Halpern, F., 88
Hammer, E.F., 89, 173
Harris, D.B., 173, 188, 190
Hartley, R.E., Goldenson, R.M., 91
Hassell, J., Smith, E., 187
Homans, G.C., 272
Holmes, Bauer, 140
Holtzman, P.S., Kringlen, E., Levy, D.L., et al., 232
Holtzman, P.S., Levy, D.L., Proctor, L.R., 232
Holtzman, P.S., Proctor, L.R., Levy, D.L., et al., 232
Huddleston, C.I., 232

WORD INDEX

socially appropriate behavior, 272, 273
society, 271
sorting shells, 265, 269
Southern California Sensory Integration Test, 191, 228, 249
space relationships, 105
spontaneous drawing, 86, 95, 99, 106, 113, 116, 119
spontaneous drawing task, 97, 99, 105, 109
stability, 165, 238
standardization, 263, 275, 321
standardize, 10
Stanford Binet Intelligence Test, 173
strokes, 129, 134
structure, 198, 309
super-symmetry, 134
surface coverage, 131, 132
symmetrical tonic neck reflex, 239
symmetry, 131, 134

T
tactile responses, 182
target ball, 198
task investment, 159
Task Oriented Assessment (TOA), 255, 258, 264
terminal interview, 25
texture, 131, 133, 201
Thematic Apperception Test, 128, 141
testing procedure, 3, 8
The Adolescent Role Assessment, 11

The Nurses Observational Scale (NOSIE), 190
The Southern California Battery, 9, 11
time, 129, 131, 135, 170, 267
tonic labyrinthine reflex, 239-240
type of object, 153

U
use of space, 132
utopian place, 157, 158

V
validity, 130, 165, 222, 228, 247, 280, 322
verbal communication, 273
verbalization, 104, 105, 107, 109, 111, 129, 135
vestibular system, 231
Vineland Social Maturity Scale, 273
visual-motor coordination, 88
visual organization, 88
visual pursuits, 238

W
Wechsler-Adult Intelligence Scale (WAIS), 88
Winterhaven Copy Forms and Visual Retention Test, 184
work group, 160
workmanship, 159
work skills, 155, 159
work with peers, 274